NCLEX-RN®
New-Format Questions
Third Edition

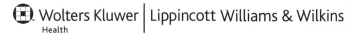
Wolters Kluwer | Lippincott Williams & Wilkins
Health
Philadelphia · Baltimore · New York · London
Buenos Aires · Hong Kong · Sydney · Tokyo

STAFF

Executive Publisher
Judith A. Schilling McCann, RN, MSN

Clinical Director
Joan M. Robinson, RN, MSN

Art Director
Elaine Kasmer

Electronic Project Manager
John Macalino

Clinical Project Manager
Beverly Ann Tscheschlog, RN, MS

Editor
Diane Labus

Associate Manufacturing Manager
Beth J. Welsh

Editorial Assistants
Karen J. Kirk, Jeri O'Shea, Linda K. Ruhf

Production Project Manager
Cynthia Rudy

RNNFQ3010110
10 9 8 7 6 5 4 3 2 1

Library of Congress Cataloging-in-Publication Data
NCLEX-RN new format questions. — 3rd ed.
    p. ; cm.
  Rev. ed. of: NCLEX-RN 250 new-format questions. 2nd ed. ©2007.
  ISBN 978-1-60547-199-0 (alk. paper)
  1. Nursing—Examinations, questions, etc. 2. Nursing—Outlines, syllabi, etc. 3. Nurses—Licenses—United States—Examinations—Study guides. I. NCLEX-RN 250 new-format questions.
  [DNLM: 1. Nursing Care—Examination Questions.
2. Nursing—Examination Questions. WX 18.2 N337 2009]
  RT55.N435 2009
  610.73076—dc22   2008047087

Contents

Contributors and consultants

Helen C. Ballestas, RN, MS, CRRN
Nursing Faculty
New York Institute of Technology
Old Westbury

Carol Blakeman, MSN, ARNP
Professor
Central Florida Community College
Ocala

Cheryl L. Brady, RN, MSN
Assistant Professor of Nursing
Kent State University
Salem, Ohio

Barbara Broome, RN, PhD
Associate Dean and Chair of Community/Mental
   Health
University of South Alabama
College of Nursing
Mobile

Marsha L. Conroy, RN, MSN, APN
Nurse Educator
Cuyahoga Community College
Cleveland
Indiana Wesleyan University
Marion

Kim Cooper, RN, MSN
Nursing Department Chair
Ivy Tech Community College
Terre Haute, Indiana

Linda Carman Copel, PhD, APRN, BC, CGP,
   NCC, DAPA
Associate Professor
Villanova (Pa.) University

Susan Denman, RN, PhD, APRN-BC, FNP
Assistant Professor
Duke University School of Nursing
Durham, N.C.

Marsha Gerdeman, RN, MS
Associate Professor
Rhodes State College
Lima, Ohio

Karla Jones, RN, MS
Associate Professor
University of Alaska
Anchorage

Kathy J. Keister, RN, PhD
Assistant Professor
Wright State University
College of Nursing
Dayton, Ohio

Elayne Sugar-Karrel, RN, MSN
Clinical Nurse Specialist Consultant/Author
Crestwood, Ky.

Allison J. Terry, RN, MSN, PhD
Director, Center for Nursing
Alabama Board of Nursing
Montgomery

Student advisory board

Susan Barnason, PhD, RN, CEN, CCRN, CS
Associate Professor
University of Nebraska Medical Center
College of Nursing
Lincoln

Michael A. Carter, DNSC, FAAN, APRN-BC
University Distinguished Professor
University of Tennessee Health Science Center
College of Nursing
Memphis

Caroline Dorsen, MSN, APRN, BC, FNP
Clinical Instructor and Coordinator, Adult Nurse
  Practitioner Program
New York University
College of Nursing

Stephen Gilliam, PhD, FNP, APRN-BC
Assistant Professor
Medical College of Georgia
School of Nursing
Athens

Margaret Mary Hansen, EdD, MSN, RN,
  NI CERTIFICATE
Associate Professor
University of San Francisco

Kathy Henley Haugh, PhD, RN
Assistant Professor
University of Virginia
School of Nursing
Charlottesville

Janice J. Hoffman, PhD, RN, CCRN
Assistant Professor and Vice Chair
Organizational Systems and Adult Health
University of Maryland School of Nursing
Baltimore

Linda Honan Pellico, PhD, MSN, APRN
Assistant Professor
Yale University
School of Nursing
New Haven, Conn.

Susan L. Woods, PhD, RN, FAAN, FAHA
Professor and Associate Dean for Academic
  Programs
University of Washington
Seattle

PART | ONE

Preparing for the NCLEX®

NCLEX basics

Passing the National Council Licensure Examination (NCLEX®) is an important landmark in your career as a nurse. The first step on your way to passing the NCLEX is to understand what it is and how it's administered.

NCLEX structure

The NCLEX is a test written by nurses who, like most of your nursing instructors, have a master's degree and clinical expertise in a particular area. Only one small difference distinguishes nurses who write NCLEX questions: They're trained to write questions in a style particular to the NCLEX.

If you've completed an accredited nursing program, you've already taken numerous tests written by nurses with backgrounds and experiences similar to those of the nurses who write for the NCLEX. The test-taking experience you've already gained will help you pass the NCLEX. So your NCLEX review should be just that—a review.

The NCLEX is designed for one purpose: to determine whether it's appropriate for you to receive a license to practice as a nurse. By passing the NCLEX, you demonstrate that you possess the minimum level of knowledge necessary to practice nursing safely.

If you completed your nursing education in a foreign country, you must follow certain guidelines to be eligible to work as a registered nurse in the United States. (See *Guidelines for international nurses*.)

In nursing school, you probably took courses organized according to the medical model. Courses were separated into such subjects as medical-surgical, pediatric, maternal-neonatal, and psychiatric nursing. In contrast, the NCLEX is integrated, meaning that different subjects are mixed together.

As you answer NCLEX questions, you may encounter patients in any stage of life, from neonatal to geriatric. These patients—clients, in NCLEX terminology—may be of any background, may be completely well or extremely ill, and may have any of a variety of disorders.

Client needs

The NCLEX draws questions from four categories of *client needs* that were developed by the National Council of State Boards of Nursing (NCSBN), the organization that sponsors and manages the NCLEX. Client needs categories ensure that a wide variety of topics appears on every NCLEX examination.

The NCSBN developed client needs categories after conducting a work-study analysis of new nurses. All aspects of nursing care observed in the study were broken down into four main categories, some of which were broken down further into subcategories. (See *Client needs categories,* page 4.)

Integrated processes

Integrated throughout the client needs categories and subcategories are four key processes that are fundamental to the practice of nursing:

- **Nursing process**—a problem-solving approach to client care that includes assessment, analysis, planning, implementation, and evaluation
- **Caring**—an atmosphere of mutual respect and trust that exists between the nurse and the client in which the nurse provides encouragement, support, hope, and compassion to help the client achieve desired outcomes
- **Communication and documentation**—nonverbal and verbal exchanges or interactions among the nurse and client, the client's significant other, and the health care team, and the validation of client care in written and electronic records that reflects standards of practice and accountability in the provision of care
- **Teaching and learning**—making possible the gaining of knowledge, attitudes, and skills to promote a change in the client's behavior.

NCLEX test plan

The four client needs categories and their corresponding subcategories provide the basic framework for the NCLEX test plan. Question-writers and the other people who compile the examination use the NCLEX test plan to ensure that the content and distribution of test questions cover the full spectrum of nursing activities and competencies across all client care settings. Although client needs categories appear in most NCLEX review and question-and-answer books (including this one), you don't need to be concerned about them as a test-taker. The categories serve only as a frame of reference; they don't actually appear on the NCLEX.

Critical thinking

Although NCLEX questions cover all levels of cognitive abilities—from basic nursing knowledge to comprehension, application, and analysis—most are written at the higher cognitive levels (such as analysis), which requires critical thinking. Critical thinking relies on the

In order to become eligible to work as a registered nurse (RN) in the United States, you will need to complete several steps. In addition to passing the NCLEX-RN, you may need to obtain a certificate and credentials evaluation from the Commission on Graduates of Foreign Nursing Schools (CGFNS®) and acquire a visa. Since requirements differ from state to state, it's important that you first contact the board of nursing in the state where you want to practice nursing.

CGFNS certification Program

Most states require that you obtain CGFNS certification. This certification requires:

■ a review and authentication of your credentials, including your nursing education, registration, and licensure

■ a passing score on the CGFNS Qualifying Examination of nursing knowledge

■ a passing score on an English language proficiency test.

In order to be eligible to take the CGFNS Qualifying Examination, you must complete a minimum number of classroom and clinical practice hours in medical-surgical nursing, maternal-neonatal nursing, pediatric nursing, and psychiatric and mental health nursing from a government-approved nursing school. You must also be registered as a first-level nurse in your country of education, and currently hold a license as an RN in some jurisdiction.

The CGFNS Qualifying Examination is a paper-and-pencil test that includes 260 multiple-choice questions. It's administered under controlled testing conditions. Because the test is designed to predict your likelihood of successfully passing the NCLEX-RN exam, it's based on the NCLEX-RN test plan.

You may select from three English proficiency examinations: Test of English as a Foreign Language (TOEFL®), Test of English for International Communication (TOEIC®), or International English Language Testing System (IELTS). Each test has different passing scores and the scores are valid for up to 2 years.

CGFNS credentials evaluation service

This evaluation is a comprehensive report that analyzes and compares your education and licensure with U.S. standards. It's prepared by the CGFNS for a state board of nursing, an immigration office, an employer, or a university. It requires that you complete an application, submit appropriate documentation, and pay a fee.

More information about the CGFNS certification program and credentials evaluation service is available at *www.cgfns.org*.

Visa

You can't legally immigrate to work in the United States without an occupational visa (temporary or permanent) from the United States Citizenship and Immigration Services (USCIS). The visa process is separate from the CGFNS certification process, although some of the same steps are involved. Some visas require prior CGFNS certification and a *VisaScreen®* Certificate from the International Commission on Healthcare Professions. The *VisaScreen* program involves:

■ a credentials review of your nursing education and current registration or licensure

■ successful completion of either the CGFNS certification program or the NCLEX-RN

■ a passing score on an approved English language proficiency examination.

Once you successfully complete all parts of the *VisaScreen* program, you will receive a certificate to present to the USCIS. The visa-granting process can take up to a year.

You can obtain more detailed information about visa application at *www.uscis.gov*.

---

nurse's knowledge, skills, and ability to problem-solve. Critical thinking strategies are provided for all rationales in this book to help you focus on where or how to find the correct answer to each question as you study for the NCLEX.

Testing by computer

Like many standardized tests today, the NCLEX is administered by computer. That means you won't be filling in empty circles, sharpening pencils, or erasing frantically. It also means that you must become famil-iar with computer tests, if you aren't already. Fortunately, the skills required to take the NCLEX on a computer are simple enough to allow you to focus on the questions, not the keyboard.

When you take the test, depending on the question format, you'll be presented with a question and four or more possible answers, a blank space in which to enter your answer, a figure on which you'll click the mouse to select the correct area of the figure, a series of charts or exhibits to view in order to select the correct response, or items you must prioritize by dragging and dropping them in place.

The NCLEX is a *computer-adaptive test*, meaning that the computer reacts to the answers you give, supplying more difficult questions if you answer correctly and slightly easier questions if you answer incorrectly. Each test is thus uniquely adapted to the individual test-taker.

You have a great deal of flexibility with the amount of time you spend on individual questions. The examination lasts a maximum of 6 hours, however, so don't waste time. If you fail to answer a set number of questions within 6 hours, the computer will determine that you lack minimum competency.

Most students have plenty of time to complete the test, so take as much time as you need to get the question right without wasting time. Keep moving at a decent pace to help maintain concentration.

If you find as you progress through the test that the questions seem to be increasingly difficult, it's a good sign. The more questions you answer correctly, the more difficult the questions become.

Some students, though, knowing that questions get progressively harder, focus on the degree of difficulty of subsequent questions to try to figure out if they're answering questions correctly. Avoid the temptation to do this, as this may get you off track. Stay focused on selecting the best answer for each question put before you.

The computer test finishes when one of these events occurs:

■ You demonstrate minimum competency, according to the computer program.

■ You demonstrate a lack of minimum competency, according to the computer program.

■ You've answered the maximum number of questions (265 total questions).

■ You've used the maximum time allowed (6 hours).

Alternate-format questions

In April of 2004, the NCSBN added alternate-format items to the exam. These include five types:

■ multiple response–multiple choice

■ fill-in-the-blank

■ hotspot

■ chart or exhibit

■ drag and drop.

However, most of the questions on the NCLEX are four-option, multiple-choice items with only one correct answer. Certain strategies can help you understand and answer any type of NCLEX question.

The NCSBN hasn't yet established a percentage of alternate-format items to be administered to each candidate. In fact, your exam may contain only one alternate-format item. So relax; the standard, four-option, multiple-choice format questions compose the bulk of the test.

Multiple-response, multiple-choice question

The first type of alternate-format item is the *multiple-response, multiple-choice question*. Unlike a traditional multiple-choice question, each multiple-response, multiple-choice question has more than one correct answer for every question, and it may contain more than four possible answer options. You'll recognize this type of question because it will ask you to select *all* answers that apply—not just the best answer (as may be requested in the more traditional multiple-choice questions).

Keep in mind that for each multiple-response, multiple-choice question, you must select at least one answer and you must select all correct answers for the item to be counted as correct. On the NCLEX, there's no partial credit in the scoring of these items.

Fill-in-the blank question

The second type of alternate-format item is the *fill-in-the-blank*. These questions require you to provide the answer yourself, rather than select it from a list of options. You will perform a calculation, then type your answer (a number without any words, units of measurement, commas, or spaces) in the blank space provided after the question. A calculator button is provided so you can easily do your calculations electronically.

Hotspot question

The third type of alternate-format item is a question that asks you to identify an area on an illustration or graphic. For these so-called *"hotspot" questions,* the computerized exam will ask you to place your cursor and click over the correct area on an illustration. Try to be as precise as possible when marking the location. As with the fill-in-the-blanks, the identification questions on the computerized exam may require extremely precise answers to be considered correct.

Chart/exhibit question

The fourth type of alternate-format item is the *chart/exhibit* format. Here you'll be given a problem, then a series of small screens containing additional information you'll need in order to answer the question. By clicking on the TAB button, you can access each screen in turn. Your answer can then be chosen from four multiple-choice answer options.

Drag-and-drop question

The final type of alternate-format item involves prioritizing, or placing in correct order, a series of statements using a drag-and-drop technique. You'll decide which of the given options is first, click and hold it with the mouse, then drag it into the first box given beneath and drop it into place. You'll repeat this process until you've placed all the available options in the lower boxes. (See *Sample NCLEX questions,* pages 6 and 7.)

Understanding the question

NCLEX questions are usually long. As a result, it's easy to feel overwhelmed with information. To focus on the question, apply proven strategies for answering NCLEX questions, including:

■ determining what the question is asking
■ determining relevant facts about the client
■ rephrasing the question in your mind
■ choosing the best option(s) before entering your answer.

Determine what the question is asking

Read the question twice. If the answer isn't apparent, rephrase the question in simpler, more personal terms. Breaking down the question into easier, less intimidating terms may help you to focus more accurately on the correct answer.

For example, a question might read: "A 74-year-old client with a history of heart failure is admitted to the coronary care unit with pulmonary edema. He's intubated and placed on a mechanical ventilator. Which parameter should the nurse monitor closely to assess the client's response to a bolus dose of furosemide (Lasix) I.V.?"

The options for this question—numbered from 1 to 4—may be:

☐ **1.** Daily weight

☐ **2.** 24-hour intake and output

☐ **3.** Serum sodium levels

☐ **4.** Hourly urine output

Read the question again, ignoring all details except what's being asked. Focus on the last line of the

Sometimes, getting used to the test format is as important as knowing the material covered. Try your hand at these sample questions and you'll have a leg up when you take the real test!

Sample four-option, multiple-choice question

A client's arterial blood gas (ABG) results are as follows: pH, 7.16; $Paco_2$, 80 mm Hg; Pao_2, 46 mm Hg; HCO_3^-, 24 mEq/L; Sao_2, 81%. This ABG result represents which condition?

☐ **1.** Metabolic acidosis

☐ **2.** Metabolic alkalosis

☐ **3.** Respiratory acidosis

☐ **4.** Respiratory alkalosis

Answer: 3

Sample multiple-response, multiple-choice question

The nurse is caring for a 45-year-old married client who has undergone hemicolectomy for colon cancer. The client has two children. Which concepts about families should the nurse keep in mind when providing care for this client? Select all that apply:

☐ **1.** Illness in one family member can affect all members.

☐ **2.** Family roles don't change because of illness.

☐ **3.** A family member may have more than one role in the family.

☐ **4.** Children typically aren't affected by adult illness.

☐ **5.** The effects of an illness on a family depend on the stage of the family's life cycle.

☐ **6.** Changes in sleeping and eating patterns may be signs of stress in a family.

Answer: 1, 3, 5, 6

Sample fill-in-the-blank calculation question

An infant who weighs 8 kg is to receive ampicillin 25 mg/kg I.V. every 6 hours. How many milligrams should the nurse administer per dose? Record your answer using a whole number.

_____ milligrams

Answer: 200

Sample hotspot question

An elderly client has a history of aortic stenosis. Identify the area where the nurse should place the stethoscope to best hear the murmur.

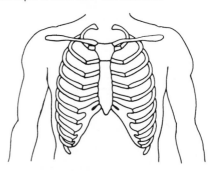

Answer:

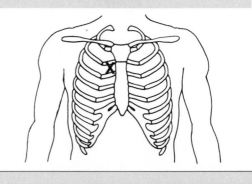

Sample chart/exhibit question

A 3-year-old client is being treated for severe status asthmaticus. After reviewing the progress notes (shown below), the nurse should determine that this client is being treated for which condition?

Progress notes

4/5/09 0600	Pt. was acutely restless, diaphoretic, and with SOB at 05:30. Dr. T. Smith notified and ordered ABG analysis. ABG drawn from Ⓡ radial artery. Stat results as follows: pH 7.28, Paco₂ 55 mm Hg, HCO₃⁻ 26 mEg/L. Dr. Smith with pt. now. ———— J. Collins, RN.

☐ **1.** Metabolic acidosis

☐ **2.** Respiratory alkalosis

☐ **3.** Respiratory acidosis

☐ **4.** Metabolic alkalosis

Answer: 3

Sample drag-and-drop question

When teaching an antepartal client about the passage of the fetus through the birth canal during labor, the nurse describes the cardinal mechanisms of labor. Place these events in the sequence in which they occur. Use all the options.

1. Flexion
2. External rotation
3. Descent
4. Expulsion
5. Internal rotation
6. Extension

Answer: 3, 1, 5, 6, 2, 4

---

question. It asks you to select the appropriate assessment for monitoring a client who received a bolus of furosemide I.V.

Determine what facts about the client are relevant

Next, sort out the relevant client information. Start by asking whether any of the information provided about the client isn't relevant. For instance, do you need to know that the client has been admitted to the coronary care unit? Probably not; his reaction to I.V. furosemide won't be affected by his location in the hospital.

Determine what you do know about the client. In the example, you know that:

■ he just received an I.V. bolus of furosemide, a crucial fact

■ he has pulmonary edema, the most fundamental aspect of the client's underlying condition

■ he's intubated and placed on a mechanical ventilator, suggesting that his pulmonary edema is serious

■ he's 74 years old and has a history of heart failure, a fact that may or may not be relevant.

Rephrase the question

After you've determined relevant information about the client and the question being asked, consider rephrasing the question to make it clearer. Eliminate jargon and put the question in simpler, more personal terms. Here's how you might rephrase the question in the example: "My client has pulmonary edema. He requires intubation and mechanical ventilation. He's 74 years old and has a history of heart failure. He received an I.V. bolus of furosemide. What assessment parameter should I monitor?"

Choose the best option

Armed with all the information you now have, it's time to select an option. You know that the client received an I.V. bolus of furosemide, a diuretic. You know that monitoring fluid intake and output is a key nursing intervention for a client taking a diuretic, a fact that eliminates options 1 and 3 (daily weight and serum sodium levels), narrowing the answer down to option 2 or 4 (24-hour intake and output or hourly urine output).

You also know that the drug was administered by I.V. bolus, suggesting a rapid effect. (In fact, furosemide administered by I.V. bolus takes effect almost immediately.) Monitoring the client's 24-hour intake and output would be appropriate for assessing the effects of repeated doses of furosemide. Hourly urine output, however, is most appropriate in this situation because it monitors the immediate effect of this rapid-acting drug.

Key strategies

Regardless of the type of question, four key strategies will help you determine the correct answer for each question. (See *Strategies for success*.) These strategies are:

- considering the nursing process
- referring to Maslow's hierarchy of needs
- reviewing patient safety
- reflecting on principles of therapeutic communication.

Strategies for success

Keeping a few main strategies in mind as you answer each NCLEX question can help ensure greater success. These four strategies are critical for answering NCLEX questions correctly:

- If the question asks what you should do in a situation, use the nursing process to determine which step in the process would be next.
- If the question asks what the client needs, use Maslow's hierarchy to determine which need to address first.
- If the question indicates that the client doesn't have an urgent physiologic need, focus on the patient's safety.
- If the question involves communicating with a patient, use the principles of therapeutic communication.

Nursing process

One of the ways to answer a question is to apply the nursing process. Steps in the nursing process include:

- assessment
- analysis
- planning
- implementation
- evaluation.

The nursing process may provide insights that help you analyze a question. According to the nursing process, assessment comes before analysis, which comes before planning, which comes before implementation, which comes before evaluation.

You're halfway to the correct answer when you encounter a four-option, multiple-choice question that asks you to assess the situation and then provides two assessment options and two implementation options. You can immediately eliminate the implementation options, which then gives you, at worst, a 50-50 chance of selecting the correct answer. Use the following sample question to apply the nursing process:

A client returns from an endoscopic procedure during which he was sedated. Before offering the client food, which action should the nurse take?

- ☐ **1.** Assess the client's respiratory status.
- ☐ **2.** Check the client's gag reflex.
- ☐ **3.** Place the client in a side-lying position.
- ☐ **4.** Have the client drink a few sips of water.

According to the nursing process, the nurse must assess a client before performing an intervention. Does the question indicate that the client has been properly assessed? No, it doesn't. Therefore, you can eliminate options 3 and 4 because they're both interventions.

That leaves options 1 and 2, both of which are assessments. Your nursing knowledge should tell you the correct answer—in this case, option 2. The sedation required for an endoscopic procedure may impair the client's gag reflex, so you would assess the gag reflex before giving food to the client to reduce the risk of aspiration and airway obstruction.

Why not select option 1, assessing the client's respiratory status? You might select this option but the question is specifically asking about offering the client food, an action that wouldn't be taken if the client's respiratory status were at all compromised. In this case, you're making a judgment based on the phrase "Before offering the client food." If the question were trying to test your knowledge of respiratory depression following an endoscopic procedure, it probably wouldn't mention a function—such as giving food to a client—that clearly occurs only after the client's respiratory status has been stabilized.

Maslow's hierarchy

Knowledge of Maslow's hierarchy of needs can be a vital tool for establishing priorities on the NCLEX. Maslow's theory states that physiologic needs are the most basic human needs of all. Only after physiologic needs have been met can safety concerns be addressed. Only after safety concerns are met can concerns involving love and belonging be addressed, and so forth. Apply the principles of Maslow's hierarchy of needs to the following sample question:

A client complains of severe pain 2 days after surgery. Which action should the nurse perform first?

☐ **1.** Offer reassurance to the client that he will feel less pain tomorrow.

☐ **2.** Allow the client time to verbalize his feelings.

☐ **3.** Check the client's vital signs.

☐ **4.** Administer an analgesic.

In this example, two of the options—3 and 4—address physiologic needs. Options 1 and 2 address psychosocial concerns. According to Maslow, physiologic needs must be met before psychosocial needs, so you can eliminate options 1 and 2.

Now, use your nursing knowledge to choose the best answer from the two remaining options. In this case, option 3 is correct because the client's vital signs should be checked before administering an analgesic (assessment before intervention). When prioritizing according to Maslow's hierarchy, remember your ABCs—airway, breathing, circulation—to help you further prioritize. Check for a patent airway before addressing breathing. Check breathing before checking the health of the cardiovascular system.

Just because an option appears on the NCLEX doesn't mean it's a viable choice for the client referred to in the question. Always examine your choice in light of your knowledge and experience. Ask yourself, "Does this choice make sense for this client?" Allow yourself to eliminate choices—even ones that might normally take priority—if they don't make sense for a particular client's situation.

Patient safety

As you might expect, patient safety takes high priority on the NCLEX. You'll encounter many questions that can be answered by asking yourself, "Which answer will best ensure the safety of this client?" Use patient safety criteria for situations involving laboratory values, drug administration, or nursing care procedures.

You may encounter a question in which some options address the client and others address the equipment. When in doubt, select an option relating to the client; never place equipment before a client.

For instance, suppose a question asks what the nurse should do first when entering a client's room where an infusion pump alarm is sounding. If two options deal with the infusion pump, one with the infusion tubing, and another with the client's catheter insertion site, select the one relating to the client's catheter insertion site. Always check the client first; the equipment can wait.

Therapeutic communication

Some NCLEX questions focus on the nurse's ability to communicate effectively with the client. Therapeutic communication incorporates verbal or nonverbal responses and involves:

■ listening to the client

■ understanding the client's needs

■ promoting clarification and insight about the client's condition.

Like other NCLEX questions, those dealing with therapeutic communication require choosing the best response. First, eliminate options that indicate the use of poor therapeutic communication techniques, such as those in which the nurse:

■ tells the client what to do without regard to the client's feelings or desires (the "do this" response)

■ asks a question that can be answered "yes" or "no," or with another one-syllable response

■ seeks reasons for the client's behavior

■ implies disapproval of the client's behavior

■ offers false reassurances

■ attempts to interpret the client's behavior rather than allowing the client to verbalize his own feelings

■ offers a response that focuses on the nurse, not the client.

When answering NCLEX questions, look for responses that:

■ allow the client time to think and reflect

■ encourage the client to talk

■ encourage the client to describe a particular experience

■ reflect that the nurse has listened to the client, such as through paraphrasing the client's response.

Avoiding pitfalls

Even the most knowledgeable students can get tripped up on certain NCLEX questions. (See *A tricky question*.) Students commonly cite three areas that can be difficult for unwary test-takers:

■ knowing the difference between the NCLEX and the "real world"

■ delegating care

■ knowing laboratory values.

NCLEX versus the real world

Some students who take the NCLEX have extensive practical experience in health care. For example, many test-takers have worked as licensed practical nurses or nursing assistants. In one of those capacities, test-takers might have been exposed to less than optimum clinical practice and may carry those experiences over to the NCLEX.

However, the NCLEX is a textbook examination—not a test of clinical skills. Take the NCLEX with the understanding that what happens in the real world may differ from what the NCLEX and your nursing school say should happen.

If you've had practical experience in health care, you may know a quicker way to perform a procedure or tricks to get by when you don't have the right equipment. Situations such as staff shortages may force you to improvise. On the NCLEX, such scenarios can lead to trouble. Always check your practical experiences against textbook nursing care, taking care to select the response that follows the textbook.

Delegating care

On the NCLEX, you may encounter questions that assess your ability to delegate care. Delegating care involves coordinating the efforts of other health care workers to provide effective care for your client. On the NCLEX, you may be asked to assign duties to:

■ licensed practical nurses or licensed vocational nurses

■ direct care workers, such as nursing assistants and personal care aides

■ other support staff, such as nutrition assistants and housekeepers.

In addition, you'll be asked to decide when to notify a physician, a social worker, or another hospital staff member. In each case, you'll have to decide when, where, and how to delegate.

As a general rule, it's okay to delegate actions that involve stable clients or standard, unchanging procedures. Bathing, feeding, dressing, and transferring clients are examples of procedures that can be delegated.

Be careful not to delegate complicated or complex activities. In addition, don't delegate activities that involve assessment, evaluation, or your own nursing judgment. On the NCLEX and in the real world, these duties fall squarely on your shoulders. Make sure that you take primary responsibility for assessing and evaluating the client and for making decisions about the client's care. Never hand off those responsibilities to someone with less training.

Deciding when to notify a physician, a social worker, or another hospital staff member is an important element of nursing care. On the NCLEX, however, choices that involve notifying the physician are usually incorrect. Remember that the NCLEX wants to see you, the nurse, at work.

If you're sure the correct answer is to notify the physician, though, make sure the client's safety has been addressed before notifying a physician or another staff member. On the NCLEX, the client's safety has a higher priority than notifying other health care providers.

Knowing laboratory values

Some NCLEX questions supply laboratory results without indicating normal levels. As a result, answering questions involving laboratory values requires you to have the normal range of the most common laboratory values memorized to make an informed decision (See *Normal laboratory values*.)

Normal laboratory values

- Blood urea nitrogen: 8 to 25 mg/dl
- Creatinine: 0.6 to 1.5 mg/dl
- Sodium: 135 to 145 mmol/L
- Potassium: 3.5 to 5.5 mEq/L
- Chloride: 97 to 110 mmol/L
- Glucose (fasting plasma): 65 to 115 mg/dl
- Hemoglobin
  Male: 13.8 to 17.2 g/dl
  Female: 12.1 to 15.1 g/dl
- Hematocrit
  Male: 40.7% to 50.3%
  Female: 36.1% to 44.3%

Study preparations

If you're like most people preparing to take the test, you're probably feeling nervous, anxious, or concerned. Keep in mind that most test-takers pass the NCLEX the first time around.

Passing the test won't happen by accident, though; you'll need to prepare carefully and efficiently. To help jump-start your preparations:

- determine your strengths and weaknesses
- create a study schedule
- set realistic goals
- find an effective study space
- think positively
- start studying sooner rather than later.

Strengths and weaknesses

Most students recognize that, even at the end of their nursing studies, they know more about some topics than others. Because the NCLEX covers a broad range of material, you should make some decisions about how intensively you'll review each topic.

Base those decisions on a list. Divide a sheet of paper in half vertically. On one side, list topics you think you know well. On the other side, list topics you need to review. Pay no attention if one side is longer than the other. When you're done studying, you'll feel strong in every area.

To make sure your list reflects a comprehensive view of all the areas you studied in school, look at the contents page in the front of this book. For each topic listed, place it in the "know well" column or "needs review" column. Separating content areas this way shows immediately which topics need less study time and which need more time.

Scheduling study time

Study when you're most alert. Most people can identify a period of the day when they feel most alert. If you feel most alert and energized in the morning, for example, set aside sections of time in the morning for topics that need a lot of review. Then you can use the evening, a time of lesser alertness, for topics that need some refreshing. The opposite is true as well; if you're more alert in the evening, study difficult topics at that time.

Set up a basic schedule for studying. Using a calendar or organizer, determine how much time remains before you'll take the NCLEX. (See *2 to 3 months before the NCLEX*, page 12.) Fill in the remaining days with specific times and topics to be studied. For example, you might schedule the respiratory system on a Tuesday morning and the GI system

With 2 to 3 months remaining before you plan to take the examination, take these steps:

- Establish a study schedule. Set aside ample time to study but also leave time for social activities, exercise, family or personal responsibilities, and other matters.

- Become knowledgeable about the NCLEX-RN examination, its content, the types of questions it asks, and the testing format.

- Begin studying your notes, texts, and other study materials.

- Take some NCLEX practice questions to help you diagnose strengths and weaknesses as well as to become familiar with NCLEX-style questions.

that afternoon. Remember to schedule difficult topics during your most alert times.

Keep in mind that you shouldn't fill each day with studying. Be realistic and set aside time for normal activities. Try to create ample study time before the NCLEX and then stick to the schedule.

Part of creating a schedule means setting goals you can accomplish. You no doubt studied a great deal in nursing school, and by now you have a sense of your own capabilities. Ask yourself, "How much can I cover in a day?" Set that amount of time aside and then stay on task. You'll feel better about yourself—and your chances of passing the NCLEX—when you meet your goals regularly.

Study space

Find a space conducive to effective learning and then study there. Whatever you do, don't study with a television on in the room. Instead, find a quiet, inviting study space that:

- is located in a quiet, convenient place, away from normal traffic patterns

- contains a solid chair that encourages good posture (Avoid studying in bed; you'll be more likely to fall asleep and not accomplish your goals.)

- uses comfortable, soft lighting with which you can see clearly without eye strain

- has a temperature between 65° and 70° F

- contains flowers or green plants, familiar photos or paintings, and easy access to soft, instrumental background music.

Consider taping positive messages around your study space. Make signs with words of encouragement, such as, "You can do it!" "Keep studying!" and "Remember the goal!" These upbeat messages can help keep you going when your attention begins to waver.

Maintaining concentration

When you're faced with reviewing the amount of information covered by the NCLEX, it's easy to become distracted and lose your concentration. When you lose concentration, you make less effective use of valuable study time. To help stay focused, keep these tips in mind:

- Alternate the order of the subjects you study during the day to add variety to your study. Try alternating between topics you find most interesting and those you find least interesting.

- Approach your studying with enthusiasm, sincerity, and determination.

- Once you've decided to study, begin immediately. Don't let anything interfere with your thought processes once you've begun.

- Concentrate on accomplishing one task at a time, to the exclusion of everything else.

- Don't try to do two things at once, such as studying and watching television or conversing with friends.

- Work continuously without interruption for a while, but don't study for such a long period that the whole experience becomes grueling or boring.

- Allow time for periodic breaks to give yourself a change of pace. Use these breaks to ease your transition into studying a new topic.

- When studying in the evening, wind down from your studies slowly. Don't progress directly from studying to sleeping.

Taking care of yourself

Never neglect your physical and mental well-being in favor of longer study hours. Maintaining physical and mental health is critical for success in taking the NCLEX. (See *4 to 6 weeks before the NCLEX*.)

You can increase your likelihood of passing the test by following these simple health rules:

- Get plenty of rest. You can't think deeply or concentrate for long periods when you're tired.

- Drink enough noncaffeinated beverages. Mild dehydration increases the effort required to concentrate and reason while distracting attention through feelings of fatigue and thirst.

- Eat nutritious meals. Maintaining your energy level is impossible when you're undernourished.
- Exercise regularly. Regular exercise helps you work harder and think more clearly. As a result, you'll study more efficiently and increase the likelihood of success.

If you're having trouble concentrating but would rather push through than take a break, try making your studying more active by reading out loud. Active studying can renew your powers of concentration. By reading review material out loud to yourself, you're engaging your ears as well as your eyes—and making your studying a more active process. Hearing the material out loud also fosters memory and subsequent recall.

You can also rewrite in your own words a few of the more difficult concepts you're reviewing. Explaining these concepts in writing forces you to think through the material and can jump-start your memory.

Study schedule

When you were creating your schedule, you might have asked yourself, "How long should I study? One hour at a stretch? Two hours? Three?" To make the best use of your study time, you'll need to answer those questions.

Optimum study time

Experts are divided about the optimum length of study time. Some say you should study no more than 1 hour at a time several times a day. Their reasoning: You remember the material you study at the beginning and end of a session best and tend to remember less material studied in the middle of the session.

Other experts say you should hold longer study sessions because you lose time in the beginning, when you're just getting warmed up, and again at the end, when you're cooling down. Therefore, say those experts, a long, concentrated study period will allow you to cover more material.

So what's the answer? It doesn't matter as long as you determine what's best for *you*. At the beginning of your NCLEX study schedule, try study periods of varying lengths. Pay close attention to those that seem more successful.

Remember that you're a trained nurse who is competent at assessment. Think of yourself as a patient, and assess your own progress. Then implement the strategy that works best for you.

Finding time to study

So does that mean that short sections of time are useless? Not at all. We all have spaces in our day that might otherwise be dead time. (See *1 week before the NCLEX*.) These are perfect times to review for the NCLEX but not to cover new material because by the time you get deep into new material, your time will be over. Always keep some flashcards or a small notebook handy for situations when you have a few extra minutes.

You'll be amazed how many short sessions you can find in a day and how much reviewing you can do in 5 minutes. The following places offer short stretches of time you can use:

- eating breakfast
- waiting for, or riding on, a train or bus
- waiting in line at the bank, post office, bookstore, or other places.

Creative studying

Even when you study in a perfect study space and concentrate better than ever, studying for the NCLEX can get a little, well, dull. Even people with terrific study habits occasionally feel bored or sluggish. That's why it's important to have some creative tricks in your study bag to liven up your studying during those down times.

Creative studying doesn't have to be hard work. It involves making efforts to alter your study habits a bit. Some techniques that might help include studying with a partner or group and creating flash cards or other audiovisual study tools.

Study partners

Studying with a partner or group of students can be an excellent way to energize your studying. Working with a partner allows you to test each other on the material you've reviewed. Your partner can give you encouragement and motivation. Perhaps most important, working with a partner can provide a welcome break from solitary studying.

Exercise some care when choosing a study partner or assembling a study group. A partner who doesn't fit your needs won't help you make the most of your study time. Look for a partner who:

- possesses similar goals to yours. For example, someone taking the NCLEX at approximately the same date who feels the same sense of urgency as you do might make an excellent partner.
- possesses about the same level of knowledge as you. Tutoring someone can sometimes help you learn, but partnering should be give-and-take so both partners can gain knowledge.
- can study without excess chatting or interruptions. Socializing is an important part of creative study, but remember, you've still got to pass the NCLEX— so stay serious!

Audiovisual tools

Flash cards and other audiovisual tools foster retention and make learning and reviewing fun.

Flash cards can provide you with an excellent study tool. The process of writing material on a flash card will help you remember it. In addition, flash cards are small and easily portable, perfect for those 5-minute slivers of time that show up during the day.

Creating a flash card should be fun. Use magic markers, highlighters, and other colorful tools to make them visually stimulating. The more effort you put into creating your flash cards, the better you'll remember the material contained on the cards.

Flowcharts, drawings, diagrams, and other image-oriented study aids can also help you learn material more effectively. Substituting images for text can be a great way to give your eyes a break and recharge your brain. Remember to use vivid colors to make your creations visually engaging.

If you learn more effectively when you hear information rather than see it, consider recording key ideas using a handheld tape recorder. Recording information helps promote memory because you say the information aloud when taping and then listen to it when playing it back. Like flash cards, tapes are portable and perfect for those short study periods during the day. (See *The day before the NCLEX*.)

The day before the NCLEX

With 1 day before the NCLEX, take these steps:

- Drive to the test site, review traffic patterns, and find out where to park. If your route to the test site occurs during heavy traffic or if you're expecting bad weather, set aside extra time to ensure prompt arrival.
- Do something relaxing during the day.
- Avoid concentrating on the test.
- Rest, eat, and drink well, and avoid dwelling on the NCLEX during nonstudy periods.
- Call a supportive friend or relative for some last-minute words of encouragement.

Practice tests

Practice questions should constitute an important part of your NCLEX study strategy. Practice questions can improve your studying by helping you review material and familiarizing yourself with the exact style of questions you'll encounter on the NCLEX.

Consider working through some practice questions as soon as you begin studying for the NCLEX. For example, you might try a half-dozen questions from each chapter in this book.

If you score well, you probably know the material contained in that chapter fairly well and can spend less time reviewing that particular topic. If you have trouble with the questions, spend extra study time on that topic.

Practice questions can also provide an excellent means of marking your progress. Don't worry if you have trouble answering the first few practice questions you take; you'll need time to adjust to the way the questions are asked. Eventually you'll become accustomed to the question format and begin to focus more on the questions themselves.

If you make practice questions a regular part of your study regimen, you'll be able to notice areas in which you're improving. You can then adjust your study time accordingly.

As you near the examination date, continue to answer practice questions, but also set aside time to take an entire NCLEX practice test. (We've included six at the back of this book.) That way, you'll know exactly what to expect. (See *The day of the NCLEX*.) The more you know ahead of time, the better you're likely to do on the NCLEX.

Taking an entire practice test is also a way to gauge your progress. When you find yourself answering questions correctly, it will give you the confidence you need to conquer the real NCLEX.

The day of the NCLEX

On the day of the NCLEX examination, take these steps:

- Get up early.
- Wear comfortable clothes, preferably with layers you can adjust to fit the room temperature.
- Drink a glass of water and eat a small nutritious breakfast.
- Leave your house early.
- Arrive at the test site early.
- Avoid looking at your notes as you wait for your test computer.
- Listen carefully to the instructions given before entering the test room.
- Succeed, succeed, *succeed!*

PART 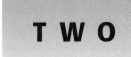 TWO

Fundamentals of nursing

Basic physical care

1. A nurse is developing a care plan for a client with an injury to the frontal lobe of the brain. Which of the following interventions should be part of the care plan? Select all that apply.

☐ **1.** Keep instructions simple and brief because the client will have difficulty concentrating.

☐ **2.** Speak clearly and slowly because the client will have difficulty hearing.

☐ **3.** Assist with bathing because the client will have vision disturbances.

☐ **4.** Orient the client to person, place, and time as needed because of memory problems.

☐ **5.** Assess vital signs frequently because vital bodily functions are affected.

Answer: 1, 4

Rationale: Damage to the frontal lobe affects personality, memory, reasoning, concentration, and motor control of speech. Damage to the temporal lobe, not the frontal lobe, causes hearing and speech problems. Damage to the occipital lobe causes vision disturbances. Damage to the brain stem affects vital functions.

Critical thinking strategy: Recall the physiologic functions of the different areas of the brain to understand what type of damage has occurred in order to plan your care.

Client needs category: Physiological integrity

Client needs subcategory: Basic care and comfort

Cognitive level: Application

Integrated process: Communication and documentation

Reference: Craven, pages 1231–1232

---

2. A nurse is caring for a client with emphysema. Which of the following nursing interventions would be appropriate? Select all that apply.

☐ **1.** Reduce fluid intake to less than 2,500 ml/day.

☐ **2.** Teach diaphragmatic, pursed-lip breathing.

☐ **3.** Administer low-flow oxygen.

☐ **4.** Keep the client in a supine position as much as possible.

☐ **5.** Encourage alternating activity with rest periods.

☐ **6.** Teach use of postural drainage and chest physiotherapy.

Answer: 2, 3, 5, 6

Rationale: Diaphragmatic, pursed-lip breathing strengthens respiratory muscles and enhances oxygenation in clients with emphysema. Low-flow oxygen should be administered because a client with emphysema has chronic hypercapnia and a hypoxic respiratory drive. Alternating activity with rest allows the client to perform activities without excessive distress. If the client has difficulty mobilizing copious secretions, the nurse should teach him and his family members how to perform postural drainage and chest physiotherapy. Fluid intake should be increased to 3,000 ml/day, if not contraindicated, to liquefy secretions and facilitate their removal. The client should be placed in high-Fowler's position to improve ventilation.

Critical thinking strategy: Recall the pathophysiology of emphysema and the client's physical needs created by the disease process.

Client needs category: Physiological integrity

Client needs subcategory: Basic care and comfort

Cognitive level: Application

Integrated process: Nursing process/planning

Reference: Smeltzer, pages 687–689

---

3. A nurse is caring for a client who underwent surgical repair of a detached retina in the right eye. Which of the following interventions should the nurse perform? Select all that apply.

☐ **1.** Place the client in a prone position.

☐ **2.** Approach the client from the left side.

☐ **3.** Encourage deep breathing and coughing.

☐ **4.** Discourage bending down.

☐ **5.** Orient the client to his environment.

☐ **6.** Administer a stool softener.

Answer: 2, 4, 5, 6

Rationale: The nurse should approach the client from the left side—the unaffected side—to avoid startling him. She should also discourage the client from bending down, deep breathing, hard coughing and sneezing, and other activities that can increase intraocular pressure during the postoperative period. The client should be oriented to his environment to reduce the risk of injury. Stool softeners should be administered to discourage straining during defecation. The client should lie on his back or on the unaffected side to reduce intraocular pressure in the affected eye.

Critical thinking strategy: Recall the pathophysiology of a detached retina and increased intraocular pressure.

Client needs category: Physiological integrity

Client needs subcategory: Reduction of risk potential

Cognitive level: Application

Integrated process: Nursing process/implementation

Reference: Smeltzer, page 2068

---

4. A nurse is planning care for a client with hyperthyroidism. Which of the following nursing interventions are appropriate? Select all that apply.

☐ **1.** Instill isotonic eyedrops as necessary.

☐ **2.** Provide several small, well-balanced meals.

☐ **3.** Provide rest periods.

☐ **4.** Keep the environment warm.

☐ **5.** Encourage frequent visitors and conversation.

☐ **6.** Weigh the client daily.

Answer: 1, 2, 3, 6

Rationale: If the client has exophthalmos (a sign of hyperthyroidism), the conjunctivae should be moistened often with isotonic eyedrops. Hyperthyroidism results in increased appetite, which can be satisfied by frequent small, well-balanced meals. The nurse should provide the client with rest periods to reduce metabolic demands. The client should be weighed daily to check for weight loss, a possible consequence of hyperthyroidism. Because metabolism is increased in hyperthyroidism, heat intolerance and excitability result. Therefore, the nurse should provide a cool and quiet environment, not a warm and busy one, to promote client comfort.

Critical thinking strategies: Recall the signs and symptoms and pathophysiology of hyperthyroidism.

Client needs category: Physiological integrity

Client needs subcategory: Basic care and comfort

Cognitive level: Application

Integrated process: Nursing process/planning

Reference: Smeltzer, page 1459

5. A client has a tumor of the posterior pituitary gland. A nurse planning his care should include which of the following interventions? Select all that apply.

☐ **1.** Weigh the client daily.

☐ **2.** Restrict fluids.

☐ **3.** Measure urine specific gravity.

☐ **4.** Encourage intake of coffee or tea.

☐ **5.** Monitor intake and output.

Answer: 1, 3, 5

Rationale: Tumors of the pituitary gland can lead to diabetes insipidus due to deficiency of antidiuretic hormone (ADH). Decreased ADH reduces the kidneys' ability to concentrate urine, resulting in excessive urination, thirst, and fluid intake. To monitor fluid balance, the nurse should weigh the client daily, measure urine specific gravity, and monitor intake and output. She should also encourage fluids to keep intake equal to output and prevent dehydration. Coffee, tea, and other fluids that have a diuretic effect should be avoided.

Critical thinking strategies: Focus on the pathophysiology and implications of a tumor of the posterior pituitary gland.

Client needs category: Physiological integrity

Client needs subcategory: Basic care and comfort

Cognitive level: Application

Integrated process: Nursing process/planning

Reference: Smeltzer, page 1446

---

6. A nurse is preparing to administer an I.M. injection in the deltoid muscle. Identify the area where the nurse would administer this injection.

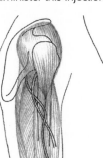

Answer:

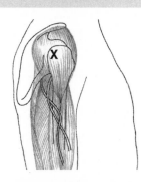

Rationale: To locate the deltoid muscle, find the lower edge of the acromial process and the point on the lateral arm in line with the axilla. The needle should be inserted 1″ to 2″ which is (usually two or three fingerbreadths) below the acromial process, and at a 90-degree angle, or slightly angled, toward the process.

Critical thinking strategies: Focus on the anatomy of the upper arm and the location of the deltoid muscle and recall the process for administering an I.M. injection.

Client needs category: Physiological integrity

Client needs subcategory: Pharmacological and parenteral therapies

Cognitive level: Application

Integrated process: Nursing process/implementation

Reference: Taylor, page 799

---

7. A nurse is performing a fecal occult blood test using a Hemoccult slide. Place the steps for performing the fecal occult blood test in the correct order.

1.	Allow the specimens to dry for 3 minutes.
2.	Put on gloves.
3.	Apply a drop of Hemoccult developing solution to boxes A and B on the slide's reverse side.
4.	Place a stool smear on box A of the slide.
5.	Apply a stool smear from another part of the specimen to box B on the slide.
6.	Put a drop of Hemoccult developing solution on each control dot on the slide's reverse side.

Answer: 2, 4, 5, 1, 6, 3

Rationale: After receiving the stool specimen from the client, the nurse should put on gloves and then follow the other steps in the order listed above. Before using the developer, the nurse should check the expiration date; she should discard the developer if the date has expired. A blue reaction after 30 to 60 seconds indicates a positive result.

Critical thinking strategy: Recall the process of standard precautions and visualize the sequence of steps to be performed.

Client needs category: Health promotion and maintenance

Client needs subcategory: None

Cognitive level: Application

Integrated process: Nursing process/implementation

Reference: Taylor, page 1564

8. A nurse is caring for a client with a hiatal hernia. The client complains of abdominal and sternal pain after eating. The pain makes it difficult for him to sleep. Which of the following instructions should the nurse recommend when teaching this client? Select all that apply.

☐ **1.** Avoid constrictive clothing.

☐ **2.** Lie down for 30 minutes after eating.

☐ **3.** Decrease intake of caffeine and spicy foods.

☐ **4.** Eat three meals per day.

☐ **5.** Sleep with the upper body elevated.

☐ **6.** Maintain a normal body weight.

Answer: 1, 3, 5, 6

Rationale: A hiatal hernia may cause abdominal and sternal pain after eating. The discomfort is associated with reflux of gastric contents. To reduce gastric reflux, the nurse should instruct the client to avoid constrictive clothing, caffeine, and spicy foods; sleep with his upper body elevated; lose weight, if obese; remain upright for 2 hours after eating; and eat small, frequent meals.

Critical thinking strategy: Focus on the pathophysiology of hiatal hernia and recall the clinical manifeststions of this disorder.

Client needs category: Physiological integrity

Client needs subcategory: Basic care and comfort

Cognitive level: Application

Integrated process: Teaching and learning

Reference: Smeltzer, pages 1163–1164

9. A nurse is assessing a client's pulses. Identify the area where the left dorsalis pedis pulse would be palpated.

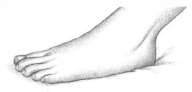

Answer:

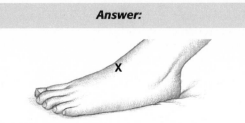

Rationale: The dorsalis pedis pulse can be palpated on the medial dorsal surface of the foot when the client's toes are pointed down. This pulse can be difficult to palpate and may seem to be absent in healthy clients.

Critical thinking strategy: Focus on the location of the dorsalis pedis pulse and recall the correct finger placement when performing the assessment.

Client needs category: Physiological integrity

Client needs subcategory: Physiological adaptation

Cognitive level: Application

Integrated thinking: Nursing process/implementation

Reference: Craven, page 430

---

10. A client with renal failure is placed on a potassium-restricted diet. For lunch, the client consumed 6 oz of hamburger on a bun, 1 cup of cooked broccoli, a raw pear, and iced tea. Using the chart provided, calculate how many milliequivalents of potassium were in this meal.

Answer: 4

Rationale: According to the chart, 4 oz of beef contain 11.2 mEq of potassium. Add 5.6 mEq for the additional 2 oz for a total of 16.8 mEq of potassium in the beef. The amount of potassium in 1 cup of broccoli is 14 mEq. A pear has 6.2 mEq. Thus, the total amount of potassium in this meal is 37 mEq. The iced tea and bun don't contain significant amounts of potassium and, therefore, aren't listed on the chart.

Critical thinking strategy: Use basic math skills to calculate the totals requested.

Client needs category: Physiological integrity

Client needs subcategory: Physiological adaptation

Cognitive level: Analysis

Integrated process: Nursing process/evaluation

Reference: Smeltzer, pages 1525–1526

Intake & output

DIETARY SOURCES OF POTASSIUM

Foods and beverages	Serving size	Amount of potassium (mEq)
Meats		
Beef	4 oz (112 g)	11.2
Chicken	4 oz	12.0
Scallops	5 large	30.0
Vegetables		
Broccoli (cooked)	1/2 cup	7.0
Carrots (raw)	1 large	8.8
Potatoes (baked)	1 small	15.4
Tomatoes (raw)	1 medium	10.4
Fruits		
Bananas	1 medium	12.8
Cantaloupe	6 oz	13.0
Pears (raw)	1 medium	6.2
Beverages		
Orange juice	1 cup	11.4
Prune juice	1 cup	14.4
Tomato juice	1 cup	11.6
Milk (whole or skim)	1 cup	8.8

☐ **1.** 24.4

☐ **2.** 30

☐ **3.** 31.4

☐ **4.** 37

---

11. A nurse is teaching a client with left leg weakness to walk with a cane. The nurse should include which of the following points about safe cane use in her client teaching? Select all that apply.

☐ **1.** Place the cane 8″ to 10″ from the base of the little toe.

☐ **2.** Hold the cane on the uninvolved side.

☐ **3.** Adjust the cane so that the handle is level with the hip bone.

☐ **4.** Walk by moving the involved leg, then the cane, and then the uninvolved leg.

☐ **5.** Shorten the stride length on the involved side.

☐ **6.** Avoid leaning on the cane to get in and out of a chair.

Answer: 2, 3, 6

Rationale: To ambulate safely, a client with leg weakness should hold the cane in the hand opposite the involved leg with the handle level with the hip bone. The client shouldn't lean on the cane to get in or out of a chair because of the risk of falls. The cane base should be placed 4″ to 6″ from the base of the little toe. When walking, the client should move the cane and involved leg simultaneously, alternating with the uninvolved leg in equal length strides and timing.

Critical thinking strategy: Recall the placement of the device in relation to the involved side and the importance of ensuring patient safety.

Client needs category: Physiological integrity

Client needs subcategory: Reduction of risk potential

Cognitive level: Application

Integrated process: Teaching and learning

Reference: Taylor, pages 1305–1306

---

12. A nurse is caring for a client who is recovering from an illness requiring prolonged bed rest. Based on the nursing documentation below, which of the procedures would the nurse implement next?

Progress notes

2/10/09	Pt. instructed in contraction of back
1015	extensors, hip extensors, knee extensors, and
	ankle flexors and extensors. Pt. able to
	demonstrate correct technique without joint
	motion or muscle lengthening. c/o being "a
	little tired" after holding each contraction 5
	seconds and repeating three times.
	Instructed to repeat exercises three times
	daily; pt. verbalized understanding of all
	information given. ————F. Brown, RN

☐ **1.** Performing active range-of-motion exercises of the legs

☐ **2.** Performing isometric exercises of the legs

☐ **3.** Providing assistance walking the client to the bathroom

☐ **4.** Performing passive range-of-motion exercises of the legs

Answer: 1

Rationale: Active range-of-motion exercises involve moving the client's joints through their full range of motion; they require some muscle strength and endurance. The client should have received passive range-of-motion exercises since admission to maintain joint flexibility and should have been taught isometric exercises to build strength and endurance for transfers and ambulation. Walking to the bathroom would be unsafe without the ability to first dangle the legs over the bedside and transfer from bed to chair.

Critical thinking strategy: Focus on the types of exercise being discussed with the client and review the correct sequence of activities when advancing the client's mobility status.

Client needs category: Physiological integrity

Client needs subcategory: Reduction of risk potential

Cognitive level: Application

Integrated process: Nursing process/planning

Reference: Craven, pages 761–764

13. The nurse is providing care for a client who has had a stroke. Since the onset of symptoms, she has been experiencing left-sided hemianopsia. Which of the following nursing interventions would be appropriate? Select all that apply.

- ☐ **1.** Place the client's belongings on the right side of the bed.
- ☐ **2.** Approach the client from the left side.
- ☐ **3.** Refuse to acknowledge the condition to promote the client's independence.
- ☐ **4.** Stand on the right side of the bed when providing care.
- ☐ **5.** Provide the client with an eye patch for the right eye.
- ☐ **6.** Dim the lights in the room to prevent eye strain.

Answer: 1, 4

Rationale: Hemianopsia is a condition in which the client has lost half of the visual field. It's most often associated with stroke. In this case, the stroke has affected the client's left side; therefore, placing her belongings on the right side of the bed will enable the client to best see them. Standing on the right side of the bed when providing care will ensure the client is able to see the nurse. Approaching the client from the left side is counterproductive because the client won't be able to adequately see the nurse. Using an eye patch or dimming the lights won't help with treating or managing the condition.

Critical thinking strategy: Recall the clincal effects of hemianopsia and consider the client's basic need to have meaningful interactions with the nursing staff and her environment.

Client needs category: Physiological integrity

Client needs subcategory: Basic needs and comfort

Cognitive level: Application

Integrated process: Nursing process/implementation

Reference: Smeltzer, page 2208

---

14. The physician writes an order that a client can have 12 ounces of clear liquids at each meal and can supplement this with 10 ounces at each shift (7-3, 3-11, and 11-7). How many milliliters should the nurse document for the day shift (7-3) if the client took in all of the ordered volumes? Record your answer using a whole number.

_____ milliliters

Answer: 1,020

Rationale: The nurse must add all the volumes together, knowing that 1 ounce (oz) equals 30 milliliters (ml). There are 2 meals in the day shift (7-3).

$$12 \text{ oz} \times 30 \text{ ml} = 360 \text{ ml}$$
$$360 \text{ ml} \times 2 \text{ meals} = 720 \text{ ml}$$
$$10 \text{ oz (supplement)} \times 30 \text{ ml} = 300 \text{ ml}$$
$$720 \text{ ml} + 300 \text{ ml} = 1,020 \text{ ml}$$

Critical thinking strategy: Focus on what the question is asking (the total volume of intake for the day shift) and review dosage equivalents.

Client needs category: Physiological integrity

Client needs subcategory: Basic care and comfort

Cognitive level: Application

Integrated process: Communication and documentation

Reference: Taylor, page 1693

15. The nurse is recording the intake and output for a client with the following: D$_5$NSS 1,000 ml; urine 450 ml; emesis 125 ml; Jackson Pratt drain #1 35 ml; Jackson Pratt drain #2 32 ml; and Jackson Pratt drain #3 12 ml. How many milliliters should the nurse document as the client's output? Record your answer using a whole number.

_____ milliliters

Answer: 654

Rationale: The nurse must add all the output volumes together:

$$450 \text{ ml} + 125 \text{ ml} + 35 \text{ ml} + 32 \text{ ml} + 12 \text{ ml} = 654 \text{ ml}$$

D$_5$NSS 1,000 ml is considered input, not output.

Critical thinking strategy: Focus on what the question is asking (the total volume of output).

Client needs category: Physiological integrity

Client needs subcategory: Basic care and comfort

Cognitive level: Application

Integrated process: Communication and documentation

Reference: Taylor, page 1693

Basic psychosocial needs

1. A nurse is caring for a client who is disoriented to time, place, and person and is attempting to get out of bed and pull out an I.V. line that's supplying hydration and antibiotics. The client has a vest restraint and bilateral soft wrist restraints. Which of the following actions by the nurse would be appropriate? Select all that apply.

☐ **1.** Perform a face-to-face behavior evaluation every hour.

☐ **2.** Tie the restraints in quick-release knots.

☐ **3.** Tie the restraints to the side rails of the bed.

☐ **4.** Document the client's condition.

☐ **5.** Document alternative methods used before the restraints were applied.

☐ **6.** Document the client's response to the intervention.

Answer: 1, 2, 4, 5, 6

Rationale: A face-to-face evaluation must be performed every hour. Restraints should be tied in knots that can be released quickly and easily. The nurse should document the client's condition, any alternative methods used before the restraints were applied, and the client's response to the interventions. Restraints should never be secured to side rails because doing so can cause injury if the side rail is lowered without untying the restraint.

Critical thinking strategy: Consider the client's safety needs and review basic care and comfort procedures for clients who are confused and at increased risk for falls.

Client needs category: Safe, effective care environment

Client needs subcategory: Safety and infection control

Cognitive level: Application

Integrated process: Nursing process/implementation

Reference: Craven, pages 665–667

2. A client has just been diagnosed with terminal cancer and is being transferred to home hospice care. The client's daughter tells the nurse, "I don't know what to say to my mother if she asks me if she's going to die." Which of the following responses by the nurse would be appropriate? Select all that apply.

☐ **1.** "Tell your mother not to worry. She still has some time left."

☐ **2.** "Let's talk about your mother's illness and how it will progress."

☐ **3.** "You sound like you have some questions about your mother dying. Let's talk about that."

☐ **4.** "Don't worry, hospice will take care of your mother."

☐ **5.** "Tell me how you're feeling about your mother dying."

Answer: 2, 3, 5

Rationale: Conveying information clearly and openly can alleviate fears and strengthen the individual's sense of control. Encouraging verbalization of feelings helps build a therapeutic relationship based on trust and reduces anxiety. Advising the daughter not to worry, or having her tell her mother that, ignores her feelings and discourages further communication.

Critical thinking strategy: Focus on the psychosocial needs of the family of a dying client and review therapeutic communication techniques.

Client needs category: Psychosocial integrity

Client needs subcategory: None

Cognitive level: Analysis

Integrated process: Caring

Reference: Taylor, pages 488–489

---

3. While providing care to a 26-year-old married client, the nurse notes multiple blue, purple, and yellow ecchymotic areas on her arms and trunk. When the nurse asks how she got these bruises, the client responds, "I tripped." What actions should the nurse take? Select all that apply.

☐ **1.** Document the client's statement and complete a body map indicating the size, color, shape, location, and type of injuries.

☐ **2.** Contact the local authorities to report suspicions of abuse.

☐ **3.** Assist the client in developing a safety plan for times of increased violence.

☐ **4.** Call the client's husband to arrange a meeting to discuss the situation.

☐ **5.** Tell the client that she needs to leave the abusive situation as soon as possible.

☐ **6.** Provide the client with telephone numbers of local shelters and safe houses.

Answer: 1, 3, 6

Rationale: The nurse should objectively document her assessment findings. A detailed description of physical findings of abuse in the medical record is essential if legal action is pursued. All women suspected of being abuse victims should be counseled on a safety plan, which consists of recognizing escalating violence within the family, formulating a plan to exit quickly, and knowing the telephone numbers of local shelters and safe houses. The nurse should not report this suspicion of abuse because the client is a competent adult who has the right to self-determination. Contacting the client's husband without her consent violates confidentiality. The nurse should respond to the client in a nonthreatening manner that promotes trust, rather than ordering her to break off her relationship.

Critical thinking strategy: Review the nurse's responsibilities when caring for a potential abuse victim and consider the client's age to determine appropriate actions.

Client needs category: Psychosocial integrity

Client needs subcategory: None

Cognitive level: Analysis

Integrated process: Communication and documentation

Reference: Smeltzer, page 1621

4. A nurse is caring for a terminally ill client. Place the following five stages of death and dying described by Elisabeth Kübler-Ross in the order in which they occur.

1. Bargaining
2. Denial and isolation
3. Acceptance
4. Anger
5. Depression

Rationale: According to Kübler-Ross, the five stages of death and dying are denial and isolation, anger, bargaining, depression, and acceptance.

Critical thinking strategy: Focus on the stages of death and dying and review the work of Elisabeth Kübler-Ross.

Client needs category: Psychosocial integrity

Client needs subcategory: None

Cognitive level: Analysis

Integrated process: Caring

Reference: Taylor, pages 987–988

5. A 26-year-old client with chronic renal failure was recently told by his physician that he is a poor candidate for a transplant because of chronic uncontrolled hypertension and diabetes mellitus. Now the client tells the nurse, "I want to go off dialysis. I'd rather not live than be on this treatment for the rest of my life." Which of the following responses is appropriate? Select all that apply.

☐ **1.** Take a seat next to the client and sit quietly to reflect on what he said.

☐ **2.** Say to the client, "We all have days when we don't feel like going on."

☐ **3.** Leave the room to allow the client privacy to collect his thoughts.

☐ **4.** Say to the client, "You're feeling upset about the news you got about the transplant."

☐ **5.** Say to the client, "The treatments are only 3 days a week. You can live with that."

Answer: 1, 4

Rationale: Silence is a therapeutic communication technique that allows the nurse and client to reflect on what has taken place or been said. By waiting quietly and attentively, the nurse encourages the client to initiate and maintain a conversation. By reflecting the client's implied feelings, the nurse promotes communication. Using such platitudes as "We all have days when we don't feel like going on" fails to address the client's needs. The nurse should not leave the client alone because he may harm himself. Reminding the client of the treatment frequency doesn't address his feelings.

Critical thinking strategy: Focus on the care of the client under emotional stress and review the principles of therapeutic communication.

Client needs category: Psychosocial integrity

Client needs subcategory: None

Cognitive level: Analysis

Integrated process: Caring

Reference: Taylor, pages 488–490

6. A nurse is caring for a client with advanced cancer. After reading the nursing note below, determine the nurse's next intervention.

Progress notes	
1/7/09	Pt. states, "The doctor says my chemotherapy
1545	isn't working anymore. They can only treat my
	symptoms now. I don't want to die in the
	hospital, I want to be in my own bed."
	———— R. Daly, RN

☐ **1.** Reread the Patient's Bill of Rights to the client.

☐ **2.** Call the client's spouse to discuss the client's statements.

☐ **3.** Tell the client that only in the hospital can he receive adequate pain relief.

☐ **4.** Explain the use of an advance directive to express the client's wishes.

Answer: 4

Rationale: An advance directive is a legal document used as a guideline for life-sustaining medical care of a client with an advanced disease or disability who can no longer indicate his own wishes. This document can include a living will, which instructs the health care provider to administer no life-sustaining treatment, and a durable power of attorney for health care, which names another person to act on the client's behalf for medical decisions if the client can't act for himself. The Patient's Bill of Rights doesn't specifically address the client's wishes regarding future care. Calling the spouse is a breach of the client's right to confidentiality. Stating that only a hospital can provide adequate pain relief in a terminal situation demonstrates inadequate knowledge of the resources available in the community through hospice and home care agencies in collaboration with the client's health care provider.

Critical thinking strategy: Focus on the needs of a client who is making difficult medical decisions, consider referrals available to the nurse, and review the use of advance directives.

Client needs category: Psychosocial integrity

Client needs subcategory: None

Cognitive level: Application

Integrated process: Caring

Reference: Taylor, pages 990–993

---

7. The nurse is caring for a client whose cultural background is different from her own. Which of the following actions are appropriate for the nurse to take? Select all that apply.

☐ **1.** Consider that nonverbal cues, such as eye contact, may have a different meaning in different cultures.

☐ **2.** Respect the client's cultural beliefs.

☐ **3.** Ask the client if he has cultural or religious requirements that should be considered in his care.

☐ **4.** Explain the nurse's beliefs so that the client will understand the differences.

☐ **5.** Understand that all cultures experience pain in the same way.

Answer: 1, 2, 3

Rationale: Nonverbal cues may have different meanings in different cultures. In one culture, eye contact may be a sign of disrespect; in another, eye contact may show respect and attentiveness. The nurse should always respect the client's cultural beliefs and ask if he has cultural or religious requirements. This may include food choices or restrictions, body coverings, or time for prayer. The nurse should attempt to understand the client's culture; it isn't the client's responsibility to understand the nurse's culture. The nurse should never impose her own beliefs on her clients. Culture influences a client's experience of pain. For example, pain may be openly expressed in one culture and quietly endured in another.

Critical thinking strategy: Recall the implications of culturally sensitive care and the nurse's responsibilities when delivering such care to clients.

Client needs category: Psychosocial integrity

Client needs subcategory: None

Cognitive level: Analysis

Integrated process: Caring

Reference: Taylor, pages 52–54

8. A nurse is caring for a 45-year-old married woman who has undergone hemicolectomy for colon cancer. The woman has two children. Which of the following concepts about families should the nurse keep in mind when providing care for this client? Select all that apply.

- ☐ **1.** Illness in one family member can affect all members.
- ☐ **2.** Family roles don't change because of illness.
- ☐ **3.** A family member may perform more than one role at a time.
- ☐ **4.** Children typically aren't affected by adult illness.
- ☐ **5.** The effects of an illness on a family depend on the stage of the family's life cycle.
- ☐ **6.** Changes in sleeping and eating patterns may be signs of stress in a family.

Answer: 1, 3, 5, 6

Rationale: Illness in one family member can affect all family members, even children. Each member of a family may have several roles to perform. A middle-aged woman, for example, may have the roles of mother, wife, wage-earner, and housekeeper. When one family member can't fulfill a role because of illness, the roles of the other family members are affected. Families move through certain predictable life cycles (such as birth of a baby, a growing family, adult children leaving home, and grandparenting). The impact of illness on the family depends on the stage of the life cycle as family members take on different roles and the family structure changes. Illness produces stress in families; changes in eating and sleeping patterns are signs of stress.

Critical thinking strategy: Concentrate on the impact of stress and illness on the family and recall the manifestations that may result from stress.

Client needs category: Health promotion and maintenance

Client needs subcategory: None

Cognitive level: Analysis

Integrated process: Nursing process/implementation

Reference: Taylor, pages 32–35

---

9. A nurse is assessing a newly admitted client. In the family assessment, whom should the nurse consider to be a part of the client's family? Select all that apply.

- ☐ **1.** People related by blood or marriage
- ☐ **2.** People whom the client views as family
- ☐ **3.** People who live in the same house
- ☐ **4.** People whom the nurse thinks are important to the client
- ☐ **5.** People of the same racial background who live in the same house as the client
- ☐ **6.** People who provide for the physical and emotional needs of the client

Answer: 2, 6

Rationale: When providing care to a client, the nurse should consider family members to be all the people whom the client views as family. Family members may also include those people who provide for the physical and emotional needs of the client. The traditional definition of a family has changed and may include people not related by blood or marriage, those of a different racial background, and those who may not live in the same house as the client. Family members are defined by the client, not by the nurse.

Critical thinking strategy: Recall the components of a family group and consider the changes that have taken place in society relating to family members. Review the definition of family.

Client needs category: Health promotion and maintenance

Client needs subcategory: None

Cognitive level: Analysis

Integrated process: Nursing process/assessment

Reference: Craven, page 295

10. A nurse is working with the family of a client who has Alzheimer's disease. The nurse notes that the client's spouse is too exhausted to continue providing care all alone. The adult children live too far away to provide relief on a weekly basis. Which nursing interventions would be most helpful? Select all that apply.

☐ **1.** Calling a family meeting to tell the absent children that they must participate in caregiving

☐ **2.** Suggesting that the spouse seek psychological counseling to help cope with exhaustion

☐ **3.** Recommending community resources for adult day care and respite care

☐ **4.** Encouraging the spouse to talk about the difficulties involved in caring for a loved one

☐ **5.** Asking whether friends or church members can help with errands or provide short periods of relief

☐ **6.** Recommending that the client be placed in a long-term care facility

Answer: 3, 4, 5

Rationale: Many community services exist for Alzheimer's clients and their families. Encouraging use of these resources may make it possible to keep the client at home and to alleviate the spouse's exhaustion. The nurse can also support the caregiver by urging her to talk about the difficulties she's facing in caring for her spouse. Friends and church members may be able to help provide care to the client, allowing the caregiver time for rest, exercise, or an enjoyable activity. Arranging a family meeting to tell the children to participate more would probably be ineffective and might evoke anger or guilt. Counseling might be helpful, but it wouldn't alleviate the caregiver's physical exhaustion or address the client's immediate needs. A long-term care facility isn't an option until the family is ready to make that decision.

Critical thinking strategy: Think of the nurse's role when offering emotional support to individuals struggling with the stressors associated with caring for the chronically ill.

Client needs category: Psychosocial integrity

Client needs subcategory: None

Cognitive level: Analysis

Integrated process: Caring

Reference: Smeltzer, page 246

---

11. The home health nurse is completing the admission paperwork for a new client diagnosed with osteomyelitits who will be receiving home service intravenous therapy for the next month. The client is 32 years old and happily married. Which of the following findings will warrant further investigation? Select all that apply.

☐ **1.** The client reports having many hobbies and interests outside of the home.

☐ **2.** The client voices concerns about recovering quickly so that she might return back to work in the next month.

☐ **3.** The client talks repeatedly about her death.

☐ **4.** The client spends a great deal of time reflecting back on her teen years.

☐ **5.** The client is talkative about her spouse and children.

Answer: 3, 4

Rationale: At age 32, the client is in the middle adult stage of life. Her repeated discussions about death and reflections back on life aren't appropriate or expected for this stage of development and should be investigated further. An interest in civic responsibilities and the establishment of hobbies is expected. During this developmental period, the greatest concern typically relates to establishing gainful employment and significant relationships. This is being demonstrated by the client's willingness to discuss her spouse and children.

Critical thinking strategy: Review Erikson's developmental stages and consider the client's age in relation to what's appropriate.

Client needs category: Psychosocial integrity

Client needs subcategory: None

Cognitive level: Application

Integrated process: Caring

Reference: Craven, pages 247–248

Medication and I.V. administration

1. A physician prescribes I.V. normal saline solution to be infused at a rate of 150 ml/hour for a client admitted with dehydration and pneumonia. How many liter(s) of solution will the client receive during an 8-hour shift? Record your answer using one decimal place.

_____ liters

Answer: 1.2

Rationale: The ordered infusion rate is 150 ml/hour. The nurse should multiply 150 ml by 8 hours to determine the total volume in milliliters the client will receive during an 8-hour shift (1,200 ml). Then she should convert milliliters to liters by dividing by 1,000. The total volume in liters that the client will receive in 8 hours is 1.2 liters.

Critical thinking strategy: Focus on what the question is asking (the volume to be received in an 8-hour period). Review basic drug calculations and basic conversions.

Client needs category: Physiological integrity

Client needs subcategory: Pharmacological and parenteral therapies

Cognitive level: Analysis

Integrated process: Nursing process/planning

Reference: _Dosage Calculations Made Incredibly Easy,_ pages 237–238

2. A client is prescribed heparin 6,000 units subcutaneously every 12 hours for deep vein thrombosis prophylaxis. The pharmacy dispenses a vial containing 10,000 units/1 ml. How many milliliter(s) of heparin should the nurse administer? Record your answer using one decimal place.

_____ milliliter(s)

Answer: 0.6

Rationale: The dose dispensed by the pharmacy is 10,000 units/1 ml, and the desired dose is 6,000 units. The nurse should use the following equations to determine the amount of heparin to administer:

Dose on hand/Quantity on hand = Dose desired/X

$$10,000 \text{ units}/1 \text{ ml} = 6,000 \text{ units}/X$$

$$10,000 \text{ units} \times X = 6,000 \text{ units} \times 1 \text{ ml}$$

$$X = 6,000 \text{ units} \times 1 \text{ ml}/10,000 \text{ units}$$

$$X = 0.6 \text{ ml}$$

Critical thinking strategy: Focus on what the question is asking (the amount of milliliters for a dose of medication), and use the calculation method of ratio and proportion to set up this problem.

Client needs category: Physiological integrity

Client needs subcategory: Pharmacological and parenteral therapies

Cognitive level: Analysis

Integrated process: Nursing process/planning

Reference: _Dosage Calculations Made Incredibly Easy,_ page 77

3. A nurse is ordered to administer ampicillin (Polycillin) 125 mg I.M. every 6 hours to a 10-kg child with a respiratory tract infection. The drug label reads, "The recommended dose for a client weighing less than 40 kg is 25 to 50 mg/kg/day I.M. or I.V. in equally divided doses at 6- to 8-hour intervals." The drug concentration is 125 mg/5 ml. Which nursing interventions are appropriate at this time? Select all that apply.

☐ **1.** Draw up 10 ml of ampicillin to administer.

☐ **2.** Administer the medication at 10 a.m., 2 p.m., 6 p.m., and 10 p.m.

☐ **3.** Assess the client for allergies to penicillin.

☐ **4.** Administer the medication because the dosage is within the recommended range.

☐ **5.** Question the prescriber about the order because it's for more than the recommended dosage.

☐ **6.** Obtain a sputum culture, if ordered, before administering the medication.

Answer: 3, 4, 6

Rationale: Because ampicillin is a penicillin antibiotic, the nurse should assess the client for penicillin allergies before administering this drug. The ampicillin dose is within the recommended range for a 10-kg client: 50 mg/kg × 10 kg = 500 mg. A dose of 500 mg divided by four (given every 6 hours) = 125 mg. Cultures should be obtained before antibiotics are given. The nurse should draw up 5 ml—not 10 ml—to administer the correct dose, according to the concentration on the label. The correct dosing schedule is every 6 to 8 hours, not every 4 hours.

Crtical thinking strategy: Focus on what the question is asking (all the appropriate interventions for a pediatric client to receive an antibiotic), and review medication administration safety practices as well as the dosage guidelines for pediatric dosing of antibiotics.

Client needs category: Physiological integrity

Client needs subcategory: Pharmacological and parenteral therapies

Cognitive level: Analysis

Integrated process: Nursing process/implementation

Reference: *Dosage Calculations Made Incredibly Easy,* pages 268–270

---

4. A cardiologist prescribes digoxin (Lanoxin) 125 mcg by mouth every morning for a client diagnosed with heart failure. The pharmacy dispenses tablets that contain 0.25 mg each. How many tablet(s) should the nurse administer in each dose? Record your answer using one decimal place.

_____ tablet(s)

Answer: 0.5

Rationale: The nurse should begin by converting 125 mcg to milligrams:

$$125 \text{ mcg}/1,000 = 0.125 \text{ mg.}$$

Then she should use the following formula to calculate the drug dosage:

Dose on hand/Quantity on hand = Dose desired/X

$$0.25 \text{ mg}/1 \text{ tablet} = 0.125 \text{ mg}/X$$

$$0.25 \times X = 0.125 \times 1 \text{ tablet}$$

$$X = 0.5 \text{ tablet}$$

Critical thinking strategy: Focus on the question being asked (the number of tablets in each dose), and use the calculation method of ratio and proportion to set up this problem.

Client needs category: Physiological integrity

Client needs subcategory: Pharmacological and parenteral therapies

Cognitive level: Analysis

Integrated process: Nursing process/implementation

Reference: *Dosage Calculations Made Incredibly Easy,* page 77

---

5. A 75-year-old client is admitted to the hospital with lower GI bleeding. His hemoglobin on admission to the emergency department is 7.3 g/dl. The physician prescribes 2 units of packed red blood cells to infuse over 2 hours each. Each unit of packed red blood cells contains 250 ml. The blood administration set has a drip factor of 10 gtt/ml. What is the flow rate in drops per minute? Round your answer to the nearest whole number.

_____ gtt/minute

Answer: 21

Rationale: Each unit of packed red blood cells contains 250 ml, which should infuse over 2 hours (120 minutes). Therefore, the rate per minute is:

250 ml/120 minutes = 2.08 ml/minute.

Multiply by the drip factor to determine the flow rate:

2.08 ml × 10 gtt = 20.8 gtt/minute
(round up to 21 gtt/minute).

Critical thinking strategy: Focus on what the question is asking (the drop rate per minute of blood), and review I.V. administration calculations, first obtaining the milliliters per hour then calculating the drops per minute.

Client needs category: Physiological integrity

Client needs subcategory: Pharmacological and parenteral therapies

Cognitive level: Analysis

Integrated process: Nursing process/implementation

Reference: _Dosage Calculations Made Incredibly Easy,_ pages 236–238

---

6. A nurse is preparing a teaching plan for a client who was prescribed enalapril maleate (Vasotec) for treatment of hypertension. Which of the following instructions should the nurse include in the teaching plan? Select all that apply.

☐ **1.** Instruct the client to avoid salt substitutes.

☐ **2.** Tell the client that light-headedness is a common adverse effect that doesn't need to be reported.

☐ **3.** Inform the client that he may have a sore throat for the first few days of therapy.

☐ **4.** Advise the client to report facial swelling or difficulty breathing immediately.

☐ **5.** Tell the client that blood tests will be necessary every 3 weeks for 2 months and periodically after that.

☐ **6.** Advise the client not to change position suddenly to minimize orthostatic hypotension.

Answer: 1, 4, 6

Rationale: The nurse should tell the client to avoid salt substitutes because they may contain potassium, which can cause light-headedness and syncope. Facial swelling or difficulty breathing should be reported immediately because they may be signs of angioedema, which would require discontinuation of the drug. The client should also be advised to change position slowly to minimize orthostatic hypotension. The nurse should tell the client to report light-headedness, especially during the first few days of therapy, so dosage adjustments can be made. The client should also report signs of infection, such as sore throat and fever, because the drug may decrease the white blood cell (WBC) count. Because this effect is generally seen within 3 months, the WBC count and differential should be monitored periodically.

Critical thinking strategy: Focus on what the question is asking (instructions for the teaching plan of a client receiving enalapril maleate), and recall the classes of ACE inhibitors and antihypertensives and what type of adverse reactions to expect.

Client needs category: Physiological integrity

Client needs subcategory: Pharmacological and parenteral therapies

Cognitive level: Application

Integrated process: Teaching and learning

Reference: Smeltzer, pages 952–953

7. After sustaining a closed head injury, a client is prescribed phenytoin (Dilantin) 100 mg I.V. every 8 hours for seizure prophylaxis. Which nursing interventions are necessary when administering phenytoin? Select all that apply.

☐ **1.** Administer phenytoin through any peripheral I.V. site.

☐ **2.** Mix I.V. doses in solutions containing dextrose 5% in water.

☐ **3.** Administer an I.V. bolus no faster than 50 mg/minute.

☐ **4.** Monitor electrocardiogram (ECG), blood pressure, and respiratory status continuously when administering phenytoin I.V.

☐ **5.** Don't use an inline filter when administering the drug.

☐ **6.** Keep in mind that early toxicity may cause drowsiness, nausea, vomiting, nystagmus, ataxia, dysarthria, tremor, and slurred speech.

Answer: 3, 4, 6

Rationale: Administer an I.V. bolus by slow (50 mg/minute) I.V. push; too rapid an injection may cause hypotension and circulatory collapse. Continuous monitoring of ECG, blood pressure, and respiratory status is essential when administering phenytoin I.V. Early toxicity may cause drowsiness, nausea, vomiting, nystagmus, ataxia, dysarthria, tremor, and slurred speech. Later effects may include hypotension, arrhythmias, respiratory depression, and coma. Death may result from respiratory and circulatory depression. Phenytoin shouldn't be administered by I.V. push in veins on the back of the hand; larger veins are needed to prevent discoloration associated with purple glove syndrome. Mix I.V. doses in normal saline solution and use the solution within 30 minutes; doses mixed in dextrose 5% in water will precipitate. Use of an inline filter is recommended.

Critical thinking strategy: Focus on what the question is asking (nursing interventions of a client prescribed phenytion [Dilantin]) and review the therapeutic class of anticonvulsants, concentrating on the nursing interventions.

Client needs category: Physiological integrity

Client needs subcategory: Pharmacological and parenteral therapies

Cognitive level: Application

Integrated process: Nursing process/implementation

Reference: Smeltzer, pages 2193–2194

---

8. A 53-year-old client returns to his room from the postanesthesia care unit after undergoing a right hemicolectomy. The physician orders 1 L of dextrose 5% in half-normal saline solution to infuse at 125 ml/hour. The drop factor of the available I.V. tubing is 15 gtt/ml. What is the drip rate in drops per minute? Round your answer to the nearest whole number.

_____ gtt/minute

Answer: 31

Rationale: The flow rate is 125 ml/hour, or 125 ml/60 minutes. Use the following equation to determine the drip rate:

125 ml/60 minutes $\times$ 15 gtt/1 ml = 31.25 gtt/minute (round down to 31 gtt/minute).

Critical thinking strategy: Focus on what the question is asking (the drip rate per minute of I.V. fluid) and review how to calculate I.V. drip rates.

Client needs category: Physiological integrity

Client needs subcategory: Pharmacological and parenteral therapies

Cognitive level: Application

Integrated process: Nursing process/implementation

Reference: _Dosage Calculations Made Incredibly Easy,_ pages 233–234

---

9. A physician prescribes I.V. heparin 25,000 units in 250 ml of normal saline solution to infuse at 600 units/hour for a client who suffered an acute myocardial infarction. After 6 hours of heparin therapy, the client's partial thromboplastin time is subtherapeutic. The physician orders the infusion to be increased to 800 units/hour. The nurse should set the infusion pump to deliver how many milliliters per hour? Record your answer using a whole number.

_____ milliliters/hour

Rationale: The nurse should calculate the infusion rate using the following formula:

Dose on hand/Quantity on hand = Dose desired/X

25,000 units/250 ml = 800 units/hour ÷ X

25,000 units × X = 250 ml × 800 units/hour

25,000 × X = 200,000 ml/hour

X = 8 ml/hour

Critical thinking strategy: Focus on what the question is asking (setting an I.V. infusion device, which delivers milliliters per hour), and review the calculation method of ratio and proportion and use of I.V. fusion delivery devices.

Client needs category: Physiological integrity

Client needs subcategory: Pharmacological and parenteral therapies

Cognitive level: Application

Integrated process: Nursing process/implementation

Reference: _Dosage Calculations Made Incredibly Easy,_ pages 246–248

---

10. After undergoing small-bowel resection, a client is prescribed metronidazole (Flagyl) 500 mg I.V. The mixed I.V. solution contains 100 ml. The nurse is to administer the drug over 30 minutes. The drop factor of the available I.V. tubing is 15 gtt/ml. What is the drip rate in drops per minute? Record your answer using a whole number.

_____ drops/minute

Answer: 50

Rationale: The nurse should use the following equation to calculate the drip rate:

Total quantity/Administration time × gtt/min = X

100 ml/30 min × 15 gtt/min = X

$$X = \frac{1500 \text{ gtt}}{30 \text{ min}}$$

X = 50 gtt/minute

Critical thinking strategy: Focus on what the question is asking (the drip rate per minute of a secondary infusion) and review the calculation of I.V. drip rates.

Client needs category: Physiological integrity

Client needs subcategory: Pharmacological and parenteral therapies

Cognitive level: Application

Integrated process: Nursing process/implementation

Reference: _Dosage Calculations Made Incredibly Easy,_ page 257

11. A client with an I.V. line in place complains of pain at the insertion site. Assessment of the site reveals a vein that's red, warm, and hard. Which of the following actions should the nurse take? Select all that apply.

☐ **1.** Slow the infusion rate while notifying the prescriber.

☐ **2.** Discontinue the infusion at the affected site.

☐ **3.** Restart the infusion distal to the discontinued I.V. site.

☐ **4.** Assess the client for skin sloughing.

☐ **5.** Apply warm soaks to the I.V. site.

☐ **6.** Document the assessment, nursing actions taken, and the client's response.

Rationale: Redness, warmth, pain, and a hard, cord-like vein at the I.V. insertion site suggest that the client has phlebitis. The nurse should discontinue the I.V. infusion and insert a new I.V. catheter proximal to or above the discontinued site or in the other arm. Applying warm soaks to the site reduces inflammation. The nurse should document the assessment of the I.V. site, the actions taken, and client's response to the situation. Slowing the infusion rate won't reduce the phlebitis. Restarting the infusion at a site distal to the phlebitis may contribute to the inflammation. Skin sloughing isn't a symptom of phlebitis; it's associated with extravasation of certain toxic medications.

Critical thinking strategy: Recall the assessment findings associated with I.V. sites and the interventions for an abnormal assessment.

Client needs category: Physiological integrity

Client needs subcategory: Pharmacological and parenteral therapies

Cognitive level: Application

Integrated process: Nursing process/planning

Reference: Craven, page 575

---

12. After suffering an acute myocardial infarction (MI), a client with a history of type 1 diabetes is prescribed metoprolol (Lopressor) I.V. Which nursing interventions are associated with I.V. administration of metoprolol? Select all that apply.

☐ **1.** Monitor glucose levels closely.

☐ **2.** Monitor for heart block and bradycardia.

☐ **3.** Monitor blood pressure closely.

☐ **4.** Mix the drug in 50 ml of dextrose 5% in water and infuse over 30 minutes.

☐ **5.** Be aware that the drug isn't compatible with morphine.

Rationale: Metoprolol masks the common signs of hypoglycemia; therefore, glucose levels should be monitored closely in diabetic clients. When used to treat an MI, metoprolol is contraindicated in clients with heart rates less than 45 beats/minute and any degree of heart block, so the nurse should monitor the client for bradycardia and heart block. Metoprolol masks common signs and symptoms of shock, such as decreased blood pressure, so blood pressure should also be monitored closely. The nurse should give the drug undiluted by direct injection. Although metoprolol shouldn't be mixed with other drugs, studies have shown that it's compatible when mixed with morphine sulfate or when administered with alteplase infusion at a Y-site connection.

Critical thinking strategy: Focus on the nursing interventions required for a client receiving I.V. metoprolol (Lopressor), and review the pharmacological and therapeutic classes of beta blockers and antihypertensives, concentrating on I.V. administration.

Client needs category: Physiological integrity

Client needs subcategory: Pharmacological and parenteral therapies

Cognitive level: Application

Integrated process: Nursing process/implementation

Reference: Smeltzer, pages 869–870

13. When administering medication, the nurse ensures client safety by following the rights of medication administration. Identity the "rights of medication administration." Select all that apply.

- ☐ **1.** Right room
- ☐ **2.** Right client
- ☐ **3.** Right dose
- ☐ **4.** Right medication
- ☐ **5.** Right time
- ☐ **6.** Right route

Rationale: A nurse must always implement safe nursing practice when administering medications. Following the rights of medication administration helps protect the client from medication errors. Safe procedure includes confirming the right client, dose, medication, time, and route. Confirming the room number doesn't guarantee that the right client will receive the correct medication.

Critical thinking strategy: Review safety guidelines for medication administration.

Client needs category: Physiological integrity

Client needs subcategory: Pharmacological and parenteral therapies

Cognitive level: Application

Integrated process: Communication and documentation

Reference: Taylor, page 784

---

14. A client is to be started on a new diuretic medication. Which of the following should be included in the teaching plan? Select all that apply.

- ☐ **1.** Advise the client to reduce his dietary sodium intake.
- ☐ **2.** Encourage the use of salt substitutes.
- ☐ **3.** Tell the client to alert the physician about any visible edema.
- ☐ **4.** Instruct the client to take the medication as directed.
- ☐ **5.** Suggest taking the medication just before bedtime to establish a routine.

Answer: 1, 3, 4

Rationale: Reducing dietary sodium intake will help increase the effectiveness of diuretic medication and may allow smaller doses to be ordered. Diuretics are commonly prescribed to control fluid accumulation in the body; therefore, the presence of edema may indicate the need for the physician to adjust the therapy. Compliance is very important with diuretics. In order to effectively monitor therapy, the nurse should encourage the client to take the medication exactly as prescribed. Salt substitutes aren't recommended because they contain potassium instead of sodium and may cause serious cardiovascular effects. Diuretics cause an increased urine output, which may interfere with the client's sleep if taken at bedtime.

Critical thinking strategy: Focus on the pharmacologic concepts and use of diuretics and the education needs of clients taking these drugs.

Client needs category: Health promotion and maintenance

Client needs subcategory: None

Cognitive level: Analysis

Integrated process: Teaching and learning

Reference: Smeltzer, page 953

15. A client receives a short-acting insulin and an intermediate-acting insulin before breakfast at 0800. Using the chart below, when should the nurse expect the intermediate insulin to start to take effect?

Medication administration record

Insulin type	Onset	Peak	Duration
Short-acting	15-30 minutes	2-3 hours	4-6 hours
Intermediate-acting	2-4 hours	4-12 hours	16-20 hours

☐ **1.** 1500

☐ **2.** 1300

☐ **3.** 1000

☐ **4.** 0900

Answer: 3

Rationale: The timing of insulin's effects varies according to the type. Referring to the chart, the nurse would note that the onset of action for the intermediate insulin is 2 to 4 hours. Because the administration time was 0800, the effects should begin 2 hours after administration, at 1000.

Critical thinking strategy: Review the pharmacologic properties of insulin and focus on what the question is asking (the onset of intermediate-acting insulin's effects).

Client needs category: Physiological integrity

Client needs subcategory: Pharmacological and parenteral therapies

Cognitive level: Application

Integrated process: Nursing process/evaluation

Reference: Smeltzer, page 1392

---

16. A client has an I.V. line in place for 3 days and begins to complain of discomfort at the insertion site. Based on the client's progress notes below, what condition has most likely occurred?

Progress notes

02/15/09 0730	I.V. site assessed and found to have blanching around the site, swelling, and coolness to the touch. Laboratory results include a white blood cell count within normal limits. —Sue Thompson, RN

☐ **1.** Infiltration

☐ **2.** Phlebitis

☐ **3.** Infection

☐ **4.** Infection and infiltration

Answer: 1

Rationale: The assessment findings of pallor, swelling, skin that's cool to the touch at the I.V. insertion site, and a normal white blood cell count all indicate infiltration. The infusion should be discontinued and restarted in a different site. Phlebitis would be evidenced by redness at the cannula tip and along the vein. Infection would be evidenced by an elevated white blood cell count.

Critical thinking strategy: Recall the signs and symptoms of I.V. complications.

Client needs category: Physiological integrity

Client needs subcategory: Pharmacological and parenteral therapies

Cognitive level: Application

Integrated process: Nursing process/analysis

Reference: Taylor, page 1714

17. A client is ordered an I.V. solution of 1,000 ml to infuse from 0800 to 2000. The nurse will use an infusion pump that delivers in milliliters per hour. At what rate should the nurse set the pump to deliver the solution? Record your answer using a whole number.

_____ milliliters/hour

Answer: 83

Rationale: First determine how many hours the infusion needs to run. 0800 to 2000 is 12 hours. Use the following equation to determine the milliliters/hour:

$$\frac{\text{Volume to infuse}}{\text{Infusion time}} = \text{Flow rate per hour}$$

$$\frac{1,000 \text{ ml}}{12 \text{ hours}} = 83.3 \text{ ml/hour (rounded to 83 ml/hour)}$$

The pump should be set to deliver 83 ml/hour.

Critical thinking strategy: Focus on what the question is asking (the milliliters per hour using an infusion device) and review calculations of I.V. drip rates.

Client needs category: Physiological integrity

Client needs subcategory: Basic care and comfort

Cognitive level: Analysis

Integrated process: Nursing process/planning

Reference: _Dosage Calculations Made Incredibly Easy,_ pages 237–238

---

18. A nurse enters a client's semiprivate room and prepares to administer the 0900 medications. Place the following steps in chronological sequence to indicate the safest to least safe measure to take when administering these medications. Use all the options.

1. Administer the medications.
2. Obtain the correct unit-dose medications.
3. Confirm the client's identity.
4. Check the client's medication administration record (MAR) for the 0900 medications.
5. Open the unit-dose packages.

Answer: 4, 2, 3, 5, 1

Rationale: Following sequential steps helps ensure safe medication administration. The nurse should first check to see which medications the client is due to receive at 0900 and then obtain them. Next, the nurse should confirm the client's identity according to facility protocol. Once the client is properly identified, the nurse should open the drug packages at the bedside, administer the medications to the client, and record that she administered them.

Critical thinking strategy: Review medication administration safety practices.

Client needs category: Physiological integrity

Client needs subcategory: Pharmacological and parenteral therapies

Cognitive level: Application

Integrated process: Nursing process/implementation

Reference: Craven, pages 510–512

19. The nurse prepares to administer medications into a client's jejunostomy tube. Identify the area where the nurse would assess the tube to be.

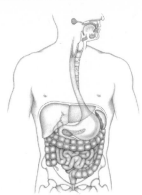

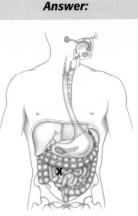

Rationale: The jejunum is the immediate portion of the small intestine that connects proximally with the duodenum and distally with the ileum.

Critical thinking strategy: Review the anatomy of the gastrointestinal system and the correct placement for a jejunostomy tube.

Client needs category: Health promotion and maintenance

Client needs subcategory: None

Cognitive level: Application

Integrated process: Nursing process/assessment

Reference: Craven, page 1117

Basic physical assessment

1. A client who was involved in a motor vehicle accident is admitted to the intensive care unit. The emergency department admission record indicates that the client was hit in the right temporal lobe. A nurse would expect the client to demonstrate which of the following abnormalities? Select all that apply.

☐ **1.** Difficulty comprehending language

☐ **2.** Decreased hearing

☐ **3.** Aphasia

☐ **4.** Amnesia for recent events

☐ **5.** Ataxic gait

☐ **6.** Personality changes

Answer: 1, 2, 4

Rationale: The temporal lobe controls hearing, language comprehension, and the storage and recall of memories; therefore, the client would likely have difficulty comprehending language, diminished hearing, and amnesia for recent events. Aphasia and personality changes might be expected from injury to the frontal lobe. An ataxic gait would indicate injury primarily to the cerebellum.

Critical thinking strategy: Recall the anatomy and physiology of the brain and the specific function of each section, focusing particularily on the temporal lobe.

Client needs category: Safe, effective care environment

Client needs subcategory: Management of care

Cognitive level: Analysis

Integrated process: Nursing process/assessment

Reference: Smeltzer, page 2131

2. A nurse is assessing a client who reports burning on urination and a low-grade fever. On physical examination, the nurse notes right-sided costovertebral tenderness. Identify the area the nurse percussed to elicit this sign.

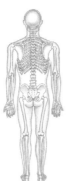

Answer:

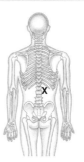

Rationale: To determine whether costovertebral tenderness (a sign of glomerulonephritis) is present, the nurse should percuss the costovertebral angle (the angle over each kidney that's formed by the lateral and downward curve of the lowest rib and the vertebral column). The costovertebral angle can be percussed by placing the palm of one hand over the costovertebral angle and striking it with the fist of the other hand.

Critical thinking strategy: Review the assessment techniques for the renal system and the clinical manifestations of the findings.

Client needs category: Physiological integrity

Client needs subcategory: Physiological adaptation

Cognitive level: Application

Integrated process: Nursing process/assessment

Reference: Smeltzer, page 1504

---

3. A nurse is assessing a client's abdomen. Identify the area where the nurse's hand should be placed to palpate the liver.

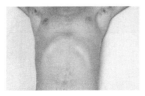

Answer:

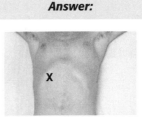

Rationale: The nurse can best palpate the liver by standing on the client's right side and placing her right hand on the client's abdomen, along the right midclavicular line. She should point the fingers of her right hand toward the client's head, just under the right rib margin.

Critical thinking strategy: Review the anatomy of the gastrointestinal system and techniques for assessing the liver.

Client needs category: Health promotion and maintenance

Client needs subcategory: None

Cognitive level: Application

Integrated process: Nursing process/assessment

Reference: Taylor, pages 638–639

4. While examining the hands of a client with osteoarthritis, a nurse notes Heberden's nodes on the second (index) finger. Identify the area on the finger where the nurse observed the node.

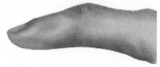

Answer:

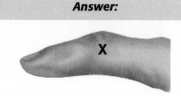

Rationale: Heberden's nodes appear on the distal interphalangeal joints. These bony and cartilaginous enlargements are usually hard and painless and typically occur in middle-aged and elderly clients with osteoarthritis.

Critical thinking strategy: Review the anatomy of the hand and the pathophysiology of osteoarthritis.

Client needs category: Physiological integrity

Client needs subcategory: Physiological adaptation

Cognitive level: Application

Integrated process: Nursing process/assessment

Reference: Smeltzer, page 1915

---

5. A nurse is percussing a client's abdomen. Identify the area where liver dullness is best percussed.

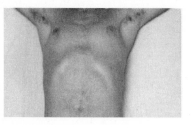

Answer:

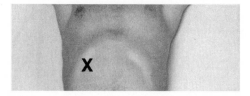

Rationale: To hear liver dullness, the nurse should percuss the abdomen at the right midclavicular line, starting at a level below the umbilicus (in an area of tympany, not dullness) and continuing upward toward the liver.

Critical thinking strategy: Review anatomy of the gastrointestinal system and techniques for assessing the liver.

Client needs category: Health promotion and maintenance

Client needs subcategory: None

Cognitive level: Application

Integrated process: Nursing process/assessment

Reference: Taylor, page 638

6. A client is diagnosed with herpes zoster. Place in chronological order the pathophysiologic changes associated with the client's disorder.

| 1. Fever, malaise, and red nodules appear in a dermatome distribution. |
| 2. The virus multiplies in the ganglia, causing deep pain, itching, and paresthesia or hyperesthesia. |
| 3. Vesicles crust and scab but no longer shed the virus. |
| 4. Residual antibodies from the initial infection mobilize but are ineffective. |
| 5. Vesicles appear, filled with either clear fluid or pus. |
| 6. Varicella-zoster virus is reactivated. |

Rationale: Herpes zoster is an acute inflammation caused by infection with the herpes virus varicella-zoster (chickenpox virus). The pathophysiologic changes associated with this disorder occur in the order described above.

Critical thinking strategy: Review the pathophysiology of herpes zoster.

Client needs category: Physiological integrity

Client needs subcategory: Physiological adaptation

Cognitive level: Application

Integrated process: Nursing process/analysis

Reference: Smeltzer, pages 1958–1959

---

7. An elderly client has a history of aortic stenosis. Identify the area where the nurse should place the stethoscope to best hear the murmur.

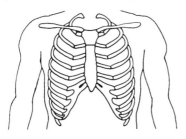

Answer:

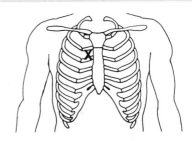

Rationale: The murmur of aortic stenosis is low-pitched, rough, and rasping. It's heard best in the second intercostal space, to the right of the sternum.

Critical thinking strategy: Review the anatomy of the cardiovascular system and techniques for assessing the heart.

Client needs category: Physiological integrity

Client needs subcategory: Physiological adaptation

Cognitive level: Application

Integrated process: Nursing process/assessment

Reference: Taylor, page 632

8. A nurse is assessing a client who has a rash on his chest and upper arms. Which questions should the nurse ask in order to gain further information about the client's rash? Select all that apply.

☐ **1.** "When did the rash start?"

☐ **2.** "Are you allergic to any medications, foods, or pollen?"

☐ **3.** "How old are you?"

☐ **4.** "What have you been using to treat the rash?"

☐ **5.** "Have you recently traveled outside the country?"

☐ **6.** "Do you smoke cigarettes or drink alcohol?"

Answer: 1, 2, 4, 5

Rationale: The nurse should first find out when the rash began; this can assist with the correct diagnosis. She should also ask about allergies; rashes can occur when a person changes medications, eats new foods, or contacts pollen. It's also important to find out how the client has been treating the rash; some topical ointments or oral medications may worsen it. The nurse should ask about recent travel; exposure to foreign foods and environments can cause a rash. The client's age and smoking and drinking habits won't provide further insight into the rash or its cause.

Critical thinking strategy: Review the anatomy and pathophysiology of the integumentary system and history-taking techniques.

Client needs category: Physiological integrity

Client needs subcategory: Physiological adaptation

Cognitive level: Application

Integrated process: Nursing process/assessment

Reference: Smeltzer, pages 1933–1935

---

9. While assessing a client's spine for abnormal curvatures, a nurse notes kyphosis. Identify the area of the spine that's affected by kyphosis.

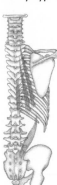

Answer:

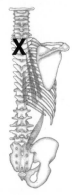

Rationale: Kyphosis is characterized by an accentuated forward curve of the thoracic area of the spine.

Critical thinking strategy: Review the anatomy of the nervous system and techniques for assessing the spinal column.

Client needs category: Health promotion and maintenance

Client needs subcategory: None

Cognitive level: Application

Integrated process: Nursing process/assessment

Reference: Smeltzer, page 2347

10. A nurse is auscultating a client's lungs. Identify the area on the client's vertebrae, representing the base of the lungs, where the nurse expects the breath sounds to stop at the end of expiration.

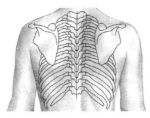

Answer:

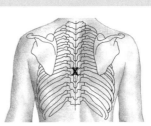

Rationale: Based on posterior landmarks, the lungs extend from the cervical area to the level of the 10th thoracic vertebrae (T10) at the end of expiration.

Critical thinking strategy: Review the anatomy of the respiratory system and techniques for assessing the lungs.

Client needs category: Health promotion and maintenance

Client needs subcategory: None

Cognitive level: Application

Integrated process: Nursing process/assessment

Reference: Smeltzer, page 574

---

11. A nurse is performing an otoscopic examination on a client with ear pain and notes that the tympanic membrane is bulging and red. Identify the structure that the nurse is assessing.

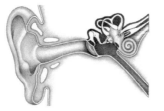

Answer:

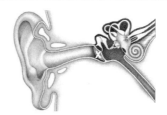

Rationale: The tympanic membrane separates the external and middle ear and may appear red and bulging in a client with otitis media.

Critical thinking strategy: Review the anatomy and pathophysiology of the ear and assessment techniques.

Client needs category: Physiological integrity

Client needs subcategory: Physiological adaptation

Cognitive level: Application

Integrated process: Nursing process/assessment

Reference: Smeltzer, page 2094

12. A nurse is performing a cardiac assessment on a client with a suspected murmur. Identify the area where the nurse should place the stethoscope to auscultate Erb's point.

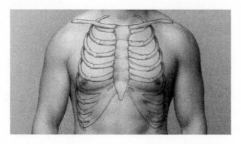

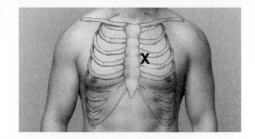

Rationale: Erb's point is located at the third intercostal space, to the left of the sternum. Murmurs of both aortic and pulmonic origin may be heard at Erb's point.

Critical thinking strategy: Review the anatomy of the cardiovascular system and techniques for assessing the heart.

Client needs category: Health promotion and maintenance

Client needs subcategory: None

Cognitive level: Application

Integrated process: Nursing process/assessment

Reference: Smeltzer, page 801

---

13. A nurse is performing a head and neck assessment on a client who reports fatigue. Identify the area that the nurse should palpate to assess the occipital lymph nodes.

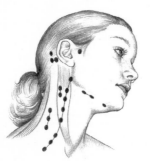

Answer:

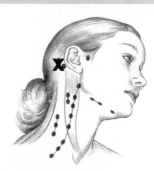

Rationale: Using the pads of the fingers, the nurse should palpate the area behind the ears bilaterally to assess the occipital lymph nodes.

Critical thinking strategy: Review the anatomy of the lymphatic system and techniques for assessing lymph nodes.

Client needs category: Physiological integrity

Client needs subcategory: Physiological adaptation

Cognitive level: Application

Integrated process: Nursing process/assessment

Reference: Taylor, pages 623–624

14. A nurse is performing a cardiovascular assessment. Identify the area where the nurse should place the stethoscope to best auscultate the pulmonic valve.

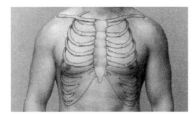

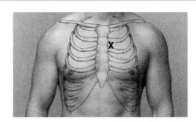

Rationale: The pulmonic valve is best heard at the second intercostal space, just left of the sternum.

Critical thinking strategy: Review the anatomy of the cardiovascular system and techniques for assessing the heart.

Client needs category: Health promotion and maintenance

Client needs subcategory: None

Cognitive level: Application

Integrated process: Nursing process/assessment

Reference: Smeltzer, page 801

---

15. A client has been admitted with severe abdominal pain that has lasted for the past 4 hours. Place in chronological order the correct sequence for conducting an abdominal assessment. Use all of the options.

1. Auscultate the client's abdomen.
2. Perform light palpation.
3. Ask client to urinate.
4. Percuss the client's abdomen.

Answer: 3, 1, 4, 2

Rationale: The nurse should begin the assessment by having the client empty his bladder first. This allows the nurse to hear abdominal sounds better during auscultation. Because the client is in pain, the nurse should auscultate the abdomen before percussing it. Also, ascultation is usually performed before palpation and percussion since bowel sounds induced by percussion or palpation may mask abdominal bruits or pleural rubs. The nurse should then perform light palpation over the abdomen, leaving the painful area for last.

Critical thinking strategy: Review techniques to use when assessing the abdomen.

Client needs category: Physiological integrity

Client needs subcategory: Basic care and comfort

Cognitive level: Knowledge

Integrated process: Nursing process/assessment

Reference: Craven, pages 402–404

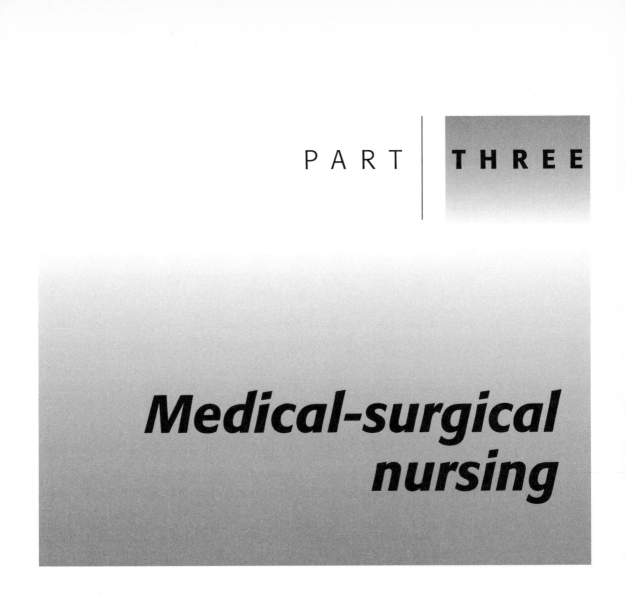

PART | THREE

Medical-surgical nursing

Cardiovascular disorders

1. A client with sepsis and hypotension is being treated with dopamine hydrochloride (Inotropin). A nurse asks a colleague to double-check the dosage that the client is receiving. The 250-ml bag contains 400 mg of dopamine, the infusion pump is running at 23 ml/hour, and the client weighs 80 kg. How many micrograms per kilogram per minute is the client receiving? Record your answer using one decimal point.

_____ micrograms/
kilogram/
minute

Answer: 7.7

Rationale: First, calculate how many milligrams per milliliter of dopamine are in the bag:

$$400 \text{ mg}/250 \text{ ml} = 1.6 \text{ mg/ml}.$$

Next, convert milligrams to micrograms:

$$1.6 \text{ mg/ml} \times 1,000 \text{ mcg/mg} = 1,600 \text{ mcg/ml}.$$

Lastly, calculate the dose:

$$\frac{1,600 \text{ mcg}}{1 \text{ ml}} \times \frac{23 \text{ ml}}{60 \text{ min}} \times \frac{1}{80 \text{ kg}} =$$

$$\frac{36,800 \text{ mcg}}{4,800 \text{ kg/min}} = 7.7 \text{ mcg/kg/minute}$$

Critical thinking strategy: Determine how many micrograms the client is receiving each minute of the infusion, and remember to convert milligrams to micrograms.

Client needs category: Physiological integrity

Client needs subcategory: Pharmacological and parenteral therapies

Cognitive level: Analysis

Integrated process: Nursing process/analysis

Reference: *Dosage Calculations Made Incredibly Easy,* pages 304–305

---

2. A client with deep vein thrombosis is receiving an I.V. infusion of heparin sodium at 1,500 units/hour. The concentration in the bag is 25,000 units/500 ml. How many milliliters should the nurse document as intake from this infusion for an 8-hour shift? Record your answer using a whole number.

_____ milliliters

Answer: 240

Rationale: First, calculate how many units are in each milliliter of the medication:

$$25,000 \text{ units}/500 \text{ ml} = 50 \text{ units/ml}.$$

Next, calculate how many milliliters the client receives each hour:

$$1 \text{ ml}/50 \text{ units} \times 1,500 \text{ units/hour} = 30 \text{ ml/hour}.$$

Lastly, multiply by 8 hours:

$$30 \text{ ml/hour} \times 8 \text{ hours} = 240 \text{ ml}.$$

Critical thinking strategy: Focus on what the question is asking (calculating infusion of fluid over an 8-hour time period), and review calculation steps for giving I.V. medications based on time.

Client needs category: Physiological integrity

Client needs subcategory: Pharmacological and parenteral therapies

Cognitive level: Analysis

Integrated process: Nursing process/analysis

Reference: *Dosage Calculations Made Incredibly Easy,* pages 235–236

3. A nurse is evaluating the following telemetry strips from two of her clients. Based on her review, which of the following statements is true?

ECG strips

☐ **1.** The ventricular rhythm is irregular in the second strip only.

☐ **2.** The PR interval in the first strip is within the normal range.

☐ **3.** Both strips show atrial abnormalities.

☐ **4.** The second strip shows sawtooth fibrillatory (F) waves.

4. A nurse is interpreting a client's telemetry strip. If the PR interval measures four small blocks, how many seconds is the PR interval?

_____ seconds

5. A nurse is caring for a client with Raynaud's phenomenon secondary to systemic lupus erythematosus. Which of the following client statements shows an understanding of the nurse's teaching about this disorder? Select all that apply.

- ☐ **1.** "My hands get pale, bluish, and feel numb and painful when I'm really stressed."
- ☐ **2.** "I can't continue to wash dishes and do my cleaning because of this problem."
- ☐ **3.** "I don't need to report any other skin problems with my fingers or hands to my practitioner."
- ☐ **4.** "I probably got this disorder because I have lupus."
- ☐ **5.** "This problem is caused by a temporary lack of circulation in my hands."
- ☐ **6.** "Medication might help treat this problem."

Answer: 1, 4, 5, 6

Rationale: Raynaud's phenomenon causes blanching, cyanosis, coldness, numbness, and throbbing pain in the hands when the client is exposed to cold or stress. It's caused by episodic vasospasm in the small peripheral arteries and arterioles and can affect the feet as well as the hands. The phenomenon is commonly associated with connective tissue diseases such as lupus and may be alleviated by calcium channel blockers or adrenergic blockers. It doesn't limit the client's ability to function, although the symptoms are bothersome. Keeping the hands warm and learning to manage stressful situations effectively reduces the frequency of episodes. The disorder can progress to skin ulcerations and even gangrene in some clients, so all skin changes should be reported to the practitioner promptly.

Critical thinking strategy: Focus on the pathophysiology of Raynaud's phenomenon.

Client needs category: Physiological integrity

Client needs subcategory: Physiological adaptation

Cognitive level: Analysis

Integrated process: Nursing process/evaluation

Reference: Smeltzer, pages 1003–1005

---

6. A nurse is evaluating the 12-lead electrocardiogram (ECG) of a client experiencing an inferior wall myocardial infarction (MI). While conferring with the team, the nurse correctly identifies which of the following ECG changes associated with an evolving MI? Select all that apply.

- ☐ **1.** Notched T wave
- ☐ **2.** Presence of a U wave
- ☐ **3.** T-wave inversion
- ☐ **4.** Prolonged PR interval
- ☐ **5.** ST-segment elevation
- ☐ **6.** Pathologic Q wave

Answer: 3, 5, 6

Rationale: T-wave inversion, ST-segment elevation, and a pathologic Q wave are all signs of tissue hypoxia that occur during an MI. Ischemia results from inadequate blood supply to the myocardial tissue and is reflected by T-wave inversion. Injury results from prolonged ischemia and is reflected by ST-segment elevation. Q waves may become evident when the injury progresses to infarction. A notched T wave may indicate pericarditis in an adult client. A U wave may be apparent on a normal ECG; it represents repolarization of the Purkinje fibers. A prolonged PR interval is associated with first-degree atrioventricular block.

Critical thinking strategy: Focus on myocardial infarction and review rhythm strip analysis.

Client needs category: Physiological integrity

Client needs subcategory: Physiological adaptation

Cognitive level: Analysis

Integrated process: Nursing process/evaluation

Reference: Smeltzer, pages 874–876

---

7. A client with a bicuspid aortic valve has severe stenosis and is scheduled for valve replacement. While teaching the client about his condition and upcoming surgery, the nurse shows him a heart illustration. Identify which valve the nurse indicates as needing replacement.

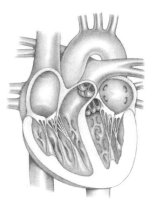

Answer:

Rationale: The aortic valve is located between the left ventricle and the aorta. It's one of the semilunar valves and normally has three cusps. A person with a bicuspid aortic valve is at risk for aortic stenosis and aortic regurgitation. This impaired blood flow through the valve leads to increased pumping pressure of the left ventricle.

Critical thinking strategy: Focus on the anatomy of the heart.

Client needs category: Physiological integrity

Client needs subcategory: Physiological adaptation

Cognitive level: Application

Integrated process: Teaching and learning

Reference: Smeltzer, page 785

---

8. A nurse is awaiting the arrival of a client from the emergency department who is being admitted with a left ventricular myocardial infarction. In caring for this client, the nurse should be alert for which of the following signs and symptoms of left-sided heart failure? Select all that apply.

☐ **1.** Jugular vein distention

☐ **2.** Hepatomegaly

☐ **3.** Dyspnea

☐ **4.** Crackles

☐ **5.** Tachycardia

☐ **6.** Right-upper-quadrant pain

Answer: 3, 4, 5

Rationale: Signs and symptoms of left-sided heart failure include dyspnea, orthopnea, and paroxysmal nocturnal dyspnea; fatigue; nonproductive cough and crackles; hemoptysis; point of maximal impulse displaced toward the left anterior axillary line; tachycardia; S_3 and S_4 heart sounds; and cool, pale skin. Jugular vein distention, hepatomegaly, and right-upper-quadrant pain are all signs of right-sided heart failure.

Critical thinking strategy: Focus on the pathophysiology of heart failure, and review the differences between right- and left-sided heart failure.

Client needs category: Physiological integrity

Client needs subcategory: Physiological adaptation

Cognitive level: Application

Integrated process: Nursing process/assessment

Reference: Smeltzer, pages 950–951

9. A client is admitted to the emergency department after complaining of acute chest pain radiating down his left arm. Which of the following laboratory studies would be indicated? Select all that apply.

☐ **1.** Hemoglobin and hematocrit

☐ **2.** Serum glucose

☐ **3.** Creatine kinase (CK)

☐ **4.** Troponin T and troponin I

☐ **5.** Myoglobin

☐ **6.** Blood urea nitrogen (BUN)

Answer: 3, 4, 5

Rationale: With myocardial ischemia or infarction, levels of CK, troponin T, and troponin I typically rise because of cellular damage. Myoglobin elevation is an early indicator of myocardial damage. Hemoglobin, hematocrit, serum glucose, and BUN levels don't provide information related to myocardial ischemia.

Critical thinking strategy: Focus on laboratory studies that diagnose cardiac problems, and review diagnostic findings for myocardial infarction.

Client needs category: Health promotion and maintenance

Client needs subcategory: None

Cognitive level: Application

Integrated process: Nursing process/application

Reference: Smeltzer, page 876

---

10. A client is prescribed lisinopril (Zestril) for treatment of hypertension. He asks a nurse about possible adverse effects. Which common adverse effects of angiotensin-converting enzyme (ACE) inhibitors should the nurse include in her teaching? Select all that apply.

☐ **1.** Constipation

☐ **2.** Dizziness

☐ **3.** Headache

☐ **4.** Hyperglycemia

☐ **5.** Hypotension

☐ **6.** Impotence

Answer: 2, 3, 5

Rationale: Dizziness, headache, and hypotension are all common adverse effects of lisinopril and other ACE inhibitors. Lisinopril may cause diarrhea, not constipation; it isn't known to cause hyperglycemia or impotence.

Critical thinking strategy: Review the pharmacological class of ACE inhibitors and focus on the common adverse effects.

Client needs category: Physiological integrity

Client needs subcategory: Pharmacological and parenteral therapies

Cognitive level: Application

Integrated process: Nursing process/implementation

Reference: Smeltzer, pages 952–953

11. A nurse is performing a 12-lead electrocardiogram (ECG) on a client who's complaining of chest pain. Identify the area where lead V_6 should be placed.

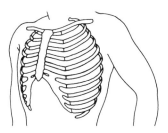

Answer:

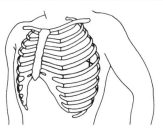

Rationale: The V_6 lead should be placed at the fifth intercostal space, at the midaxillary line. Correct lead placement is essential when performing a 12-lead ECG in order to accurately document the electrical potential of the heart. V_6 is one of the precordial leads and, combined with the other leads, records potential in the horizontal plane.

Critical thinking strategy: Review the placement of electrodes for an ECG, keeping in mind that V_1 is placed medially and, as the numbers progress higher, the electrodes are placed more laterally.

Client needs category: Physiological integrity

Client needs subcategory: Reduction of risk potential

Cognitive level: Application

Integrated process: Nursing process/implementation

Reference: Smeltzer, page 826

---

12. A nurse is counseling a client about risk factors for hypertension. Which of the following should the nurse list as risk factors for primary hypertension? Select all that apply.

☐ **1.** Obesity

☐ **2.** Glomerulonephritis

☐ **3.** Head injury

☐ **4.** Stress

☐ **5.** Hormonal contraceptive use

☐ **6.** High intake of sodium or saturated fat

Answer: 1, 4, 6

Rationale: Obesity, stress, high intake of sodium or saturated fat, and family history are all risk factors for primary hypertension. Diabetes mellitus, head injury, and hormonal contraceptive use are risk factors for secondary hypertension.

Critical thinking strategy: Focus on key words (in this question, the key words are *risk factors* and *primary*), and review the risk factors and types of hypertension.

Client needs category: Health promotion and maintenance

Client needs subcategory: None

Cognitive level: Application

Integrated process: Nursing process/assessment

Reference: Smeltzer, page 1023

13. A nurse is caring for a client with first-degree atrioventricular (AV) block. Identify the area in the conduction cycle of the heart where this block occurs.

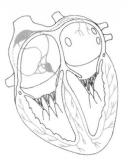

Answer:

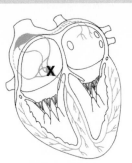

Rationale: First-degree AV block is a conduction disturbance in which electrical impulses flow normally from the sinoatrial node through the atria but are delayed at the AV node.

Critical thinking strategy: Review first-degree AV block and the anatomy of the heart and how it relates to cardiac electrical activity.

Client needs category: Physiological integrity

Client needs subcategory: Physiological adaptation

Cognitive level: Analysis

Integrated process: Nursing process/assessment

Reference: Smeltzer, pages 838–839

---

14. A client has just returned from a cardiac catheterization. Which of the following interventions should the nurse include in the client's care? Select all that apply.

☐ **1.** Monitor vital signs every 15 minutes.

☐ **2.** Assess all peripheral pulses frequently.

☐ **3.** Restrict the client to bed rest for 4 to 6 hours.

☐ **4.** Assess the insertion site.

☐ **5.** Perform range-of-motion exercises.

Answer: 1, 3, 4

Rationale: After cardiac catheterization, the client's vital signs are typically monitored every 15 minutes for the first hour, then every 30 minutes for 2 hours or until vital signs are stable, and then every 4 hours or according to facility policy. All peripheral pulses don't need to be assessed frequently. The pulses in the affected extremity are usually assessed with every vital signs check. Clients typically remain in bed for 4 to 6 hours unless a special closure is used. The insertion site extremity is kept straight following the procedure, so range-of-motion exercises wouldn't be performed.

Critical thinking strategy: Focus on postcatheterization care.

Client needs category: Safe, effective care environment

Client needs subcategory: Management of care

Cognitive level: Application

Integrated process: Nursing process/planning

Reference: Smeltzer, page 815

15. A nurse is caring for a client who has been pre-scribed digoxin (Lanoxin). Which of the following guidelines should the nurse include when teaching the client about digoxin? Select all that apply.

☐ **1.** Establish a set time to take your digoxin every day.

☐ **2.** Take digoxin at the same time as your antacids.

☐ **3.** Take your pulse before each dose of digoxin.

☐ **4.** If you forget a dose, you may take the missed dose with your usual dose the following day.

☐ **5.** Notify your practitioner if you experience increasing fatigue or muscle weakness.

Answer: 1, 3, 5

Rationale: It's usually helpful for a client to take digoxin at a specific time each day because doing so serves as a reminder to take the medication. The nurse should teach the client to take his pulse before each dose of digoxin and to notify the practitioner if the rate or rhythm changes, specifically if the rate drops to less than 60 beats/minute. The client should also be instructed to report increasing fatigue or muscle weakness immediately, as these are signs of digitalis (digoxin) toxicity. Antacids inhibit the absorption of digoxin, so digoxin shouldn't be taken with these drugs. If the client forgets to take a dose of digoxin, he may take the missed dose only up to 12 hours later.

Critical thinking strategy: Focus on the safe administration of digoxin and review cardiac glycosides.

Client needs category: Health promotion and maintenance

Client needs subcategory: None

Cognitive level: Application

Integrated process: Teaching and learning

Reference: Smeltzer, page 956

---

16. A nurse is interpreting a cardiac monitor strip and notes an abnormality in the QRS wave on lead II. Identify the area in the conduction cycle of the heart where this abnormality occurs.

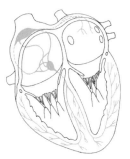

Answer:

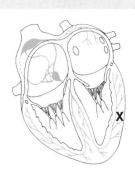

Rationale: An abnormality in the ventricular conduction will be reflected in the QRS wave.

Critical thinking strategy: Review the anatomy and electrical activity of the heart, and focus on the QRS wave of the cardiac cycle.

Client needs category: Physiological integrity

Client needs subcategory: Physiological adaptation

Cognitive level: Analysis

Integrated process: Nursing process/assessment

Reference: Smeltzer, page 826

17. A client exhibits the following rhythm on the cardiac monitor. Which of the following interventions should the nurse do first?

ECG strips

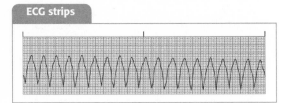

☐ **1.** Place the client on oxygen.

☐ **2.** Confirm the rhythm with a 12-lead electrocardiogram.

☐ **3.** Administer amiodarone (Cordarone) I.V. as prescribed.

☐ **4.** Assess the client's airway, breathing, and circulation.

Answer: 4

Rationale: The rhythm the client is experiencing is ventricular tachycardia (VT). Although all of the options listed are appropriate for someone with stable VT, it's not yet known whether the client's VT is stable, unstable, or pulseless. Therefore, the nurse must first assess the airway, breathing, circulation, and level of consciousness to establish the client's stability. Different actions are required if the client's VT is unstable or pulseless.

Critical thinking strategy: Remember to treat the client, not the rhythm strip.

Client needs category: Physiological integrity

Client needs subcategory: Reduction of risk potential

Cognitive level: Analysis

Integrated process: Nursing process/implementation

Reference: Smeltzer, pages 835–836

---

18. A client is hospitalized following a report of dizziness, shortness of breath, and chest pain. Based on the following electrocardiogram rhythm, the client is scheduled for a transesophageal echocardiogram (TEE) today. Which of the following nursing interventions would be appropriate at this time?

ECG strips

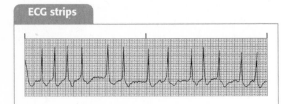

☐ **1.** Allow the client to eat.

☐ **2.** Encourage the client to ambulate to the bathroom.

☐ **3.** Prepare the client for immediate electrical cardioversion.

☐ **4.** Administer oxygen as prescribed.

Answer: 4

Rationale: The client is experiencing atrial fibrillation and is symptomatic; therefore, because of the client's symptoms, the nurse would administer oxygen. The client should be given nothing by mouth before undergoing a TEE. To ensure safety, the nurse shouldn't encourage ambulation when the client is experiencing dizziness, shortness of breath, or chest pain. A TEE is sometimes prescribed before electrical cardioversion to ensure there are no clots in the atria; if none are found, then the cardioversion can be safely performed.

Critical thinking strategy: Focus on identifying the rhythm and its clinical mainfestations, and review atrial fibrillation and TEE.

Client needs category: Physiological integrity

Client needs subcategory: Reduction of risk potential

Cognitive level: Analysis

Integrated process: Nursing process/implementation

Reference: Smeltzer, pages 832–833

19. A client who underwent cardiac surgery has been prescribed morphine sulfate 2 mg I.V. for pain. The morphine sulfate is packaged as 2 mg/ml. The nurse dilutes the medication in 4 ml of sterile water and prepares to administer the medication over 5 minutes. If the nurse administers 1 ml of fluid every minute, how many milligrams of morphine will be administered per minute? Record your answer using one decimal point.

_____ milligrams/minute

Answer: 0.4

Rationale: The nurse should first determine how much fluid the medication is in.

1 ml of morphine + 4 ml of sterile water = 5 ml of fluid

$$\frac{2 \text{ mg}}{5 \text{ mg}} = \frac{X \text{ ml}}{1 \text{ ml}} = 2 \text{ mg/ml} = 5X$$

$$\frac{2 \text{ mg/ml} = 5X}{5} = 0.4 \text{ mg/ml}$$

Since the nurse is administering 1 ml of fluid every minute, she is administering 0.4 mg of morphine every minute.

Critical thinking strategy: Focus on what the question is asking (how many milliliters you will administer in 1 minute after diluting 1 ml of morphine with 4 ml of sterile water) and review dosage calculations formulas.

Client needs category: Physiological integrity

Client needs subcategory: Pharmacological and parenteral therapies

Cognitive level: Analysis

Integrated process: Nursing process/implementation

Reference: _Dosage Calculations Made Incredibly Easy,_ page 311

---

20. The nurse is preparing to interpret an electrocardiogram (ECG) rhythm strip. Place the following steps for ECG rhythm analysis from first to last, in chronological order. Use all of the options.

1.	Measure the QRS duration.
2.	Interpret the rhythm.
3.	Analyze the P waves.
4.	Determine the rate and rhythm.
5.	Measure the P-R interval.

Answer: 4, 3, 5, 1, 2

Rationale: ECG rhythm strip analysis requires a systematic approach using a 5-step method. First, determine the rate and rhythm of both the atria and the ventricles. Then, analyze the P waves for consistency. Next, measure the P-R interval and then the QRS duration. Finally, you can interpret the rhythm with all of the information that has been collected.

Critical thinking strategy: Recall rhythm strip analysis, which includes analyzing the rate and rhythm (regular or irregular) and then the waves, complexes, and intervals.

Client needs category: Safe, effective care environment

Client needs subcategory: Management of care

Cognitive level: Application

Integrated process: Nursing process/analysis

Reference: Smeltzer, pages 825–828

21. A nurse is presenting health information at a community organization when one of the attendees passes out. The nurse assesses the attendee as being unresponsive. Indicate how the nurse should respond by placing the following actions in chronological order. Use all of the options.

1. Appoint a person to call 911.
2. Use the available automatic external defibrillator.
3. Deliver 2 rescue breaths.
4. Check for normal breathing.
5. Perform chest compressions.
6. Perform a head tilt-chin lift maneuver.

Answer: 1, 4, 6, 3, 5, 2

Rationale: Following American Heart Association (AHA) guidelines for cardiopulmonary resuscitation (CPR), the rescuer should first call for help (if alone) or appoint another person to call 911 for emergency medical services. The next step is to check for normal breathing. If breathing isn't detected, the rescuer performs a head tilt-chin lift maneuver followed by 2 rescue breaths. Next, the rescuer checks for a pulse. If none is present, the rescuer begins a cycle of chest compressions. After 5 cycles of 30 chest compressions and 2 rescue breaths, the rescuer (in this case, the nurse) should use an automatic external defibrillator, if one is available.

Critical thinking strategy: Recall the AHA guidelines for CPR.

Client needs category: Safe, effective care environment

Client needs subcategory: Management of care

Cognitive level: Application

Integrated process: Nursing process/implementation

Reference: Smeltzer, pages 970–972

Respiratory disorders

1. A nurse is caring for a client with pneumonia who was prescribed ceftriaxone (Rocephin) oral suspension 600 mg once daily. The medication label indicates that the strength is 125 mg/5 ml. How many milliliters of medication should the nurse pour to administer the correct dose? Record your answer as a whole number.

_____ milliliters

Answer: 24

Rationale: Use the following formula to calculate the drug dosage:

Dose on hand/Quantity on hand = Dose desired/X.

Plug in the values for this equation and solve for X:

$$125 \text{ mg/5 ml} = 600 \text{ mg}/X$$

$$X = 24 \text{ ml}$$

Critical thinking strategy: Focus on what the question is asking (the total amount of milliliters to be administered for the prescribed dose), and review dosage calculations using the ratio-and-proportion method.

Client needs category: Physiological integrity

Client needs subcategory: Pharmacological and parenteral therapies

Cognitive level: Application

Integrated process: Nursing process/planning

Reference: *Dosage Calculations Made Incredibly Easy,* pages 169–172

2. A nurse is caring for a client who has a chest tube connected to a three-chamber drainage system without suction. On the illustration below, identify the chamber that collects drainage from the client.

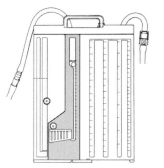

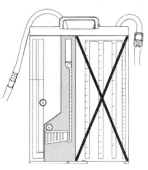

Rationale: The drainage system is on the right. It has three calibrated chambers that show the amount of drainage collected. When the first chamber fills, drainage empties into the second; when the second chamber fills, drainage flows into the third. The water seal chamber is located in the center. The suction control chamber is on the left.

Critical thinking strategy: Recall chest tube drainage systems

Client needs category: Physiological integrity

Client needs subcategory: Reduction of risk potential

Cognitive level: Comprehension

Integrated process: Nursing process/implementation

Reference: Smeltzer, pages 758–764

---

3. A client comes to the emergency department with status asthmaticus. Based on the documentation note below, the nurse suspects that the client has what abnormality?

Progress notes	
2/1/09	Pt. wheezing. RR 44, BP 140/90, P 104, T
1830	98.4° F. ABG results show pH 7.52, $PaCO_2$
	30 mm Hg, HCO_3^- 26 mEg/L, and PO_2
	77 mm Hg. —————— C. Wynn, RN

☐ **1.** Respiratory acidosis

☐ **2.** Respiratory alkalosis

☐ **3.** Metabolic acidosis

☐ **4.** Metabolic alkalosis

Answer: 2

Rationale: Respiratory alkalosis results from alveolar hyperventilation. It's marked by an increase in pH to more than 7.45 and a concurrent decrease in partial pressure of arterial carbon dioxide ($PaCO_2$) to less than 35 mm Hg. Metabolic alkalosis shows the same increase in pH but also an increased bicarbonate level and normal $PaCO_2$ (may be elevated also if compensatory mechanisms are working). Acidosis of any type means a low pH (below 7.35). Respiratory acidosis shows an elevated $PaCO_2$ and a normal to high bicarbonate level. Metabolic acidosis is characterized by a decreased bicarbonate level and a normal to low $PaCO_2$.

Critical thinking strategy: Review criteria for blood gas values, acid-base disturbances, and compensation and the disease process of status asthmaticus.

Client needs category: Physiological integrity

Client needs subcategory: Physiological adaptation

Cognitive level: Analysis

Integrated process: Nursing process/analysis

Reference: Smeltzer, pages 338–339, 717–718

4. A nurse is preparing a staff education program about pulmonary circulation. Place the following structures in chronological order to trace the pathway of normal pulmonary circulation. Use all of the options.

1. Pulmonary vein
2. Right ventricle
3. Pulmonary artery
4. Arterioles
5. Alveoli
6. Left atrium

Answer: 2, 3, 4, 5, 1, 6

Rationale: Deoxygenated blood is ejected from the right ventricle into the pulmonary artery and then into the lungs via the arterioles and alveoli. The pulmonary vein then carries oxygenated blood back to the left atrium for circulation throughout the body.

Critical thinking strategy: Recall the anatomy of the heart and lungs and pulmonary circulation.

Client needs category: Physiological integrity

Client needs subcategory: Physiological adaptation

Cognitive level: Comprehension

Integrated process: Nursing process/analysis

Reference: Craven, pages 880–881

---

5. A client with a suspected pulmonary embolus is brought to the emergency department complaining of shortness of breath and chest pain. Which of the following additional signs and symptoms would the nurse expect to assess in this client? Select all that apply.

☐ **1.** Low-grade fever

☐ **2.** Thick green sputum

☐ **3.** Bradycardia

☐ **4.** Frothy sputum

☐ **5.** Tachycardia

☐ **6.** Blood-tinged sputum

Answer: 1, 5, 6

Rationale: In addition to pleuritic chest pain and dyspnea, a client with a pulmonary embolus may present with a low-grade fever, tachycardia, and blood-tinged sputum. Thick green sputum would indicate infection, and frothy sputum would indicate pulmonary edema. A client with a pulmonary embolus is tachycardic (to compensate for decreased oxygen supply), not bradycardic.

Critical thinking strategy: Recall the pathophysiology and clinical manifestations of pulmonary embolism.

Client needs category: Physiological integrity

Client needs subcategory: Physiological adaptation

Cognitive level: Application

Integrated process: Nursing process/assessment

Reference: Smeltzer, pages 662–663

6. A client with chronic obstructive pulmonary disease (COPD) is being evaluated for a lung transplant. Which signs and symptoms would the nurse expect to find during the initial physical assessment? Select all that apply.

☐ **1.** Decreased respiratory rate

☐ **2.** Dyspnea on exertion

☐ **3.** Barrel chest

☐ **4.** Shortened expiratory phase

☐ **5.** Clubbed fingers and toes

☐ **6.** Fever

Answer: 2, 3, 5

Rationale: Typical findings for clients with COPD include dyspnea on exertion, a barrel chest, and clubbed fingers and toes. Clients with COPD are usually tachypneic with a prolonged expiratory phase. Fever isn't associated with COPD, unless an infection is also present.

Critical thinking strategy: Review the anatomy and physiology of the respiratory system, and focus on the pathophysiology and clincal manifestations of COPD.

Client needs category: Physiological integrity

Client needs subcategory: Physiological adaptation

Cognitive level: Application

Integrated process: Nursing process/assessment

Reference: Smeltzer, pages 686–690

---

7. A client with a wound infection develops septic shock. An arterial blood gas analysis reveals pH of 7.25, partial pressure of arterial carbon dioxide ($PaCO_2$) of 43 mm Hg, partial pressure of arterial oxygen (PaO_2) of 70 mm Hg, and bicarbonate (HCO_3^-) of 18 mEq/L. According to the following oxyhemoglobin dissociation curve, which statement is correct?

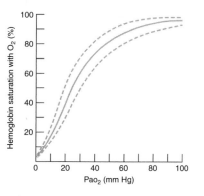

☐ **1.** The client's profile reflects alkalosis.

☐ **2.** The client's hemoglobin saturation is close to 100%.

☐ **3.** The client's oxyhemoglobin curve is shifted to the left.

☐ **4.** The client's hemoglobin saturation is close to 85%.

Answer: 4

Rationale: The acidic condition of the blood shifts the oxyhemoglobin dissociation curve to the right. This enables oxygen molecules to unload more easily from the hemoglobin. According to the client's PaO_2 value of 70 mm Hg and pH value of 7.25, his hemoglobin saturation is close to 85%.

Critical thinking strategy: Review concepts of arterial blood gases, oxyhemoglobin dissociation curve, and gas exchange and respiratory system physiology.

Client needs category: Physiological integrity

Client needs subcategory: Physiological adaptation

Cognitive level: Analysis

Integrated process: Nursing process/analysis

Reference: Smeltzer, pages 560–561

8. A client with a traumatic injury who is in the intensive care unit develops a tension pneumothorax. The nurse knows to assess the client for which of the following signs and symptoms of tension pneumothorax? Select all that apply.

☐ **1.** Decreased cardiac output

☐ **2.** Flattened neck veins

☐ **3.** Tracheal deviation to the affected side

☐ **4.** Hypotension

☐ **5.** Tracheal deviation to the opposite side

☐ **6.** Bradypnea

Answer: 1, 4, 5

Rationale: Tension pneumothorax results when air in the pleural space is under higher pressure than air in the adjacent lung. The site of the rupture of the pleural space acts as a one-way valve, allowing the air to enter on inspiration but not to escape on expiration. The air presses against the mediastinum, causing a tracheal shift to the opposite side and decreased venous return (reflected by decreased cardiac output and hypotension). Neck veins bulge with tension pneumothorax. This also leads to compensatory tachycardia and tachypnea.

Critical thinking strategy: Recall the pathophysiology and clinical manifestations of tension pneumothorax, and review respiratory system physiology and assessment techniques.

Client needs category: Physiological integrity

Client needs subcategory: Physiological adaptation

Cognitive level: Application

Integrated process: Nursing process/assessment

Reference: Smeltzer, pages 679–680

---

9. A nurse is caring for a client with right-middle-lobe pneumonia in the intensive care unit. On the anterior view of the lungs below, identify the area where the nurse may expect to hear associated adventitious breath sounds such as crackles.

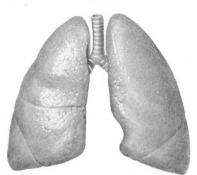

Answer:

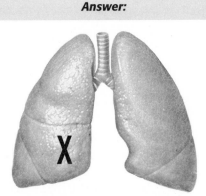

Rationale: The right lung is made up of three lobes: the right upper lobe, right middle lobe, and right lower lobe. The left lung is made up of only two lobes: the left upper lobe and left lower lobe. When assessing the anterior chest, the right lung is on the examiner's left.

Critical thinking strategy: Focus on the anatomy of the respiratory system and review breath sound assessment techniques.

Client needs category: Health promotion and maintenance

Client needs subcategory: None

Cognitive level: Analysis

Integrated process: Nursing process/assessment

Reference: Smeltzer, pages 571–575

---

10. A client is prescribed continuous positive airway pressure (CPAP) therapy for sleep apnea. Identify on the illustration below where the mechanism maintaining the positive end-expiratory pressure is located.

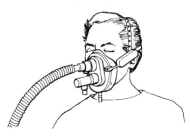

Answer:

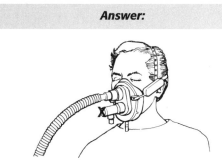

Rationale: CPAP ventilation maintains positive pressure in the airways throughout the respiratory cycle. The inlet valve attaches the oxygen tubing to the face mask, and the positive end-expiratory pressure valve maintains the pressure. CPAP can be used with or without a ventilator in intubated and nonintubated clients and can be administered just nasally for a less constrictive feeling. In addition to sleep apnea, CPAP is used to treat respiratory distress syndrome, pulmonary edema, pulmonary emboli, bronchiolitis, pneumonitis, viral pneumonia, and postoperative atelectasis.

Critical thinking strategy: Focus on the function and mechanics of CPAP therapy, and review types of respiratory care modalities.

Client needs category: Physiological integrity

Client needs subcategory: Physiological adaptation

Cognitive level: Application

Integrated process: Nusing process/planning

Reference: Smeltzer, page 743

---

11. A client with primary pulmonary hypertension is being evaluated for a heart-lung transplant. The nurse would expect the client to be receiving which of the following treatments? Select all that apply.

☐ **1.** Oxygen

☐ **2.** Aminoglycosides

☐ **3.** Diuretics

☐ **4.** Vasodilators

☐ **5.** Antihistamines

☐ **6.** Sulfonamides

Answer: 1, 3, 4

Rationale: Oxygen, diuretics, and vasodilators are among the common therapies used to treat pulmonary hypertension. Others include fluid restriction, digoxin, calcium channel blockers, beta-adrenergic blockers, and bronchodilators. Aminoglycosides and sulfonamides are antibiotics used to treat infections. Antihistamines are indicated to treat allergies, pruritus, vertigo, nausea, and vomiting; to promote sedation; and to suppress cough.

Critical thinking strategy: Review the pathophysiology of pulmonary hypertension, and focus on the clinical manifestations and treaments associated with primary pulmonary hypertension.

Client needs category: Physiological integrity

Client needs subcategory: Pharmacological and parenteral therapies

Cognitive level: Application

Integrated process: Nursing process/implementation

Reference: Smeltzer, pages 659–660

12. A nurse is performing a respiratory assessment on a client with right-lower-lobe atelectasis. Identify the area where she may hear the fine crackles associated with this condition.

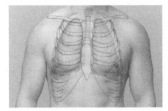

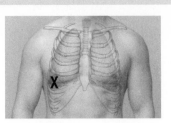

Rationale: To auscultate the right lower lobe from the anterior chest, the nurse should place the stethoscope between the fifth and sixth intercostal spaces to the left of the anterior axillary line.

Critical thinking strategy: Focus on the anatomy of the lungs related to breath sounds, and review breath sound assessment techniques.

Client needs category: Physiological integrity

Client needs subcategory: Reduction of risk potential

Cognitive level: Application

Integrated process: Nursing process/assessment

Reference: Smeltzer, pages 574–575

---

13. A fireman is admitted to the unit following an intense fire with superficial skin wounds and a sprained back. He denies respiratory complaints. Nearly 24 hours after admission, he reports shortness of breath and dyspnea on mild exertion. The nurse recognizes that the client may have an inhalation injury. Priority nursing interventions should include which of the following? Select all that apply.

☐ **1.** Monitor for fever.

☐ **2.** Make sure the client's oxygen saturation level remains below 98%.

☐ **3.** Auscultate the lungs for adventitious breath sounds.

☐ **4.** Assess for increased pulse rate.

☐ **5.** Monitor for increased anxiety levels.

Answer: 3, 4, 5

Rationale: More than half of all clients with pulmonary involvement following inhalation injury don't immediately demonstrate pulmonary signs and symptoms. Any client with possible inhalation injury must be observed for at least 24 hours for possible respiratory complications. Maintaining increased oxygen saturation levels is essential, especially following a carbon monoxide inhalation injury, to prevent the development of carboxyhemoglobin, which competes with oxygen for available hemoglobin. The client doesn't typically develop a fever with inhalation injury, but he may progress to acute respiratory syndrome with bilateral lung infiltrates, cardiac involvement with tachycardia, and increasing anxiety due to oxygen starvation.

Critical thinking strategy: Focus on the information gathered during the nursing assessment and the clinical manifestations of inhalation injury, and review the pathophysiology of inhalation injury and acute respiratory syndrome.

Client needs category: Physiological integrity

Client needs subcategory: Physiological adaptation

Cognitive level: Application and analysis

Integrated process: Nursing process/implementation

Reference: Smeltzer, pages 2001–2002

14. A client admitted with a diagnosis of pulmonary embolism (PE) also has a history of heart failure. Assessment findings reveal sudden shortness of breath and immobility. Indicate which of the following nursing diagnoses support the nursing care of a client with PE. Select all that apply.

☐ **1.** Activity intolerance related to inadequate oxygenation

☐ **2.** Anxiety related to breathlessness

☐ **3.** Disturbed sleep pattern related to inability to assume recumbent position

☐ **4.** Ineffective breathing pattern related to hypoxia

☐ **5.** Risk for decreased cardiac output related to failure of the left ventricle

Answer: 1, 2, 4, 5

Rationale: When planning care, the nurse should select nursing diagnoses that anticipate pulmonary compromise secondary to reduction of air, blood, and gas exchange because these are ensuing complications that can develop from PE, particularly in a client with a history of heart failure. The prudent nurse should analyze the client's condition and anticipate the need for safe, supportive nursing interventions related to the client's activity intolerance, anxiety, ineffective breathing, and risk for decreased oxygen output. The client history does not indicate that this client has difficulty sleeping.

Critical thinking strategy: Focus on the pathophysiology and clinical manifestations of PE, and review applicable nursing diagnoses and nursing management.

Client needs category: Physiological integrity

Client needs subcategory: Basic care and comfort

Cognitive level: Comprehension

Integrated process: Nursing process/planning

Reference: Smeltzer, pages 662–667

---

15. The nurse knows that the anatomy of the right lung differs from the left lung and keeps this in mind when auscultating a client. Identify the area where the nurse should place the stethoscope to best auscultate the middle portion of the right lung lobe.

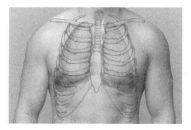

Answer:

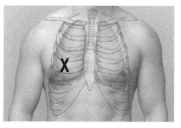

Rationale: To auscultate the right middle lobe of the lung from the anterior chest, the nurse should place the stethoscope in the fourth intercostal space.

Critical thinking strategy: Focus on the anatomy and physiology of the respiratory sytem, and review ausculation techniques.

Client needs category: Health promotion and maintenance

Client needs subcategory: None

Cognitive level: Application

Integrated process: Nursing process/assessment

Reference: Taylor, pages 627–629

16. The nurse has been assigned to care for the following six clients. Which of the clients would the nurse expect to be at risk for development of pulmonary embolism (PE)? Select all that apply.

☐ **1.** A client who is on complete bed rest following extensive spinal surgery

☐ **2.** A client who has a large venous stasis ulcer on the right ankle area

☐ **3.** A client who has recently been admitted with a broken femur and is awaiting surgery

☐ **4.** A client who has a pleural effusion secondary to lung cancer

☐ **5.** A client who is receiving supplemental oxygen following shoulder surgery

☐ **6.** A client who has undergone a total vaginal hysterectomy and is now on estrogen replacement therapy

Answer: 1, 2, 3, 6

Rationale: Bed rest, poor venous circulation, fractures, and hormone replacement therapy can cause formation of a thromboembolus, placing these clients at risk for developing PE. A deep vein thrombosis could break loose in the leg and travel to the lungs as a pulmonary embolus. The clot would then lodge somewhere in the pulmonary arteries or arterioles and impede blood flow. The client who is on complete bed rest is at risk for venous stasis, and the client who has a venous stasis ulcer is already demonstrating this condition. The client with a broken femur is at risk for a fat embolus, another form of pulmonary embolism. The client on estrogen replacement therapy is at increased risk for thromboembolic disorders. Pleural effusion and lung cancer usually have no effect on thrombus formation, and oxygen therapy doesn't cause venous stasis or increase the risk of PE.

Critical thinking strategy: Recall the pathophysiology of PE.

Client needs category: Physiological integrity

Client needs subcategory: Physiological adaptation

Cognitive level: Application

Integrated process: Nursing process/analysis

Reference: Smeltzer, page 662

---

17. The nurse is caring for several clients on the respiratory unit who are receiving the beta-adrenergic agonist bronchodilator albuterol (Accuneb) in the prescribed nebulizer treatments. Which of the following side effects would the nurse expect to assess following the respiratory treatments? Select all that apply.

☐ **1.** Increased tachypnea

☐ **2.** Irritability and nervousness

☐ **3.** Tachycardia

☐ **4.** Increased somnolence

☐ **5.** Insomnia

☐ **6.** Anxiety

Answer: 2, 3, 5, 6

Rationale: Irritability, nervousness, tachycardia, insomnia, and anxiety are common side effects of beta-adrenergic agonist bronchodilators that result from sympathetic nervous system stimulation. The expected therapeutic effect of a bronchodilator is decreased dyspnea and slower (not increased) breathing. Increased somnolence doesn't occur with sympathetic nervous system stimulation.

Critical thinking strategy: Review the action of a beta-adrenergic agonist

Client needs category: Physiological integrity

Client needs subcategory: Pharmacological and parenteral therapies

Cognitive level: Application

Integrated process: Nursing process/application

Reference: *Nursing2009 Drug Handbook,* page 841

18. A client is exhibiting signs and symptoms of pulmonary edema. Place the following nursing interventions in chronological order to show how the nurse would prioritize care for a client in respiratory distress. Use all the options.

| 1. Administer oxygen via nasal cannula at 2 L/minute. |
| 2. Call the physician. |
| 3. Position the client upright at a 45-degree angle. |
| 4. Prepare suctioning equipment at the bedside. |
| 5. Administer furosemide (Lasix) 40 mg I.V. STAT. |
| 6. Insert an indwelling urinary catheter. |

Answer: 3, 1, 4, 2, 5, 6

Rationale: The order of priority moves from the simple to the complex for bedside interventions when a client is in respiratory distress. The nurse should first attempt to maximize respiratory excursion as much as possible by sitting the client up, and then provide supplemental oxygen to minimize impending hypoxia. It's also important to have suction equipment readily available because the client may choke on his oral secretions due to the pulmonary edema. After performing these interventions, the nurse should notify the physician and anticipate orders for administration of a diuretic (such as Lasix) and insertion of an indwelling urinary catheter to measure eventual output.

Critical thinking strategy: Focus on the clincal manifestations of pulmonary edema and prioritization of care, and review emergency procedures for acute respiratory disorders.

Client needs category: Physiological integrity

Client needs subcategory: Reduction of risk potential

Cognitive level: Application

Integrated process: Nursing process/implementation

Reference: Smeltzer, pages 964–965

---

19. The physician orders additional hydration secondary to pneumonia, a urinary tract infection, dehydration, and fever of 101.4° F (38.6° C) for a client. He orders 1,000 ml of D_5W to infuse over 8 hours. The available drop factor is 20 gtt/ml. The nurse should regulate the I.V. flow rate to deliver how many drops per hour? Round your answer to the nearest whole number.

_____ gtt/hour

Answer: 42

Rationale: Calculate the flow rate using the formula below:

$$\frac{\text{Total volume ordered}}{\text{Number of hours}} = \text{Flow rate}$$

$$\frac{1,000 \text{ ml}}{8 \text{ hours}} = 125 \text{ ml/hour}$$

Then calculate the drip rate using the drop factor:

$$\frac{125 \text{ ml}}{60 \text{ min}} \times \frac{20 \text{ gtt}}{1 \text{ ml}} = 41.66$$

Rounded off, this is 42 gtt/hour.

Critical thinking strategy: Focus on what the question is asking (the drip rate per minute for the amount to be infused), and review calculations for the I.V. flow rate and drip rate.

Client needs category: Physiological integrity

Client needs subcategory: Pharmacological and parenteral therapies

Cognitive level: Application

Integrated process: Nursing process/implementation

Reference: *Dosage Calculations Made Incredibly Easy,* pages 235–237

---

20. The nurse is performing a purified protein derivative (PPD) test on a client. Which of the following statements about this test are correct? Select all that apply.

☐ **1.** A PPD test is done to test for allergies.

☐ **2.** Always aspirate before injecting the PPD solution.

☐ **3.** The PPD test is an intradermal test.

☐ **4.** Hold the syringe at a 45-degree angle to the skin.

☐ **5.** The preferred injection site is the ventral surface of the forearm.

☐ **6.** No wheal should appear at the site following injection.

Answer: 3, 5

Rationale: The PPD test is used to determine whether a person has been infected with the *Tuberculosis* bacillus. PPD tests should be injected intradermally in the ventral forearm, unless contraindicated, without aspiration prior to injecting. The syringe should be held at a 10- to 15-degree angle from the site so the needle enters the dermis as nearly parallel to the skin as possible. A small wheal should appear; this indicates that the medication has been injected into the dermis.

Critical thinking strategy: Focus on the procedure for intradermal injections, and review the disease process of tuberculosis.

Client needs category: Physiological integrity

Client needs subcategory: Pharmacological and parenteral therapies

Cognitive level: Application

Integrated process: Nursing process/analysis

Reference: Taylor, pages 832–834

Neurosensory disorders

1. A nurse is preparing a female client with tonic-clonic seizure disorder for discharge. Which instructions should the nurse include about phenytoin (Dilantin)? Select all that apply.

☐ **1.** Monitor for skin rash.

☐ **2.** Maintain adequate amounts of fluid and fiber in the diet.

☐ **3.** Perform good oral hygiene, including daily brushing and flossing.

☐ **4.** Receive necessary periodic blood work.

☐ **5.** Report to the physician any problems with walking or coordination, slurred speech, or nausea.

☐ **6.** Feel safe about taking this drug, even during pregnancy.

Answer: 1, 3, 4, 5

Rationale: If a rash appears 10 to 14 days after starting phenytoin, the client should notify the physician and discontinue the medication. Because it may cause gingival hyperplasia, the client must practice good oral hygiene and see a dentist regularly. Periodic blood work is necessary to monitor complete blood counts, platelet count, hepatic function, and drug levels. Signs and symptoms of phenytoin toxicity include problems with walking or coordination, slurred speech, and nausea. Other signs are lethargy, diplopia, nystagmus, and disturbances in balance. These must be reported to the physician immediately. Although adequate amounts of fluid and fiber are part of a healthy diet, they aren't required for a client taking phenytoin. Phenytoin must be used cautiously during pregnancy because it poses an increased risk of birth defects; phenobarbital is safer to take during pregnancy.

Critical thinking strategy: Focus on the common side effects of phenytoin, and review the adverse and toxic effects of antiseizure medications.

Client needs category: Physiological integrity

Client needs subcategory: Pharmacological and parenteral therapies

Cognitive level: Application

Integrated process: Nursing process/implementation

Reference: Smeltzer, pages 2193–2196

---

2. A nurse assesses a 21-year-old client who is diagnosed with bacterial meningitis. Which of the following signs and symptoms of meningeal irritation is the nurse likely to observe? Select all that apply.

☐ **1.** Generalized seizures

☐ **2.** Nuchal rigidity

☐ **3.** Positive Brudzinski's sign

☐ **4.** Positive Kernig's sign

☐ **5.** Babinski's reflex

☐ **6.** Photophobia

Answer: 2, 3, 4, 6

Rationale: Signs of meningeal irritation include nuchal rigidity, positive Brudzinski's and Kernig's signs, and photophobia. Other signs of meningeal irritation are exaggerated and symmetrical deep tendon reflexes as well as opisthotonos (a spasm in which the back and extremities arch backward so that the body rests on the head and heals). Generalized seizures may accompany meningitis, but they're caused by irritation to the cerebral cortex, not the meninges. Babinski's reflex is a reflex action of the toes that reflects corticospinal tract disease in adults.

Critical thinking strategy: Focus on the pathophysiology and clinical manifestations of bacterial meningitis, and review central nervous system anatomy and related assessment techniques.

Client needs category: Physiological integrity

Client needs subcategory: Physiological adaptation

Cognitive level: Application

Integrated process: Nursing process/assessment

Reference: Craven, page 1041

---

3. A nurse is preparing to administer phenytoin (Dilantin) to a client with a seizure disorder. The order is for phenytoin 5 mg/kg/day to be administered in divided doses. The client weighs 99 lb, and the medication will be administered three times per day. How many milligrams of phenytoin should be administered in the first dose? Record your answer as a whole number.

_____ milligrams

Answer: 75

Rationale: First, convert the client's weight to kilograms:

$$1 \text{ kg} = 2.2 \text{ lb}$$
$$99 \text{ lb} \div 2.2 \text{ lb/kg} = 44 \text{ kg}.$$

Then calculate the total daily dosage:

$$44 \text{ kg} \times 5 \text{ mg/kg} = 220 \text{ mg/day}.$$

Finally, divide the total daily dosage into three parts:

$$220 \text{ mg} \div 3 \text{ doses} = 75 \text{ mg/dose}.$$

Critical thinking strategy: Focus on what the question is asking (dosage in milligrams according to body weight), and review dosage calculations for dosage per kilogram of body weight.

Client needs category: Physiological integrity

Client needs subcategory: Pharmacological and parenteral therapies

Cognitive level: Application

Integrated process: Nursing process/implementation

Reference: *Dosage Calculations Made Incredibly Easy*, pages 266–270

4. A nurse is assessing a client's extraocular eye movements as part of the neurologic examination. Which of the following cranial nerves is the nurse assessing? Select all that apply.

☐ **1.** Optic (II)

☐ **2.** Oculomotor (III)

☐ **3.** Trochlear (IV)

☐ **4.** Trigeminal (V)

☐ **5.** Abducens (VI)

☐ **6.** Acoustic (VIII)

Answer: 2, 3, 5

Rationale: Assessing extraocular eye movements helps evaluate the function of cranial nerves III (oculomotor), IV (trochlear), and VI (abducens). The oculomotor nerve originates in the brain stem and controls the movement of the eyeball up, down, and inward; raises the eyelid; and constricts the pupil. The trochlear nerve rotates the eyeball downward and outward. The abducens nerve originates in the pons and rotates the eyeball laterally. Assessing the client's vision helps evaluate cranial nerve II (optic). Cranial nerve V (trigeminal), has three branches: assessing the corneal reflex helps the nurse evaluate the ophthalmic branch functions; assessing sensation to the cheek, upper jaw, teeth, lips, hard palate, maxillary sinus, and part of the nasal mucosa helps evaluate the maxillary branch functions; and assessing sensation to the lower lip, chin, ear, mucous membrane, lower teeth, and tongue helps evaluate the mandibular branch functions. Assessing hearing and balance helps evaluate the cochlear and vestibular branches of cranial nerve VIII (acoustic).

Critical thinking strategy: Recall the anatomy and physiology of the cranial nerves and the eye and cranial nerve assessment technique.

Client needs category: Physiological integrity

Client needs subcategory: Physiological adaptation

Cognitive level: Analysis

Integrated process: Nursing process/assessment

Reference: Craven, pages 392–393

---

5. A nurse assesses the level of consciousness of a client who suffered a head injury. Using the Glasgow Coma Scale, she determines that the client's score is 15. Which of the following responses did the nurse assess in this client? Select all that apply.

☐ **1.** Spontaneous eye opening

☐ **2.** Tachypnea, bradycardia, and hypotension

☐ **3.** Unequal pupil size

☐ **4.** Orientation to person, place, and time

☐ **5.** Pain localization

☐ **6.** Incomprehensible sounds

Answer: 1, 4

Rationale: To achieve a perfect score of 15 on the Glasgow Coma Scale, the client would have to open his eyes spontaneously (4), obey verbal commands (6), and be oriented to person, place, and time (5). Vital signs and pupil size aren't assessed with the Glasgow Coma Scale. The ability to localize pain earns a motor response score of 5, not the top score of 6. Making incomprehensible sounds earns a verbal response score of 2, not a 5.

Critical thinking strategy: Focus on the physiology of the brain and motor and sensory response, and recall the Glasgow Coma Scale and neurological assessment techniques.

Client needs category: Physiological integrity

Client needs subcategory: Physiological adaptation

Cognitive level: Analysis

Integrated process: Nursing process/analysis

Reference: Craven, pages 391–392

6. A nurse assesses a client using the Glasgow Coma Scale (shown below). The client complains of pain in his abdominal area, is confused about person, place, and time, and anxiously watches the nurse as she performs the assessment. Using the scale provided, what score should this client receive?

Flow sheet

Glasgow Coma Scale

Test	Client's reaction	Score
Eye opening response	Opens spontaneously	4
	Opens to verbal command	3
	Opens to pain	2
	No response	1
Best motor response	Obeys verbal command	6
	Localizes painful stimuli	5
	Flexion-withdrawal	4
	Flexion-abnormal (decorticate rigidity)	3
	Extension (decerebrate rigidity)	2
	No response	1
Best verbal response	Oriented and converses	5
	Disoriented and converses	4
	Inappropriate words	3
	Incomprehensible sounds	2
	No response	1

☐ **1.** 9

☐ **2.** 11

☐ **3.** 13

☐ **4.** 15

Rationale: The Glasgow Coma Scale assesses level of consciousness by testing and scoring the client's best eye opening, motor, and verbal responses. The highest score is 15. In this case, the client spontaneously keeps his eyes open as he watches the actions of the nurse (eye opening score of 4), can express and localize the area of his pain (motor response score of 5), and is disoriented about person, place, and time (verbal response score of 4) for a total score of 13.

Critical thinking strategy: Focus on the physiology and assessment of the neurologic system, and recall the Glasgow Coma Scale and neurologic assessment techniques.

Client needs category: Physiological integrity

Client needs subcategory: Physiological adaptation

Cognitive level: Analysis

Integrated process: Nursing process/assessment

Reference: Craven, page 391

7. A nurse is caring for a client with a T5 complete spinal cord injury. Upon assessment, the nurse notes flushed skin, diaphoresis above T5, and blood pressure of 162/96 mm Hg. The client reports a severe, pounding headache. Which of the following nursing interventions would be appropriate for this client? Select all that apply.

☐ **1.** Elevate the head of the bed to 90 degrees.

☐ **2.** Loosen constrictive clothing.

☐ **3.** Use a fan to reduce diaphoresis.

☐ **4.** Assess for bladder distention and bowel impaction.

☐ **5.** Administer antihypertensive medication.

☐ **6.** Place the client in a supine position with legs elevated.

Answer: 1, 2, 4, 5

Rationale: The client is exhibiting signs and symptoms of autonomic dysreflexia, a potentially life-threatening emergency caused by an uninhibited response from the sympathetic nervous system resulting from a lack of control over the autonomic nervous system. The nurse should immediately elevate the head of the bed to 90 degrees and place the legs in a dependent position to decrease venous return to the heart and increase venous return from the brain. Because tactile stimuli can trigger autonomic dysreflexia, any constrictive clothing should be loosened. The nurse should also assess for distended bladder and bowel impaction—which may trigger autonomic dysreflexia—and correct any problems. Elevated blood pressure is the most life-threatening complication of autonomic dysreflexia because it can cause stroke, myocardial infarction, or seizure activity. If removing the triggering event doesn't reduce the client's blood pressure, I.V. antihypertensives should be administered. A fan shouldn't be used because a cold draft may trigger autonomic dysreflexia.

Critical thinking strategy: Focus on the pathophysiology of spinal cord injury and the clinical manifestations of complications, and review autonomic dysreflexia and emergency treatment procedures.

Client needs category: Physiological integrity

Client needs subcategory: Reduction of risk potential

Cognitive level: Application

Integrated process: Nursing process/implementation

Reference: Smeltzer, pages 2256–2260

---

8. A client has a cerebral aneurysm. The physician orders hydralazine (Apresoline) 15 mg I.V. every 4 hours as needed to keep the systolic blood pressure less than 140 mm Hg. The label on the hydralazine vial reads "hydralazine 20 mg/ml." To administer the correct dose, how many milliliters of medication should the nurse draw up in the syringe? Record your answer using two decimal places.

_____ milliliters

Answer: 0.75

Rationale: The following formula is used to calculate drug dosages:

Dose on hand/Quantity on hand = Dose desired/X

20 mg/ml ÷ 15 mg/X = 0.75 ml.

Critical thinking strategy: Focus on what the question is asking (the total amount of milliliters of medication to adminster), and review dosage calculations using the ratio-and-proportion method to solve for X.

Client needs category: Physiological integrity

Client needs subcategory: Pharmacological and parenteral therapies

Cognitive level: Application

Integrated process: Nursing process/implementation

Reference: *Dosage Calculations Made Incredibly Easy,* pages 58–61

---

9. A nurse is preparing to teach students in a health class about hearing pathways. Place the following steps in chronological order to match how the nurse should describe the normal pathway of sound wave transmission and hearing to the class. Use all of the options.

1.	Interpretation of sound by the cerebral cortex

2.	Transmission of vibrations through the air and bone

3.	Stimulation of nerve impulses in the inner ear

4.	Transmission of vibrations to the auditory area of the cerebral cortex

Answer: 2, 3, 4, 1

Rationale: Vibrations transmitted through air and bone stimulate nerve impulses in the inner ear. The cochlear branch of the acoustic nerve transmits these vibrations to the auditory area of the cerebral cortex. The cerebral cortex then interprets the sound.

Critical thinking strategy: Focus on the anatomy and physiology of the ear and the physiology of the nervous system related to hearing.

Client needs category: Health promotion and maintenance

Client needs subcategory: None

Cognitive level: Application

Integrated process: Nursing process/implementation

Reference: Smeltzer, page 2096

10. A community nurse is leading a support group discussion on the progressive nature of multiple sclerosis (MS). Arrange the following degenerative changes in the order in which they occur. Use all of the options.

1.	Degeneration of axons

2.	Demyelination throughout the central nervous system

3.	Periodic and unpredictable exacerbations and remissions

4.	Plaque formation that interrupts nerve impulses

Answer: 2, 1, 4, 3

Rationale: MS produces patches of demyelination throughout the central nervous system, resulting in myelin loss from the axis cylinders and degeneration of the axons. Plaques form in the involved area and become sclerosed, interrupting the flow of nerve impulses and resulting in a variety of symptoms. Periodic and unpredictable exacerbations and remissions occur. The prognosis varies.

Critical thinking strategy: Focus on the pathophysiology of MS and review the physiology of the nervous system.

Client needs category: Physiological integrity

Client needs subcategory: Physiological adaptation

Cognitive level: Application

Integrated process: Nursing process/implementation

Reference: Smeltzer, pages 2277–2278

11. A nurse is monitoring a client's intracranial pressure (ICP) after a traumatic head injury. Based on the documentation below, how should the nurse interpret this client's ICP reading?

Flow sheet				
	0800	0805	0810	0815
ICP	20	18	18	16

☐ **1.** ICP is elevated.

☐ **2.** ICP is decreased.

☐ **3.** ICP is within normal limits.

☐ **4.** ICP was elevated but returned to normal.

Answer: 1

Rationale: A normal ICP is between 0 and 15 mm Hg. The documentation at left shows pressures greater than 15 mm Hg.

Critical thinking strategy: Focus on the pathophysiology and clinical manifestations of intracranial pressure releated to head injury, and review normal values of intracranial pressure.

Client needs category: Physiological integrity

Client needs subcategory: Reduction of risk potential

Cognitive level: Analysis

Integrated process: Nursing process/assessment

Reference: Smeltzer, pages 2233–2234

---

12. A client is experiencing problems with balance as well as fine and gross motor function. Indicate on the illustration below which area of the brain is malfunctioning.

Answer:

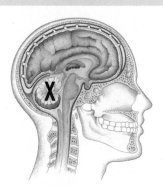

Rationale: The cerebellum is the portion of the brain that controls balance and fine and gross motor function.

Critical thinking strategy: Focus on the anatomy and physiology of the brain.

Client needs category: Physiological integrity

Client needs subcategory: Physiological adaptation

Cognitive level: Comprehension

Integrated process: Nursing process/assessment

Reference: Smeltzer, page 2133

13. A nurse is performing a neurologic assessment during a client's routine physical examination. To assess Babinski's reflex, indicate the point where the nurse should place the tongue blade to begin stroking the foot.

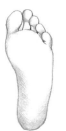

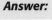

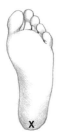

Rationale: To test for Babinski's reflex, use a tongue blade to slowly stroke the side of the sole of the foot. Start at the heel and move toward the great toe. The normal response in an adult is plantar flexion of the toes. Upward movement of the great toe and fanning of the little toes—Babinski's reflex—is abnormal.

Critcal thinking strategy: Focus on the anatomy and physiology of the nervous system, and review neurological assessment techniques.

Client needs category: Health promotion and maintenance

Client needs subcategory: None

Cognitive level: Comprehension

Integrated process: Nursing process/assessment

Reference: Smeltzer, pages 2149–2150

---

14. The nurse is caring for a client who is experiencing an exacerbation of gout. Which of the following dietary modifications are applicable to this client? Select all that apply.

☐ **1.** Eat a low-purine diet.

☐ **2.** Limit fluid intake to no more than 1 liter/day.

☐ **3.** Eat a high-protein diet, with at least two servings of lean meat per day.

☐ **4.** Eat a high-purine diet.

☐ **5.** Consume very limited amounts of baked goods containing yeast.

☐ **6.** Increase fluid intake to at least 3 liters/day.

Answer: 1, 5, 6

Rationale: The client who suffers from gout should be placed on a low-purine, alkaline-ash diet with fluid intake increased to 3 liters/day. Alcohol intake should also be limited.

Critical thinking strategy: Recall dietary modifications and nursing interventions for gout.

Client needs category: Physiological integrity

Client needs subcategory: Basic care and comfort

Cognitive level: Application

Integrated process: Nursing process/planning

Reference: Smeltzer, pages 1918–1919

15. The nurse is caring for a client who is scheduled to undergo a computerized tomography (CT) scan to assess recent symptoms of muscle weakness and tingling in her extremities. Which of the following information should the nurse include in a preprocedural teaching plan? Select all that apply.

☐ **1.** The test requires standing alone without assistance.

☐ **2.** A contrast dye may be given before the test.

☐ **3.** Throat irritation and facial flushing may occur if contrast dye is used.

☐ **4.** All medications must be withheld for 12 hours prior to the procedure.

☐ **5.** The CT scan is considered an invasive procedure, but it isn't dangerous.

☐ **6.** It's necessary to report any known allergies to iodine or seafood prior to the procedure.

Answer: 2, 3, 6

Rationale: The nurse should inform the client who is scheduled to undergo a CT scan that she may be given a contrast medium before the procedure and that the dye can cause throat irritation and facial flushing. Because the dye is iodine-based, it's essential for the client to report any known allergies to iodine or seafood before testing begins. The CT scan isn't invasive or dangerous. The client will need to lie still (not stand) during the procedure, and she won't be able to take her medications for 24 hours beforehand.

Critical thinking strategies: Focus on the CT procedure and any required nursing interventions.

Client needs category: Physiological integrity

Client needs subcategory: Reduction of risk potential

Cognitive level: Application

Integrated process: Teaching and learning

Reference: Smeltzer, pages 812–813

---

16. A physician wants to evaluate a client's temporal lobe because of recent changes in short-term memory. Identify the area where the temporal lobe is located on the illustration below.

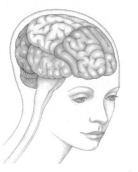

Answer:

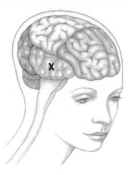

Rationale: The temporal lobe, which contains the auditory receptive areas, is located around the temples.

Critical thinking strategy: Focus on the anatomy of the brain, and review the basic functions of each lobe.

Client needs category: Physiological integrity

Client needs subcategory: Physiological adaptation

Cognitive level: Comprehension

Integrated process: Nursing process/assessment

Reference: Smeltzer, page 2131

17. A client is scheduled to undergo cerebral angiography to allow for examination of the cerebral arteries. Place the following interventions in the order in which the nurse would perform them. Use all of the options.

1. Administer anti-anxiety medication if ordered.

2. Ask the client about allergies to iodine, seafood, or radiopaque dyes.

3. Make sure the client has signed an informed consent form.

4. Maintain the affected extremity in straight alignment for 6 hours as ordered.

5. Encourage the client to verbalize questions about the procedure.

Answer: 5, 3, 2, 1, 4

Rationale: It's important to provide the client with an opportunity to ask questions about the procedure before obtaining his informed consent. The nurse should ask about allergies to iodine, seafood, or radiopaque dyes because the procedure uses an iodine-based contrast medium. This should be done before administering anti-anxiety medication to the client. After the procedure, the affected extremity should be maintained in straight alignment for 6 hours.

Critical thinking strategy: Focus on client safety and informed consent procedures, and review nursing inteventions for cerebral angiography.

Client needs category: Physiological integrity

Client needs subcategory: Reduction of risk potential

Cognitive level: Analysis

Integrated process: Nursing process/implementation

Reference: Smeltzer, page 2154

Gastrointestinal disorders

1. A nurse is reviewing the causes of gastroesophageal reflux disease (GERD) with a client. Locate on the GI tract the area the nurse should identify as the cause of reduced pressure associated with GERD.

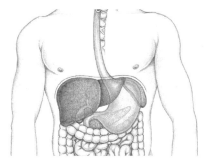

Answer:

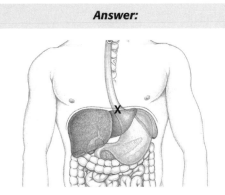

Rationale: Reflux occurs when the pressure around the cardiac or lower esophageal sphincter (LES) is deficient or when pressure in the stomach exceeds LES pressure.

Critical thinking strategy: Focus on the anatomy of the gastrointestinal system and the pathophysiology of the disorder.

Client needs category: Health promotion and maintenance

Client needs subcategory: None

Cognitive level: Application

Integrated process: Nursing process/implementation

Reference: Smeltzer, pages 1165–1166

2. As part of a routine screening for colorectal cancer, a client must undergo fecal occult blood testing. Which foods should the nurse instruct the client to avoid for 48 to 72 hours before the test and throughout the collection period? Select all that apply.

☐ **1.** High-fiber foods

☐ **2.** Red meat

☐ **3.** Turnips

☐ **4.** Cantaloupe

☐ **5.** Tomatoes

☐ **6.** Peas

Answer: 2, 3, 4

Rationale: The client should avoid red meat, poultry, and fish as well as beets, broccoli, cauliflower, horseradish, mushrooms, and turnips. Such fruits as cantaloupe, melons, and grapefruit also are prohibited. Tomatoes and peas are acceptable. The client should be taught to maintain a high-fiber diet in order to promote colonic emptying time and fecal bulk, which aid in obtaining specimens.

Critical thinking strategy: Focus on preparation for fecal occult blood test and the role of foods in the digestive tract.

Client needs category: Health promotion and maintenance

Client needs subcategory: None

Cognitive level: Application

Integrated process: Nursing process/implementation

Reference: Taylor, pages 1561–1563

---

3. A client returns from the operating room after undergoing extensive abdominal surgery. He is receiving 1,000 ml of lactated Ringer's solution via a central line infusion. The physician orders the I.V. fluid to be infused at 125 ml/hour plus the total output of the previous hour. The drip factor of the tubing is 15 gtt/ml and the output for the previous hour was 75 ml via Foley catheter, 50 ml via nasogastric tube, and 10 ml via Jackson Pratt tube. For how many drops (gtt) per minute should the nurse set the I.V. flow rate to deliver the correct amount of fluid? Record your answer as a whole number.

_____ gtt/minute

Answer: 65

Rationale: First, calculate the volume to be infused (in milliliters):

75 ml + 50 ml + 10 ml = 135 ml total output for the previous hour

135 ml + 125 ml ordered as a constant flow = 260 ml to be infused over the next hour.

Next, use the formula:

Volume to be infused/Total minutes to be infused × Drop factor = Drops/minute.

In this case:

260 ml × 60 minutes × 15 gtt/ml = 65 gtt/minute.

Critical thinking strategy: Focus on what the question is asking (I.V. flow rate in drops/minute), and review how to calculate drip rates.

Client needs category: Physiological integrity

Client needs subcategory: Pharmacological and parenteral therapies

Cognitive level: Analysis

Integrated process: Nursing process/implementation

Reference: *Dosage Calculations Made Incredibly Easy,* pages 233–234

4. A client with a retroperitoneal abscess is receiving gentamicin (Garamycin). Which of the following should the nurse monitor? Select all that apply.

☐ **1.** Hearing

☐ **2.** Urine output

☐ **3.** Hematocrit (HCT)

☐ **4.** Blood urea nitrogen (BUN) and serum creatinine levels

☐ **5.** Serum calcium level

Answer: 1, 2, 4

Rationale: Adverse effects of gentamicin include ototoxicity and nephrotoxicity; consequently, the nurse must monitor the client's hearing and instruct him to report any hearing loss or tinnitus. Signs of nephrotoxicity include decreased urine output and elevated BUN and serum creatinine levels. Gentamicin doesn't affect the serum calcium level or HCT.

Critical thinking strategy: Focus on the common side effects and potential toxicity of antibiotics, and review the therapeutic class of aminoglycosides.

Client needs category: Physiological integrity

Client needs subcategory: Pharmacological and parenteral therapies

Cognitive level: Analysis

Integrated process: Nursing process/assessment

Reference: Craven, page 506

---

5. A nurse is assessing the abdomen of a client who was admitted to the emergency department with suspected appendicitis. Identify the area of the abdomen that the nurse should palpate last.

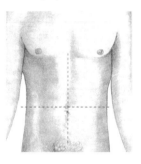

Answer:

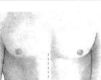

Rationale: An acute attack of appendicitis localizes as pain and tenderness in the lower right quadrant, midway between the umbilicus and the crest of the ilium. This area should be palpated last in order to determine if pain is also present in other areas of the abdomen.

Critical thinking strategy: Focus on the anatomy of the abdomen and review abdominal assessment techniques.

Client needs category: Physiological integrity

Client needs subcategory: Physiological adaptation

Cognitive level: Application

Integrated process: Nursing process/assessment

Reference: Craven, page 404

6. While preparing a client for an upper GI endoscopy (esophagogastroduodenoscopy), the nurse should implement which of the following interventions? Select all that apply.

☐ **1.** Administer a preparation to cleanse the GI tract, such as Golytely or Fleets Phospha-Soda.

☐ **2.** Tell the client he shouldn't eat or drink for 6 to 12 hours before the procedure.

☐ **3.** Tell the client he must be on a clear liquid diet for 24 hours before the procedure.

☐ **4.** Inform the client that he'll receive a sedative before the procedure.

☐ **5.** Tell the client that he may eat and drink immediately after the procedure.

Answer: 2, 4

Rationale: The client shouldn't eat or drink for 6 to 12 hours before the procedure to ensure that his upper GI tract is clear for viewing. Before the endoscope is inserted, the client will receive a sedative that will help him relax, but leave him conscious. GI tract cleansing and a clear liquid diet are interventions for a client having a lower GI tract procedure, such as a colonoscopy. Food and fluids must be withheld until the gag reflex returns after the procedure.

Critical thinking strategy: Focus on client safety and GI tract preparation, and review pre- and postendoscopy nursing interventions.

Client needs category: Physiological integrity

Client needs subcategory: Reduction of risk potential

Cognitive level: Application

Integrated process: Nursing process/implementation

Reference: Taylor, page 1564

---

7. A nurse is caring for a client who recently had a bowel resection. The client has a hemoglobin level of 8 g/dl and hematocrit of 30%. Dextrose 5% in half-normal saline solution ($D_5\frac{1}{2}NS$) is infusing through a triple-lumen central catheter at 125 ml/hour. The physician's orders include:

■ gentamicin 80 mg I.V. piggyback in 50 ml D_5W over 30 minutes

■ ranitidine (Zantac) 50 mg I.V. in 50 ml D_5W piggyback over 30 minutes

■ one unit of 250 ml of packed red blood cells (RBCs) over 3 hours

■ nasogastric tube flushes with 30 ml of normal saline solution every 2 hours.

How many milliliters should the nurse document as the total intake for the 8-hour shift? Record your answer as a whole number.

_____ milliliters

Answer: 1,470

Rationale: Add up the total intake as follows:

I.V. of $D_5\frac{1}{2}NS$ at 125 ml $\times$ 8 hr = 1,000 ml
gentamicin piggyback = 50 ml
ranitidine piggyback = 50 ml
packed RBCs = 250 ml
+ nasogastric flushes 30 ml $\times$ 4 = 120 ml
_____
Total = 1,470 ml

Critical thinking strategy: Focus on what the question is asking (the total fluid intake for 8 hours, which includes I. V. infusion, medications and transfusions), and review I.V. infusion calculations.

Client needs category: Physiological integrity

Client needs subcategory: Physiological adaptation

Cognitive level: Analysis

Integrated process: Communication and documentation

Reference: *Dosage Calculations Made Incredibly Easy,* page 257

8. Indicate the location where a client could have an ostomy that eventually might not require wearing an ostomy bag?

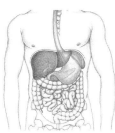

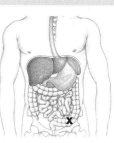

Rationale: With a sigmoid colostomy, the feces are solid; therefore, the client might eventually gain enough control that he wouldn't need to wear a colostomy bag. With a descending colostomy, the feces are semi-soft. With a transverse colostomy, the feces are soft. With an ascending colostomy, the feces are fluid. In these three latter cases, the client would be unlikely to gain control of elimination and consequently would need to continue wearing an ostomy bag.

Critical thinking strategy: Focus on the anatomy of the gastrointestinal system and review ostomy care.

Client needs category: Physiological integrity

Client needs subcategory: Basic care and comfort

Cognitive level: Application

Integrated process: Nursing process/planning

Reference: Smeltzer, page 1270

---

9. Which of the following findings are common in clients with acute diverticulitis? Select all that apply.

☐ **1.** Vomiting

☐ **2.** Cramping pain in the left lower abdominal quadrant

☐ **3.** Bowel irregularity

☐ **4.** Heartburn

☐ **5.** Intervals of diarrhea

☐ **6.** Hiccuping

Answer: 2, 3, 5

Rationale: Signs and symptoms of acute diverticulitis include bowel irregularity, intervals of diarrhea, abrupt onset of cramping pain in the left lower abdomen, and a low-grade fever. Vomiting, heartburn, and hiccuping aren't signs of the disorder.

Critical thinking strategy: Focus on the pathophysiology of diverticulitis.

Client needs category: Physiological integrity

Client needs subcategory: Physiological adaptation

Cognitive level: Analysis

Integrated process: Nursing process/assessment

Reference: Smeltzer, page 1243

10. A 28-year-old client is admitted with inflammatory bowel syndrome (Crohn's disease). Which measures would the nurse expect to be included in the client's care plan? Select all that apply.

☐ **1.** Lactulose therapy

☐ **2.** High-fiber diet

☐ **3.** High-protein milkshakes

☐ **4.** Corticosteroid therapy

☐ **5.** Antidiarrheal medications

Answer: 4, 5

Rationale: Corticosteroids such as prednisone reduce the signs and symptoms of diarrhea, pain, and bleeding by decreasing inflammation. Antidiarrheals such as diphenoxylate (Lomotil) combat diarrhea by decreasing peristalsis. Lactulose is used to treat chronic constipation and would aggravate the symptoms of Crohn's disease. A high-fiber diet and milk and milk products are contraindicated in clients with Crohn's disease because they may promote diarrhea.

Critical thinking strategy: Review the pathophysiology and treatment of Crohn's disease, and focus on clinical manifestations and nursing interventions.

Client needs category: Safe, effective care environment

Client needs subcategory: Management of care

Cognitive level: Analysis

Integrated process: Nursing process/planning

Reference: Smeltzer, pages 1248–1254

---

11. The nurse is caring for a client admitted with cirrhosis. Which of the following findings should the nurse expect when reviewing his laboratory results? Select all that apply.

☐ **1.** Prothrombin time 22 seconds

☐ **2.** Potassium 4.0 mEq/L

☐ **3.** Albumin 7.2 grams/dl

☐ **4.** Ammonia 96 micrograms/dl

☐ **5.** Platelets 75,000 cells/mm^3

☐ **6.** Amylase 250 units/L

Answer: 1, 4, 5

Rationale: The client with cirrhosis has liver dysfunction and impaired coagulation and rising ammonia levels. The prothrombin time is prolonged (normal is 9.5 to 11.0 seconds), and the platelet count is low (normal is 150,000 to 450,000 cells/mm^3). A normal ammonia level is 35 to 65 micrograms/dl, and this client's level is elevated, placing him at risk for hepatic encephalopathy. A client with cirrhosis typically has hypokalemia because of the diuretic therapy used to treat the fluid retention associated with the disease. Here, the potassium level is within normal limits (3.8 to 5.5 mEq/L). In cirrhosis, the albumin level is also typically low (normal is 3.4 to 5.0 grams/dl) due to alterations in protein metabolism in the liver. Levels of amylase, a pancreatic enzyme, typically increase with peancreatitis, not cirrhosis (normal level is 25 to 151 units/L).

Critical thinking strategy: Review the pathophysiology of cirrhosis, and focus on normal and abnormal laboratory values.

Client needs category: Physiological integrity

Client needs subcategory: Reduction of risk potential

Cognitive level: Analysis

Integrated process: Nursing process/analysis

Reference: Smeltzer, pages 1290–1291, 1319–1320

12. The nurse is evaluating how a client with hepatitis A understands the discharge teaching she has given him. Which of the following client statements indicate that further teaching is needed? Select all that apply

☐ **1.** "I can have an occasional glass of wine with my meal as I recover."

☐ **2.** "My family and I don't need to take any special precautions as long as I take my medication."

☐ **3.** "My bath towels shouldn't be used by any other family members."

☐ **4.** "My family members should receive the hepatitis A vaccine to prevent them from getting the disease."

☐ **5.** "My spouse and I can have intercourse and kiss."

☐ **6.** "I should wear a mask when visitors come."

Answer: 1, 2, 5, 6

Rationale: Clients with hepatitis should abstain from alcohol to prevent exacerbation of the disease. Standard precautions and meticulous hand washing should be practiced by all family members. All family members should avoid close contact with the client; this includes avoiding intercourse, kissing, and the use of any personal items (such as bath towels and eating utensils) that may be contaminated with the client's feces. Because hepatitis A is transmitted by the oral-fecal route, not the respiratory route, wearing a mask isn't necessary. The hepatitis A vaccine should be given prophylactically to all family members and close contacts to prevent disease transmission.

Critical thinking strategy: Focus on the transmission route for hepatitis A, and review the pathophysiology of disease.

Client needs category: Health promotion and maintenance

Client needs subcategory: None

Cognitive level: Application

Integrated process: Nursing process/evaluation

Reference: Smeltzer, pages 1309–1310

---

13. A client has continuous liquid output from his ostomy. Identify the area where the nurse would expect this type of ostomy to be located.

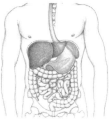

Answer:

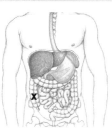

Rationale: An ostomy located in the ascending colon would likely produce continuous liquid output because feces in this section contain the most water and, therefore, have a liquid consistency. Fecal content becomes more solid as it travels through the large intestine. Feces in the sigmoid colon are usually solid. In the transverse and descending colons, the feces are generally semi-soft and soft, respectively.

Critical thinking strategy: Focus on various types of ostomies and their output, and review normal physiology of the intestinal tract.

Client needs category: Physiological integrity

Client needs subcategory: Basic care and comfort

Cognitive level: Application

Integrated process: Nursing process/implementation

Reference: Smeltzer, page 1270

14. A client has been admitted to the emergency department with severe right upper quadrant pain. Based on the signs and symptoms and laboratory data documented in the chart below, the nurse would expect the client to have which diagnosis?

Progress notes	
03/12/09 0730	Client admitted to the emergency department with severe right upper quadrant pain radiating to the back, nausea and vomiting, and fever. Laboratory results received via telephone as follows: glucose 462 mg/dl, WBC 14,000 cells/mm³, lipase 214 units/L, and calcium 6.5 mg/dl. ———Andrea Nichols, RN

☐ **1.** Peptic ulcer

☐ **2.** Crohn's disease

☐ **3.** Pancreatitis

☐ **4.** Irritable bowel syndrome

Answer: 3

Rationale: The assessment findings combined with the laboratory results suggest pancreatitis. Signs and symptoms of pancreatitis include severe right upper quadrant pain, fever, nausea, and vomiting. Inflammation of the pancreas results in leukocytosis. Injured beta cells are unable to produce insulin, leading to hyperglycemia, which may be as high as 500 to 900 mg/dl. Lipase and amylase levels become elevated as the pancreatic enzymes leak from injured pancreatic cells. Calcium becomes trapped as fat necrosis occurs, leading to hypocalcemia. Peptic ulcer, Crohn's disease, and irritable bowel syndrome don't cause amylase or lipase levels to increase.

Critical thinking strategy: Focus on the pathophysiology of pancreatitis, and review normal and abnormal laboratory values.

Client needs category: Physiological integrity

Client needs subcategory: Reduction of risk potential

Cognitive level: Analysis

Integrated process: Nursing process/analysis

Reference: Smeltzer, page 1359

---

15. The nurse is preparing to administer a 75% strength tube-feeding formula. The full-strength formula is available. To prepare 500 milliliters (ml) of feeding, the nurse should plan to dilute how many milliliters of the full-strength formula with water? Record your answer as a whole number.

_____ milliliters

Answer: 375

Rationale: To determine the amount of formula to use, multiply the 500 ml of full-strength formula by 75% (0.75):

$$500 \text{ ml} \times 0.75 = 375 \text{ ml}.$$

Critical thinking strategy: Focus on what the question is asking (how much of the 500 ml of full-strength formula to dilute to make the formula 75% strength), and review dosage calculations based on percentages.

Client needs category: Physiological integrity

Client needs subcategory: Pharmacological and parenteral therapies

Cognitive level: Application

Integrated process: Nursing process/planning

Reference: *Dosage Calculations Made Incredibly Easy*, pages 40–42

16. The nurse is assisting a client to ambulate following a bowel resection for diverticulitis. Suddenly, the client complains of sharp abdominal pain. The nurse assesses the client and determines the wound has eviscerated. Prioritize the following nursing actions in chronological order to show how the nurse should respond. Use all of the options.

1. Assess the client's response.

2. Call for assistance from other nursing personnel.

3. Cover the wound with sterile, nonadherent dressing moistened with sterile normal saline solution.

4. Document the incident, including the client's condition.

5. Place the client in low-Fowler's position.

Answer: 2, 5, 3, 1, 4

Rationale: When evisceration of an abdominal wound occurs, the nurse should remain with the client and summon help to bring necessary supplies to the client's room. The client should be placed in low-Fowler's position to lessen tension on the abdomen. The nurse shouldn't attempt to reinsert protruding organs. Instead, she should moisten sterile, nonadherent dressings with warm, sterile normal saline solution and cover the wound. It's important to conduct an ongoing client assessment until the surgeon arrives because the client is at risk for shock. Documentation of the incident and the client's condition should be completed immediately after the incident.

Critical thinking strategy: Focus on nursing interventions related to postoperative wound dehiscence, and review emergency care protocols.

Client needs category: Physiological integrity

Client needs subcategory: Physiological adaptation

Cognitive level: Analysis

Integrated process: Nursing process/implementation

Reference: Taylor, pages 1192–1193

Genitourinary disorders

1. A 176-lb client with minimal urine output has been prescribed dopamine at 5 mcg/kg/minute. The premixed medication bag contains 800 mg of dopamine in 500 ml dextrose 5% in water. How many milliliters of solution should the nurse administer each hour? Record your answer as a whole number.

_____ milliliters

Answer: 15

Rationale: Factor analysis is the easiest way to solve this problem. Identify the information you have, and then use conversion factors to obtain the information you need.

$$\frac{176 \text{ lb}}{1} \times \frac{1 \text{ kg}}{2.2 \text{ lb}} \times \frac{5 \text{ mcg}}{1 \text{ kg/min}} \times \frac{1 \text{ mg}}{1,000 \text{ mcg}}$$

$$\times \frac{500 \text{ ml}}{800 \text{ mg}} \times \frac{60 \text{ min}}{1 \text{ hr}}$$

$$\frac{26,400,000 \text{ ml}}{1,760,000 \text{ hr}} = 15 \text{ ml/hr}$$

Critical thinking strategy: Focus on what the question is asking (number of milliliters per hour to administer), and recall the steps for factor analysis and I.V. flow rate calculations.

Client needs category: Physiological integrity

Client needs subcategory: Pharmacological and parenteral therapies

Cognitive level: Application

Integrated process: Nursing process/implementation

Reference: _Dosage Calculations Made Incredibly Easy,_ pages 267–270

2. A client with marked oliguria is ordered a test dose of 0.2 g/kg of 15% mannitol solution I.V. over 5 minutes. The client weighs 132 lb. How many grams should the nurse administer? Record your answer as a whole number.

_____ grams

Answer: 12

Rationale: First, convert the client's weight from grams to kilograms:

132 lb ÷ 2.2 kg/lb = 60 kg.

Then, to calculate the number of grams to administer, multiply the ordered number of grams by the client's weight in kilograms:

0.2 g/kg ÷ 60 kg = 12 g.

Critical thinking strategy: Focus on what the question is asking (the amount of grams to administer according to the client's weight), and review I.V. calculations.

Client needs category: Physiological integrity

Client needs subcategory: Pharmacological and parenteral therapies

Cognitive level: Analysis

Integrated process: Nursing process/implementation

Reference: *Dosage Calculations Made Incredibly Easy,* pages 267–270

---

3. A nurse is providing health teaching to a client with benign prostatic hyperplasia. Identify the area where the nurse would indicate that the prostate gland is located.

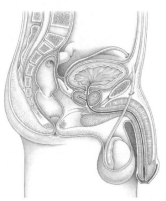

Answer:

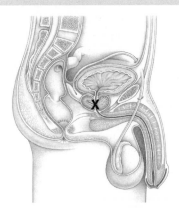

Rationale: The walnut-sized prostate gland lies beneath the bladder and surrounds the urethra.

Critical thinking strategy: Focus on the anatomy of the male genitourinary system.

Client needs category: Physiological integrity

Client needs subcategory: Physiological adaptation

Cognitive level: Application

Integrated process: Teaching and learning

Reference: Smeltzer, page 1741

4. After a retropubic prostatectomy, a client needs continuous bladder irrigation. The client has an I.V. line with dextrose in 5% water infusing at 40 ml/hour and a triple-lumen urinary catheter with normal saline solution infusing at 200 ml/hour. The nurse empties the urinary catheter drainage bag three times during an 8-hour period for a total of 2,780 ml. How many milliliters should the nurse calculate as urine? Record your answer as a whole number.

_____ milliliters

Answer: 1,180

Rationale: During 8 hours, 1,600 ml of bladder irrigant has been infused (200 ml × 8 hours = 1,600 ml/8 hours). The nurse should subtract this amount from the total volume in the drainage bag to determine the urine output (2,780 ml − 1,600 ml = 1,180 ml).

Critical thinking strategy: Focus on what the question is asking (the total amont of urine minus the amount of bladder irrigation), and review basic calculations.

Client needs category: Physiological integrity

Client needs subcategory: Basic care and comfort

Cognitive level: Analysis

Integrated process: Nursing process/implementation

Reference: Smeltzer, pages 1765–1767

---

5. A nurse is caring for a client with chronic renal failure. The laboratory results indicate hypocalcemia and hyperphosphatemia. When assessing the client, the nurse should be alert for which of the following? Select all that apply.

☐ **1.** Trousseau's sign

☐ **2.** Cardiac arrhythmias

☐ **3.** Constipation

☐ **4.** Decreased clotting time

☐ **5.** Drowsiness and lethargy

☐ **6.** Fractures

Answer: 1, 2, 6

Rationale: Hypocalcemia is a calcium deficit that causes nerve fiber irritability and repetitive muscle spasms. Signs and symptoms of hypocalcemia include Trousseau's sign, cardiac arrhythmias, diarrhea, increased clotting times, anxiety, and irritability. The calcium-phosphorus imbalance leads to brittle bones and pathologic fractures. Drowsiness and lethargy aren't typically associated with hypercalcemia.

Critical thinking strategy: Focus on the signs and symptoms of hypocalcemia and hyperphosphatemia, and review fluids and electrolyte imbalances and chronic renal failure.

Client needs category: Physiological integrity

Client needs subcategory: Reduction of risk potential

Cognitive level: Application

Integrated process: Nursing process/assessment

Reference: Smeltzer, pages 325–327, 332–333

6. A nurse is explaining menstruation to a class. Place the pathophysiologic steps of the menstrual cycle listed below in the correct sequential order. Use all of the options.

1.	The level of estrogen in the blood peaks.
2.	Peak endometrial thickening occurs.
3.	Increased estrogen and progesterone levels inhibit luteinizing hormone.
4.	The top layer of the endometrium breaks down and sloughs.
5.	A follicle matures and ovulation occurs.
6.	The endometrium begins thickening.

Rationale: The menstrual cycle begins with the first day of menstruation, when the top layer of endometrium breaks down and begins to slough off. As the endometrium thickens, the level of estrogen in the blood begins to rise and eventually peak. The follicle matures and ovulation occurs when estrogen levels peak. After ovulation, the endometrium continues to thicken to its peak level. Increased estrogen and progesterone levels inhibit follicle-stimulating hormone, which causes a feedback loop that then decreases estrogen and progesterone production. This causes the top layer of the endometrium to break down and slough, restarting the cycle in a nonpregnant female.

Critical thinking strategy: Focus on normal growth and development and the menstrual cycle.

Client needs category: Health promotion and maintenance

Client needs subcategory: None

Cognitive level: Application

Integrated process: Teaching and learning

Reference: Smeltzer, pages 1615–1616

---

7. A client requires bladder retraining for incontinence. Which procedures would the nurse expect to include in the teaching plan for this client? Select all that apply.

☐ **1.** Kegel exercises

☐ **2.** Prompted voiding

☐ **3.** External catheters

☐ **4.** Habit training

☐ **5.** Bladder training

☐ **6.** Self-catherization devices

Answer: 2, 4, 5

Rationale: Prompted voiding, habit training, and bladder training are used to correct frequent urination, keep the client dry, and promote improved voiding habits. Kegal exercises are used to strengthen bladder and pelvic muscles, and both external catheters and self-catheterization devices are used to collect urine without bladder training.

Critical thinking strategy: Focus on bladder training activities rather than devices or appliances, and review procedures for bladder training and behavioral training.

Client needs category: Health promotion and maintenance

Client needs subcategory: None

Cognitive level: Comprehension

Integrated process: Teaching and learning

Reference: Smeltzer, pages 1582–1583

8. A nurse is explaining self-catheterization to a female client who has been diagnosed with urogenic bladder. Which instructions should the nurse include in her teaching? Select all that apply.

☐ **1.** Tampons may remain in place during menstruation.

☐ **2.** The meatus should be cleaned with a towlette or soapy washcloth and then rinsed.

☐ **3.** Sterile technique isn't required.

☐ **4.** A new intermittent catherization set should be used each time.

☐ **5.** Finding the urinary meatus always requires visualization with a mirror.

Answer: 2, 3

Rationale: Cleaning the meatus with a towelette or soapy washcloth decreases the risk of introducing bacteria into the bladder. Sterile technique isn't required during self-catherization. Leaving a tampon in place can restrict the urethra and impede catheter insertion. It isn't necessary to use a new intermittent catheter each time; washing the catheter and allowing it to air-dry after each use is usually sufficient. The urinary meatus can be found using visual or tactile techniques.

Critical thinking strategy: Focus on catheter care and self-catherization technique, and review normal flora and microbiology related to the genitourinary sytem.

Client needs category: Health promotion and maintenance

Client needs subcategory: None

Cognitive level: Application

Integrated process: Teaching and leanring

Reference: Smeltzer, page 216

---

9. The nurse is reviewing a client's urine culture and sensitivity test results. Which of the following would the nurse expect to see in normal urine? Select all that apply.

☐ **1.** Ketones

☐ **2.** Protein

☐ **3.** White blood cells

☐ **4.** Crystals

☐ **5.** Nitrates

☐ **6.** Bilirubin

Answer: 2, 3

Rationale: Small amounts of protein and white blood cells are normal. Ketones, crystals, nitrates, and bilirubin are all abnormal findings

Critical thinking strategy: Focus on normal urinalysis findings, and review routine urinalysis and laboratory tests.

Client needs category: Physiological integrity

Client needs subcategory: Physiological adaptation

Cognitive level: Knowledge

Integrated process: Nursing process/analysis

Reference: Smeltzer, pages 1505–1506

10. A client returns from prostate surgery with continuous bladder irrigation that's set to irrigate the bladder with 150 ml/hour for 24 hours. The order reads: *Postoperative day 2—irrigate at rate of 100 ml/hr for 24 hours.* The output is 3,725 ml on day 1 and 3,800 on day 2. Of the output recorded, how much is urine? Record your answer as a whole number.

_____ milliliters

Answer: 1,525

Rationale: Total output is 7,525 ml. Total irrigation is as follows:

Day 1 150 × 24 = 3,600
Day 2 100 × 24 = 2,400

Total

To find the urine output, subtract the irrigation output from the total output: 7,525–6,000 = 1,525

Critical thinking strategy: Focus on basic mathematical concepts, and review calculation of intake and output.

Client needs subcategory: Health promotion and maintenance

Client needs subcategory: None

Cognitive level: Knowledge

Integrated process: Nursing process/analysis

Reference: Smeltzer, pages 1765–1767

---

11. A nurse is providing health teaching on female sexuality. Identify the area where the nurse should indicate is the site of sexual stimulation.

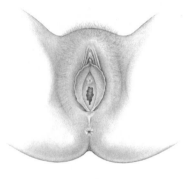

Answer:

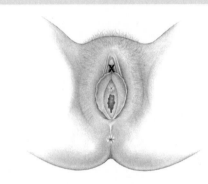

Rationale: The clitoris is directly associated with engorgement and climax.

Critical thinking strategy: Focus on anatomy of the female reproductive system and female sexuality.

Client needs category: Health promotion and maintenance

Client needs subcategory: None

Cognitive level: Knowledge

Integrated process: Teaching and learning

Reference: Smeltzer, pages 1614–1615

12. The nurse is assisting in cystometrography. Place in chronological order the sequence of events for this procedure. Use all the options.

| 1. Client is asked to void normally. |
| 2. Urinary catheter is inserted. |
| 3. Any residual urine is noted. |
| 4. Fluid is instilled into the urinary catheter. |
| 5. Client is asked to void following instillation. |
| 6. Urge to void is recorded. |

Answer: 1, 2, 4, 6, 5, 3

Rationale: First, the client is asked to void normally. Then a urinary catheter is inserted, and fluid is instilled. The first urge to void is recorded. Following the procedure, the client is instructed to void and any residual urine is noted. Finally, the catheter is removed.

Critical thinking strategy: Focus on the physiology of the genitourinary system and the cystometrography procedure.

Client needs category: Health promotion and maintenance

Client needs subcategory: None

Cognitive level: Analysis

Integrated process: Nursing process/implementation

Reference: Smeltzer, pages 1511–1512

Musculoskeletal disorders

1. A client is diagnosed with osteoporosis. Which statements should the nurse include when teaching the client about the disease? Select all that apply.

☐ **1.** Osteoporosis is common in females after menopause.

☐ **2.** Osteoporosis is a degenerative disease characterized by a decrease in bone density.

☐ **3.** The disease is congenital, caused by poor dietary intake of milk products.

☐ **4.** Osteoporosis can cause pain and injury.

☐ **5.** Passive range-of-motion exercises can promote bone growth.

☐ **6.** Weight-bearing exercise should be avoided.

Answer: 1, 2, 4

Rationale: Osteoporosis is a degenerative metabolic bone disorder in which the rate of bone resorption accelerates and the rate of bone formation decelerates, thus decreasing bone density. Postmenopausal women are at increased risk for this disorder because of their loss of estrogen. The decrease in bone density can cause pain and injury. Osteoporosis isn't a congenital disorder; however, low calcium intake does contribute to it. Passive range-of-motion exercises may be performed, but they won't promote bone growth. The client should be encouraged to participate in weight-bearing exercise because it promotes bone growth.

Critical thinking strategy: Focus on nursing inteventions and treatments for osteoporosis, and review the pathophysiology of bone disorders.

Client needs category: Physiological integrity

Client needs subcategory: Physiological adaptation

Cognitive level: Application

Integrated process: Teaching and learning

Reference: Smeltzer, pages 2404–2410

2. A client is preparing for discharge after undergoing an above-the-knee amputation. Which of the following instructions should the nurse include in the client's teaching plan? Select all that apply.

☐ **1.** Massage the residual limb in a motion away from the suture line.

☐ **2.** Avoid using heat application to ease pain.

☐ **3.** Immediately report twitching, spasms, or phantom limb pain.

☐ **4.** Avoid exposing the skin around the residual limb to excessive perspiration.

☐ **5.** Be sure to perform the prescribed exercises.

☐ **6.** Rub the residual limb with a dry washcloth for 4 minutes three times daily if the limb is sensitive to touch.

Answer: 4, 5, 6

Rationale: The nurse should advise the client that perspiration on the residual limb may cause irritation. The client should exercise as instructed to minimize complications. In addition, rubbing the limb as described with a dry washcloth helps desensitize the skin. The nurse should instruct the client to massage the residual limb toward the suture line—not away from it—to mobilize the scar and prevent its adherence to bone. Twitching, spasms, or phantom limb pain are normal reactions to an amputation and don't need to be reported. The nurse should inform the client that these symptoms might be eased by heat, massage, or gentle pressure.

Critical thinking strategy: Focus on postoperative care and nursing interventions to promote self-care and wound healing, and review postamputation rehabilitation.

Client needs category: Physiological integrity

Client needs subcategory: Reduction of risk potential

Cognitive level: Application

Integrated process: Teaching and learning

Reference: Smeltzer, pages 2464–2469

---

3. A client complains of an acute exacerbation of rheumatoid arthritis. The nurse plans care based on which of the following facts about rheumatoid arthritis? Select all that apply.

☐ **1.** Onset is acute and usually occurs between ages 25 and 40.

☐ **2.** The client experiences stiff, swollen joints bilaterally.

☐ **3.** The client may not exercise once the disease is diagnosed.

☐ **4.** Erythrocyte sedimentation rate (ESR) is elevated, and X-rays show erosions and decalcification of involved joints.

☐ **5.** Inflamed cartilage triggers complement activation, which stimulates the release of additional inflammatory mediators.

☐ **6.** The first-line treatment is gold salts and methotrexate.

Answer: 2, 4, 5

Rationale: Clients with rheumatoid arthritis experience stiff, swollen joints due to a severe inflammatory reaction. Elevated ESR and X-ray evidence of bony destruction are indicative of severe involvement. Rheumatoid arthritis starts insidiously, with fatigue, persistent low-grade fever, anorexia, and vague skeletal symptoms, usually between ages 35 and 50. Maintaining range of motion by a prescribed exercise program is essential, but clients must rest between activities. Salicylates and nonsteroidal anti-inflammatory drugs are considered the first-line treatments.

Critical thinking strategy: Focus on the pathophysiology and treatment of rheumatoid arthritis, and review commonly prescribed medications.

Client needs category: Physiological integrity

Client needs subcategory: Physiological adaptation

Cognitive level: Application

Integrated process: Nursing process/planning

Reference: Smeltzer, pages 1906–1909

4. An elderly client fell and fractured the neck of his femur. Identify the area where the fracture occurred.

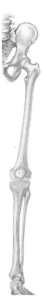

Answer:

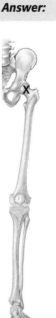

Rationale: The femur's neck connects the femur's round ball head to the shaft.

Critical thinking strategy: Focus on the anatomy of the upper leg, and review types of fractures.

Client needs category: Physiological integrity

Client needs subcategory: Physiological adaptation

Cognitive level: Comprehension

Integrated process: Nursing process/assessment

Reference: Smeltzer, page 2446

---

5. A client is in the emergency department with a suspected fracture of the right hip. Which assessment findings of the right leg would the nurse expect to assess? Select all that apply.

☐ **1.** The right leg is longer than the left leg.

☐ **2.** The right leg is shorter than the left leg.

☐ **3.** The right leg is abducted.

☐ **4.** The right leg is adducted.

☐ **5.** The right leg is externally rotated.

☐ **6.** The right leg is internally rotated.

Answer: 2, 4, 5

Rationale: In a hip fracture, the affected leg is shorter, adducted, and externally rotated.

Critical thinking strategy: Focus on the clinical manifestations of fractures, specifically the femur.

Client needs category: Physiological integrity

Client needs subcategory: Physiological adaptation

Cognitive level: Application

Integrated process: Nursing process/assessment

Reference: Smeltzer, page 2446

6. A client is scheduled for a laminectomy of the L1 and L2 vertebrae. Identify the area that's involved in the client's surgery.

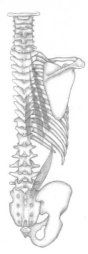

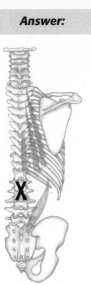

Rationale: In a laminectomy, one or more of the bony laminae that cover the vertebrae are removed. There are five lumbar vertebrae that are numbered from top to bottom. L5 is the closest to the sacrum. Count up from the sacrum to locate L1 and L2.

Critical thinking strategy: Focus on the anatomy of the spinal column and review the laminectomy surgical procedure.

Client needs category: Physiological integrity

Client needs subcategory: Physiological adaptation

Cognitive level: Comprehension

Integrated process: Nursing process/implementation

Reference: Smeltzer, page 2325

---

7. A client is diagnosed with gout. Which foods should the nurse instruct the client to avoid? Select all that apply.

☐ **1.** Green leafy vegetables

☐ **2.** Liver

☐ **3.** Cod

☐ **4.** Chocolate

☐ **5.** Sardines

☐ **6.** Eggs

Answer: 2, 3, 5

Rationale: Clients with gout should avoid foods that are high in purines, such as liver, cod, and sardines. They should also avoid anchovies, kidneys, sweetbreads, lentils, and alcoholic beverages—especially beer and wine. Green leafy vegetables, chocolate, and eggs aren't high in purines.

Critical thinking strategy: Focus on the pathophysiology of gout, and review associated nursing interventions.

Client needs category: Physiological integrity

Client needs subcategory: Basic care and comfort

Cognitive level: Application

Integrated process: Nursing process/implementation

Reference: Smeltzer, pages 1918–1919

8. A client is suspected of having carpal tunnel syndrome. The nurse assesses for Tinel's sign. Identify the area where the nurse should percuss in an attempt to elicit Tinel's sign.

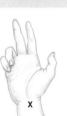

Rationale: Tinel's sign may be used to help identify carpal tunnel syndrome. It's elicited by percussing lightly over the median nerve, located on the inner aspect of the wrist. If the client reports tingling, numbness, and pain, the test is considered positive.

Critical thinking strategy: Focus on the anatomical basis for carpal tunnel syndrome, and review diagnostic clinical findings.

Client needs category: Safe, effective care environment

Client needs subcategory: Management of care

Cognitive level: Comprehension

Integrated process: Nursing process/assessment

Reference: Smeltzer, page 2398

---

9. A client is admitted with a possible diagnosis of osteomyelitis. Based on the documentation below, which laboratory result is the priority for the nurse to report to the physician?

Progress notes	
01/11/09 0900	Pt admitted with elevated temperature, complaining of bone pain and muscle spasms. Laboratory called with the following Results: rheumatoid factor negative; blood culture positive for Staphylococcus aureus; alkaline phosphatase 60 International Units/liter; erythrocyte sedimentation rate 10 mm/hr.————————Susan Wright, RN

☐ **1.** Rheumatoid factor

☐ **2.** Blood culture

☐ **3.** Alkaline phosphatase

☐ **4.** Erythrocyte sedimentation rate

Answer: 2

Rationale: Osteomyelitis is a bacterial infection of the bone and soft tissue that occurs by extension of soft tissue infection, direct bone contamination following surgery, or spreading from other infection sites in the body. A positive blood culture should be reported immediately to the physician so that specific antibiotic therapy can begin or be adjusted based on the positive culture. A negative rheumatoid factor would be expected in a possible diagnosis of osteomyelitis. An alkaline phosphatase level of 60 International Units/liter is within the normal range, and an erythrocyte sedimentation rate of 10 mm/hour is also within the normal range.

Critical thinking strategies: Focus on the pathophysiology of osteomyelitis and infections, and review the clinical manifestations of osteomyelitis.

Client needs category: Safe, effective care environment

Client needs subcategory: Management of care

Cognitive level: Comprehension

Integrated process: Nursing process/analysis

Reference: Smeltzer, page 2413

10. A client has been prescribed indomethacin (Indocin) for treatment of gouty arthritis. The orders says to give 25 mg t.i.d. for first 5 days, then increase by 25 mg per dose at weekly intervals until the daily dose reaches a maximum of 250 mg. The client is on week 3 of his treatment and has tolerated the medication without incident thus far. By week 3, what would his daily dose of medication be? Record your answer as a whole number.

_____ milligrams

Answer: 225

Rationale: First determine the first week's daily dosage: 25 mg × 3 = 75 mg. This dosage is increased by 25 mg per dose to equal the second week's daily dosage:

25 mg + 25 mg = 50 mg × 3 = 150 mg. The dosage is then increased by an additional 25 mg to equal the third week's daily dosage: 25 mg + 25 mg + 25 mg = 75 mg × 3 = 225 mg.

Critical thinking strategy: Focus on the amount of medication per dosage, the number of daily doses, and the amount to increase the dosage weekly; review dosage calculations and interpretation of medication orders.

Client needs category: Physiological integrity

Client needs subcategory: Pharmacological and parenteral therapies

Cognitive level: Application

Integrated process: Nursing process/analysis

Reference: *Dosage Calculations Made Incredibly Easy,* pages 120–122, 187

---

11. A client is scheduled for an open reduction internal fixation of the right hip. Place the following nursing interventions in chronological order to show the sequence in which the nurse should perform them. Use all of the options.

1. Develop a home care teaching plan.
2. Complete a preoperative checklist.
3. Make sure the client has signed an informed consent form.
4. Encourage coughing, turning, and deep breathing.
5. Monitor vital signs every 15 minutes × 4, every 30 minutes × 2, and every hour × 2.
6. Complete a history and physical examination.

Answer: 6, 3, 2, 5, 4, 1

Rationale: Initially, the nurse will complete the history and physical as part of the admission process. As part of the preoperative interventions, the nurse will witness the signing of the informed consent and complete a preoperative checklist. Postoperatively, the nurse will monitor vital signs frequently and, once the client is awake, alert, and oriented, she'll encourage him to turn, cough, and deep-breathe. Finally, a home care teaching plan must be developed before discharge.

Critical thinking strategy: Review the surgical procedure and related nursing interventions, and recall that client safety is paramount.

Client needs category: Health promotion and maintenance

Client needs subcategory: None

Cognitive level: Analysis

Integrated process: Nursing process/planning

Reference: Smeltzer, pages 482–483

Immune and hematologic disorders

1. A nurse is preparing a client with systemic lupus erythematosus (SLE) for discharge. Which instructions should the nurse include in the teaching plan? Select all that apply.

☐ **1.** Stay out of direct sunlight.

☐ **2.** Don't limit activity between flare-ups.

☐ **3.** Monitor body temperature.

☐ **4.** Taper the corticosteroid dosage as prescribed when symptoms are under control.

☐ **5.** Apply cold packs to relieve joint pain and stiffness.

Answer: 1, 3, 4

Rationale: A client with SLE should stay out of direct sunlight and avoid other sources of ultraviolet light because they may trigger severe skin reactions and exacerbate the symptoms. The client's body temperature should be monitored and fevers reported to the primary health care provider. The corticosteroid dosage must be tapered gradually once symptoms are relieved because stopping these drugs abruptly can cause adrenal insufficiency, a potentially life-threatening condition. Fatigue can cause an SLE flare-up, so the client should pace activities and plan for rest periods. The client should apply heat, not cold, to relieve joint pain. Cold packs may aggravate Raynaud's phenomenon, which commonly occurs in clients with SLE.

Critical thinking strategy: Focus on the nursing interventions and clinical manifestations for SLE.

Client needs category: Physiological integrity

Client needs subcategory: Reduction of risk potential

Cognitive level: Application

Integrated process: Teaching and learning

Reference: Smeltzer, pages 1909–1912

---

2. A client is to receive a blood transfusion of packed red blood cells for severe anemia. Place the following steps in the order a nurse would follow to administer this product. Use all the options.

1. Flush the I.V. tubing and line with normal saline solution.
2. Verify the blood bag identification, ABO group, and Rh compatibility against the client information.
3. Remain with the client and watch for signs of a transfusion reaction.
4. Record vital signs.
5. Put on gloves, a gown, and a face shield.
6. Check the packed cells for abnormal color, clumping, gas bubbles, and expiration date.

Answer: 4, 6, 2, 5, 1, 3

Rationale: To administer a blood transfusion, the nurse should follow the steps as listed above. Note that the transfusion may be withheld if the client's temperature is 100° F (37.8° C) or greater. Two client identifiers must be checked before the transfusion.

Critical thinking strategy: Focus on client safety and blood product administration.

Client needs category: Physiological integrity

Client needs subcategory: Pharmacological and parenteral therapies

Cognitive level: Application

Integrated process: Nursing process/implementation

Reference: Smeltzer, page 1107

3. A nurse is planning care for a client with human immunodeficiency virus (HIV). She's being assisted by a licensed practical nurse (LPN). Which statements by the LPN indicate her understanding of HIV transmission? Select all that apply.

☐ **1.** "I'll wear a gown, mask, and gloves for all client contact."

☐ **2.** "I don't need to wear any personal protective equipment because nurses have a low risk of occupational exposure."

☐ **3.** "I'll wear a mask if the client has a cough caused by an upper respiratory infection."

☐ **4.** "I'll wear a mask, gown, and gloves when splashing of body fluids is likely."

☐ **5.** "I'll wash my hands after client care."

Answer: 4, 5

Rationale: Standard precautions include wearing gloves for any known or anticipated contact with blood, body fluids, tissue, mucous membranes, or nonintact skin. If the task may result in splashing or splattering of blood or body fluids, a mask and goggles or a face shield and a fluid-resistant gown or apron should be worn. Hands should be washed before and after client care and after removing gloves.

Critical thinking strategy: Focus on universal precautions and review Centers for Disease Control and Prevention isolation guidelines.

Client needs category: Safe, effective care environment

Client needs subcategory: Safety and infection control

Cognitive level: Comprehension

Integrated process: Nursing process/planning

Reference: Taylor, page 716

---

4. Which nonpharmacologic interventions should a nurse include in the care plan for a client who has moderate rheumatoid arthritis? Select all that apply.

☐ **1.** Massaging inflamed joints

☐ **2.** Avoiding range-of-motion exercises

☐ **3.** Applying splints to inflamed joints

☐ **4.** Using assistive devices at all times

☐ **5.** Selecting clothing that has Velcro fasteners

☐ **6.** Applying moist heat to joints

Answer: 3, 5, 6

Rationale: Supportive, nonpharmacologic measures for the client with rheumatoid arthritis include applying splints to rest inflamed joints, using Velcro fasteners on clothing to aid in dressing, and applying moist heat to joints to relax muscles and relieve pain. Inflamed joints should never be massaged because doing so can aggravate inflammation. A physical therapy program, including range-of-motion exercises and carefully individualized therapeutic exercises, prevents loss of joint function. Assistive devices should only be used when marked loss of range of motion occurs.

Critical thinking strategy: Focus on the nursing interventions and pain management for rheumatoid arthritis, and review nonpharmacologic pain management therapies.

Client needs category: Physiological integrity

Client needs subcategory: Basic care and comfort

Cognitive level: Application

Integrated process: Nursing process/planning

Reference: Smeltzer, pages 1908–1909

5. A nurse is assessing a client with a suspected Epstein-Barr viral infection. Identify the quadrant of the abdomen where the nurse is best able to palpate the spleen.

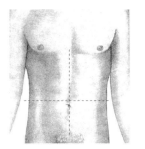

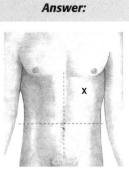

Rationale: The spleen is located in the left upper quadrant of the abdomen. It's posterior and slightly inferior to the stomach. The nurse should stop palpating immediately if she feels the spleen because compression can cause rupture.

Critical thinking strategy: Focus on the anatomy of the immune and hematologic systems, and review abdominal assessment techniques.

Client needs category: Physiological integrity

Client needs subcategory: Physiological adaptation

Cognitive level: Application

Integrated process: Nursing process/assessment

Reference: Taylor, page 639

---

6. A client has a viral infection and swollen lymph nodes. Identify the area where the nurse should place her hand to palpate the submandibular lymph nodes.

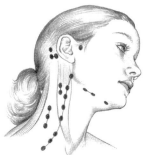

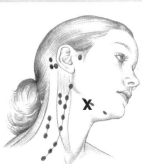

Rationale: The submandibular lymph nodes are found halfway between the angle and tip of the mandible.

Critical thinking strategy: Focus on the anatomy of the lymphatic system and the face, and review palpation techniques.

Client needs category: Physiological integrity

Client needs subcategory: Physiological adaptation

Cognitive level: Application

Integrated process: Nursing process/assessment

Reference: Taylor, pages 623–626

7. The nurse is caring for a client who is scheduled to undergo a bone marrow aspiration to assess the progression of a hematologic disorder. Which of the following interventions should the nurse include as part of her preprocedural teaching plan? Select all that apply.

☐ **1.** Explain the procedure to the client.

☐ **2.** Maintain a pressure dressing over the aspiration site.

☐ **3.** Encourage the client to ask questions before obtaining his signed informed consent.

☐ **4.** Explain that the client will receive an analgesic prior to the procedure.

☐ **5.** Administer an anxiety-relieving medication prior to the procedure.

☐ **6.** Instruct the client to save all voided urine for 24 hours after the procedure.

Rationale: The client should understand the procedure that he is undergoing and the reason why it's necessary before signing an informed consent form. He also should be advised that he'll receive some type of local analgesia before the procedure begins. Although the client may receive an anxiety-relieving medication before the procedure, administering the drug isn't part of the teaching plan. Likewise, maintaining pressure over the insertion site is a nursing intervention performed after the procedure; it's not a part of the preoperative teaching. Instructing the client to save voided urine would be part of the postprocedural discharge plan.

Critical thinking strategies: Focus on what the question is asking (preprocedure client teaching), and review guidelines on obtaining informed consent and preparation for bone marrow aspiration.

Client needs category: Physiological integrity

Client needs subcategory: Basic care and comfort

Cognitive level: Application

Integrated process: Teaching and learning

Reference: Smeltzer, page 1045

---

8. The nurse is assessing a client who is suspected of having Hodgkin's disease. The client has been admitted with swollen left-sided inguinal lymph nodes. Identify the area where the nurse would be best able to palpate for these lymph nodes.

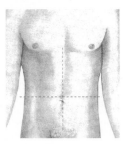

Answer:

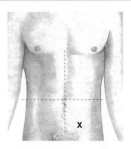

Rationale: Hodgkin's disease is a type of neoplasm involving cells of lymphoid origin. It usually begins as a painless enlargement of one or more lymph nodes. Most commonly, the lymph node enlargement involves the nodes in the neck area but it can also involve the inguinal nodes as well. The inguinal nodes are located in the groin area.

Critical thinking strategy: Focus on the anatomy of the lymphatic system and abdomen, and review the pathophysiology of Hodgkin's disease.

Client needs category: Physiological integrity

Client needs subcategory: Physiological adaptation

Cognitive level: Application

Integrated process: Nursing process/analysis

Reference: Smeltzer, pages 1080, 1784

9. A physician notes that a client who has been undergoing chemotherapy for cancer is now experiencing pancytopenia. Which laboratory values would the nurse expect the cllient to have supporting this diagnosis? Select all that apply.

☐ **1.** Decreased white blood cells

☐ **2.** Increased white blood cells

☐ **3.** Decreased platelets

☐ **4.** Increased platelets

☐ **5.** Decreased red blood cells

☐ **6.** Increased red blood cells

Answer: 1, 3, 5

Rationale: Pancytopenia is a state of simultaneous leukopenia (decreased white blood cells), thrombocytopenia (decreased platelets), and anemia (decreased red blood cells).

Critical thinking strategy: Focus on laboratory values for the disorder, and review pertinent medical terminology (such as *pan,* meaning *universal,* and *penia,* meaning *decreased*).

Client needs category: Physiological integrity

Client needs subcategory: Physiological adaptation

Cognitive level: Application

Integrated process: Nursing process/analysis

Reference: Smeltzer, page 1036

---

10. A client is scheduled to undergo Schilling's test as part of treatment for pernicious anemia. Place the following interventions in the order in which the nurse would perform them. Use all the options.

| **1.** Withhold all food and fluids after midnight before the test. |
| **2.** Instruct the client to save all voided urine for 24 hours. |
| **3.** Keep the client's urine at room temperature. |
| **4.** Explain the procedure to the client. |
| **5.** Place the signed informed consent form in the client's chart. |
| **6.** Obtain the client's informed consent. |

Answer: 4, 1, 6, 5, 2, 3

Rationale: The preprocedure steps consist of explaining the procedure to the client, withholding food and fluids after midnight, obtaining the client's informed consent, and placing the signed forms in the client's chart. Postprocedural nursing interventions include instructing the client to save all voided urine for 24 hours and then keeping the urine at room temperature.

Critical thinking strategy: Focus on routine preprocedural and postprocedural nursing care, and review the procedure for Schilling's test.

Client needs category: Health promotion and maintenance

Client needs subcategory: None

Cognitive level: Analysis

Integrated process: Nursing process/implementation

Reference: Smeltzer, page 1053

11. The nurse is caring for a client who has just been diagnosed with systemic lupus erythematosus (SLE). Which information should be included in a teaching plan that focuses on home care? Select all that apply.

☐ **1.** Avoid exposure to sunlight.

☐ **2.** Keep exercise to a minimal level.

☐ **3.** Report development of a butterfly rash on the face.

☐ **4.** Avoid over-the-counter medications unless approved by the physician.

☐ **5.** Take rest periods as needed.

Answer: 1, 2, 4, 5

Rationale: The client who suffers from systemic lupus erythematosus has a tendency toward photosensitivity; therefore, he should avoid exposure to sunlight. The client should also be advised to keep exercise to a minimum, to avoid over-the-counter medications unless directed by the physician, and to rest as needed. Because the butterfly rash associated with lupus is an initial sign, the client would already have the rash; he would not be reporting its development after discharge.

Critical thinking strategy: Focus on the pathophysiology of SLE, and review related clinical manifestations and nursing interventions.

Client needs category: Physiological integrity

Client needs subcategory: Basic care and comfort

Cognitive level: Application

Integrated process: Teaching and learning

Reference: Smeltzer, pages 1909–1912

Endocrine and metabolic disorders

1. A client is being discharged after having a thyroidectomy. Which of the following discharge instructions would be appropriate for this client? Select all that apply.

☐ **1.** Report signs and symptoms of hypoglycemia.

☐ **2.** Take thyroid replacement medication as ordered.

☐ **3.** Watch for changes in body functioning, such as lethargy, restlessness, sensitivity to cold, and dry skin, and report these changes to the physician.

☐ **4.** Avoid all over-the-counter (OTC) medications.

☐ **5.** Carry injectable dexamethasone at all times.

Answer: 2, 3

Rationale: After removal of the thyroid gland, the client needs to take thyroid replacement medication. The client also needs to report such changes as lethargy, restlessness, cold sensitivity, and dry skin, which may indicate the need for a higher dosage of medication. The thyroid gland doesn't regulate blood glucose level; therefore, signs and symptoms of hypoglycemia aren't relevant for this client. Injectable dexamethasone isn't needed for this client. Some OTC medications (such as non-aspirin products) are allowable.

Critical thinking strategy: Focus on the physiology of the thyroid gland, and review nursing interventions related to promoting rest, managing pain, and monitoring for potential complications.

Client needs category: Physiological integrity

Client needs subcategory: Physiological adaptation

Cognitive level: Application

Integrated process: Teaching and learning

Reference: Smeltzer, pages 1469–1470

2. A client is admitted with a diagnosis of diabetic ketoacidosis. An insulin drip is initiated with 50 units of insulin in 100 ml of normal saline solution administered via an infusion pump set at 10 ml/hour. The nurse determines that the client is receiving how many units of insulin each hour? Record your answer using a whole number.

_____ units/hour

Answer: 5

Rationale: To determine the number of insulin units the client is receiving per hour, first determine the number of units in each milliliter of fluid (50 units ÷ 100 ml = 0.5 unit/ml). Next, multiply the units per milliliter by the rate of milliliters per hour (0.5 unit × 10 ml/hour = 5 units).

Critical thinking strategy: Focus on what the question is asking (the amount of units of insulin being administered per hour) and then calculate the number of units per milliliter. Review solving for X and ratio and proportion.

Client needs category: Physiological integrity

Client needs subcategory: Pharmacological and parenteral therapies

Cognitive level: Application

Integrated process: Nursing process/analysis

Reference: _Dosage Calculations Made Incredibly Easy_, pages 52, 311

---

3. A client's glucose level is 365 mg/dl. His physician orders 10 units of regular insulin to be administered. The bottle of regular insulin is labeled 100 units/ml. How many milliliters of insulin should the nurse administer? Record your answer using one decimal place.

_____ milliliters

Answer: 0.1

Rationale: To find the correct administration amount, use the cross-product principle to set up the following equation:

$$\frac{X}{10 \text{ units}} = \frac{1 \text{ ml}}{100 \text{ units}}$$

Next, cross-multiply:

$$100 \times X \text{ units} = 10 \text{ units} \times 1 \text{ ml.}$$

Then divide both sides of the equation by 100 units to solve for X:

$$X = 0.1 \text{ ml.}$$

Critical thinking stategy: Focus on what the question is asking (the total number of milliliters to be administered), and review ratio-and-proportion calculations.

Client needs category: Physiological integrity

Client needs subcategory: Pharmacological and parenteral therapies

Cognitive level: Application

Integrated process: Nursing process/implementation

Reference: _Dosage Calculations Made Incredibly Easy,_ pages 52, 220–221

4. A nurse is performing an admission assessment on a client who has been diagnosed with diabetes insipidus. Which of the following findings should the nurse expect to note during the assessment? Select all that apply.

☐ **1.** Extreme polyuria

☐ **2.** Excessive thirst

☐ **3.** Elevated systolic blood pressure

☐ **4.** Low urine specific gravity

☐ **5.** Bradycardia

☐ **6.** Elevated serum potassium level

Answer: 1, 2, 4

Rationale: Signs and symptoms of diabetes insipidus include an abrupt onset of extreme polyuria, excessive thirst, dry skin and mucous membranes, tachycardia, and hypotension. Diagnostic studies reveal low urine specific gravity and osmolarity and an elevated serum sodium level. The serum potassium level is likely to be decreased, not increased.

Critical thinking strategy: Focus on the pathophysiology and clinical manifestations of diabetes insipidus.

Client needs category: Physiological integrity

Client needs subcategory: Physiological adaptation

Cognitive level: Comprehension

Integrated process: Nursing process/assessment

Reference: Smeltzer, page 1447

---

5. A client is being treated for hypothyroidism. Which of the following findings indicate that thyroid replacement therapy has been inadequate? Select all that apply.

☐ **1.** Prolonged QT interval on electrocardiogram

☐ **2.** Tachycardia

☐ **3.** Low body temperature

☐ **4.** Nervousness

☐ **5.** Bradycardia

☐ **6.** Dry mouth

Answer: 1, 3, 5

Rationale: In hypothyroidism, the body is in a hypometabolic state. Therefore, a prolonged QT interval with bradycardia and subnormal body temperature would indicate that replacement therapy was inadequate. Tachycardia, nervousness, and dry mouth are symptoms of an excessive level of thyroid hormone; these findings would indicate that the client has received an excessive dose of thyroid hormone.

Critical thinking strategy: Focus on the physiology of the thyroid gland, and review the clinical manifestations of hypothyroidism.

Client needs category: Physiological integrity

Client needs subcategory: Reduction of risk potential

Cognitive level: Analysis

Integrated process: Nursing process/analysis

Reference: Smeltzer, page 1453

6. A 55-year-old diabetic client is admitted with hypoglycemia. Which of the following information should the nurse include in her client teaching? Select all that apply.

☐ **1.** Hypoglycemia can result from excessive alcohol consumption.

☐ **2.** Skipping meals can cause hypoglycemia.

☐ **3.** Symptoms of hypoglycemia include thirst and excessive urination.

☐ **4.** Strenuous activity may result in hypoglycemia.

☐ **5.** Symptoms of hypoglycemia include shakiness, confusion, and headache.

☐ **6.** Hypoglycemia is a relatively harmless condition.

Answer: 1, 2, 4, 5

Rationale: Alcohol consumption, missed meals, and strenuous activity may lead to hypoglycemia. Symptoms of hypoglycemia include shakiness, confusion, headache, sweating, and tingling sensations around the mouth. Thirst and excessive urination are symptoms of hyperglycemia. Hypoglycemia can become a life-threatening disorder involving seizures and death of brain cells; the client shouldn't be told that the condition is relatively harmless.

Critical thinking strategy: Focus on the clinical manifestations of and nursing interventions for hypoglycema, and review the disease process of diabetes mellitus.

Client needs category: Physiological integrity

Client needs subcategory: Reduction of risk potential

Cognitive level: Application

Integrated process: Teaching and learning

Reference: Smeltzer, pages 1411–1412

---

7. A nurse is caring for a client with a low calcium level. Place the following options in chronological order to indicate the regulatory feedback mechanism of parathyroid hormone (PTH) release in relation to calcium levels. Use all of the options.

1. High serum calcium level inhibits PTH secretion.
2. Low serum calcium level stimulates parathyroid gland.
3. Calcium is reabsorbed.
4. Parathyroid gland releases PTH.

Answer: 2, 4, 3, 1

Rationale: Simple feedback occurs when the level of one substance regulates the secretion of hormones. A low calcium level stimulates the parathyroid gland to release PTH, which promotes resorption of calcium, resulting in normalized calcium levels. When calcium levels are elevated, PTH secretion is inhibited.

Critical thinking strategy: Focus on the physiology of the parathyroid gland and PTH, and review the normal physiology of endocrine glands.

Client needs category: Physiological integrity

Client needs subcategory: Physiological adaptation

Cognitive level: Analysis

Integrated process: Nursing process/analysis

Reference: Smeltzer, page 1470

8. A client with Addison's disease is scheduled for discharge after being hospitalized for an adrenal crisis. Which statements by the client would indicate that the nurse's teaching has been effective? Select all that apply.

☐ **1.** "I have to take my steroids for 10 days."

☐ **2.** "I need to weigh myself daily to be sure I don't eat too many calories."

☐ **3.** "I need to call my doctor to discuss my steroid needs before I have dental work."

☐ **4.** "I will call the doctor if I suddenly feel very weak or dizzy."

☐ **5.** "If I feel like I have the flu, I'll carry on as usual because this is an expected response."

☐ **6.** "I need to obtain and wear a Medic Alert bracelet."

Answer: 3, 4, 6

Rationale: Dental work can be a cause of physical stress; therefore, the client's physician needs to be informed about the dental work so he can adjust the dosage of steroids if necessary. Fatigue, weakness, and dizziness are symptoms of inadequate steroid therapy; the physician should be notified if these symptoms occur. A Medic Alert bracelet allows health care providers to access the client's history of Addison's disease if the client is unable to communicate this information. A client with Addison's disease doesn't produce enough steroids, so routine administration of steroids is a lifetime treatment. Daily weight should be monitored to monitor changes in fluid balance, not calorie intake. Influenza is an added physical stressor that may require an increased dosage of steroids. The client should notify the physician, not "carry on as usual."

Critical thinking strategy: Focus on the clinical manifestations and nursing interventions for Addison's disease, and review the physiology of the adrenal glands.

Client needs category: Physiological integrity

Client needs subcategory: Reduction of risk potential

Cognitive level: Analysis

Integrated process: Nursing process/evaluation

Reference: Smeltzer, pages 1477–1479

---

9. A client comes to the clinic because she has experienced a weight loss of 20 lb over the last month, even though her appetite has been "ravenous" and she hasn't changed her activity level. She's diagnosed with Graves' disease. For which other signs and symptoms of Graves' disease should the nurse assess the client? Select all that apply.

☐ **1.** Rapid, bounding pulse

☐ **2.** Bradycardia

☐ **3.** Heat intolerance

☐ **4.** Mild tremors

☐ **5.** Nervousness

☐ **6.** Constipation

Answer: 1, 3, 4, 5

Rationale: Graves' disease, or hyperthyroidism, is a hypermetabolic state that's associated with a rapid, bounding pulse; heat intolerance; tremors; and nervousness. Bradycardia and constipation are signs and symptoms of hypothyroidism.

Critical thinking strategy: Focus on the physiology of the thyroid gland and the pathophysiology of hyperthyroidism (Graves' disease).

Client needs category: Health promotion and maintenance

Client needs subcategory: None

Cognitive level: Analysis

Integrated process: Nursing process/analysis

Reference: Smeltzer, pages 1459–1463

10. A client who suffered a brain injury after falling off a ladder has recently developed syndrome of inappropriate antidiuretic hormone (SIADH). Which findings indicate that the treatment he's receiving for SIADH is effective? Select all that apply.

□ **1.** Decrease in body weight

□ **2.** Rise in blood pressure and drop in heart rate

□ **3.** Absence of wheezing

□ **4.** Increase in urine output

□ **5.** Decrease in urine osmolarity

Answer: 1, 4, 5

Rationale: SIADH is an abnormality involving an excessive release of antidiuretic hormone. The predominant feature is water retention with oliguria, edema, and weight gain. Successful treatment should result in a reduction in weight, increased urine output, and a decrease in urine osmolarity (concentration). Wheezes aren't typically associated with SIADH. The client's blood pressure should remain the same or decrease after treatment.

Critical thinking strategy: Focus on the clinical manifestations and treatment of SIADH.

Client needs category: Physiological integrity

Client needs subcategory: Physiological adaptation

Cognitive level: Analysis

Integrated process: Nursing process/evaluation

Reference: Smeltzer, pages 315–319

---

11. A nurse is about to administer a client's morning dose of insulin. The client's order is for 5 units of regular insulin and 10 units of NPH insulin given as a basal dose. He also is to receive an amount prescribed from his medium-dose sliding scale (shown below) based on his morning blood glucose level. The nurse performs a bedside blood glucose measurement and the result is 264 mg/dl. How many total units of insulin should the nurse administer to the client?

Plasma glucose (mg/dl)	Low dose (regular insulin)	Medium dose (regular insulin)	High dose (regular insulin)	Very high dose (regular insulin)
< 70	← Call physician →			
71-140	0 units	0 units	0 units	0 units
141-180	1 unit	2 units	4 units	10 units
181-240	2 units	4 units	8 units	15 units
241-300	4 units	6 units	12 units	20 units
301-400	6 units	9 units	16 units	25 units
> 400	8 units	12 units	20 units	30 units
	← and call physician →			

_____ units

Answer: 21

Rationale: The basal dose for this client is 5 units of regular insulin and 10 units of NPH insulin. The medium-dose sliding scale indicates that, based on his glucose reading of 264 mg/dl, he should receive an additional 6 units of regular insulin, totaling 21 units (5 units + 10 units + 6 units = 21 units).

Critical thinking strategy: Focus on what the question is asking (the total amount of insulin to be given).

Client needs category: Physiological integrity

Client needs subcategory: Pharmacological and parenteral therapies

Cognitive level: Application

Integrated process: Nursing process/implementation

Reference: *Dosage Calculations Made Incredibly Easy,* pages 217–221

12. A client arrives in the clinic with a possible parathyroid hormone (PTH) deficiency. Diagnosis of this condition includes the analysis of serum electrolytes. Which of the following electrolytes would the nurse expect to be abnormal? Select all that apply.

☐ **1.** Sodium

☐ **2.** Potassium

☐ **3.** Calcium

☐ **4.** Chloride

☐ **5.** Glucose

☐ **6.** Phosphorus

Answer: 3, 6

Rationale: A client with a PTH deficiency has abnormal calcium and phosphorus values because PTH regulates these two electrolytes. Sodium, chloride, potassium, and glucose aren't affected by a PTH deficiency.

Critical thinking strategy: Focus on the physiology of the parathyroid gland and its effect on serum electrolytes, and review parathyroid deficiency.

Client needs category: Health promotion and maintenance

Client needs subcategory: None

Cognitive level: Analysis

Integrated process: Nursing process/evaluation

Reference: Smeltzer, pages 1472–1473

---

13. Two weeks after a partial thyroidectomy, a client is being seen for his postoperative follow-up appointment. The nurse is aware that the client is at increased risk for hypothyroidism. Which signs and symptoms would the nurse expect to find in a client with hypothyroidism? Select all that apply.

☐ **1.** Heat intolerance

☐ **2.** Hair loss

☐ **3.** Increased energy

☐ **4.** Dry skin

☐ **5.** Cold intolerance

☐ **6.** Fatigue

Answer: 2, 4, 5, 6

Rationale: Hypothyroidism refers to suboptimal levels of thyroid hormone. A client with this condition typically has hair loss, dry skin, cold intolerance, and fatigue.

Critical thinking strategy: Focus on the physiology of the thyroid gland and hormones, and review the pathophysiology of hypothyroidism.

Client needs category: Physiological integrity

Client needs subcategory: Physiological adaptation

Cognitive level: Comprehension

Integrated process: Nursing process/analysis

Reference: Smeltzer, pages 1452–1453

14. The nurse is caring for a client following a thyroidectomy and assesses him for a possible low calcium level related to inadvertent removal of parathyroid glands. Identify the part of the body the nurse should assess to determine a positive or negative Chvostek's sign.

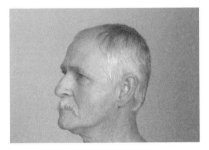

Answer:

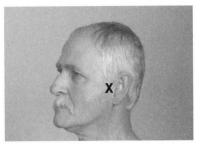

Rationale: When the facial nerve is stimulated in someone with hypocalcemia, the facial muscles contract, causing twitching of the cheek, mouth, and nose (Chvostek's sign). To elicit Chvostek's sign, tap the nerve about 2 cm anterior to the earlobe, just below the zygomatic arch.

Critical thinking strategy: Focus on postthyroidectomy care and assessment techniques, and review thyroid and parathyroid gland physiology.

Client needs category: Physiological integrity

Client needs subcategory: Physiological adaptation

Cognitive level: Analysis

Integrated process: Nursing process/analysis

Reference: Smeltzer, page 326

---

15. The nurse is preparing the morning insulin for a diabetic client on the unit. The order is for 20 units of Humulin 70/30. The nurse knows that this dose contains a mixture of intermediate-acting insulin and fast-acting insulin. How many units of intermediate-acting insulin does this dose contain? Record your answer using a whole number.

_____ units

Answer: 14

Rationale: Recall that Humulin 70/30 insulin contains both intermediate-acting insulin and fast-acting insulin. The 70 and 30 represent the percentages of each kind (the first number always pertains to the percentage of intermediate-acting insulin; the second, to the fast-acting insulin). Therefore, to calculate the amount of intermediate-acting insulin, the nurse must multiply the total number of units to be given by 0.7:

0.7×20 units $= 14$ units of intermediate-acting insulin.

Critical thinking strategy: Focus on what the question is asking (the amount of intermediate units contained in a dose of combined intermediate- and fast-acting insulin), and review calculations involving percentages.

Client needs category: Physiological integrity

Client needs subcategory: Pharmacological and parenteral therapies

Cognitive level: Application

Integrated process: Nursing process/planning

Reference: *Dosage Calculations Made Incredibly Easy,* pages 40–41, 218

16. To properly care for clients with diabetes insipidus, the nurse should be aware of the disorder's pathophysiology. Place the following events in chronological sequence to show the pathophysiologic process. Use all of the options.

1.	Thirst occurs.

2.	Dehydration occurs.

3.	Body has insufficient level of antidiuretic hormone.

4.	Polyuria occurs.

5.	Distal renal tubules are unable to absorb water.

Answer: 3, 5, 4, 2, 1

Rationale: The pathophysiology of diabetes insipidus begins with a decrease in antidiuretic hormone (ADH) or with the kidneys' inability to respond to ADH. Without ADH, the distal kidney tubules and collecting ducts can't absorb water and polyuria occurs. This leads to dehydration and then thirst.

Critical thinking strategy: Focus on the pathophysiology of diabetes insipidus, and review the anatomy and physiology of the kidney.

Client needs category: Physiological integrity

Client needs subcategory: Physiological adaptation

Cognitive level: Analysis

Integrated process: Nursing process/analysis

Reference: Smeltzer, pages 1447, 1493–1495

---

17. The nurse is admitting a client with newly diagnosed diabetes mellitus and left-sided heart failure. Assessment reveals low blood pressure, increased respiratory rate and depth, drowsiness, and confusion. The client complains of headache and nausea. Based on the serum laboratory results below, how would the nurse interpret the client's acid-base balance?

Lab results

pH	7.34
HCO_3^-	19 mEq/L
$PaCO_2$	35 mm Hg
PaO_2	88 mm Hg
Potassium	5.3 mEq/L
Chloride	102 mEq/L
Calcium	10.4 mg/dl
Anion gap	30 mEq/L

☐ **1.** Metabolic alkalosis

☐ **2.** Metabolic acidosis

☐ **3.** Respiratory acidosis

☐ **4.** Respiratory alkalosis

Answer: 2

Rationale: This client has metabolic acidosis, which typically manifests with a low pH, low bicarbonate level, normal to low $PaCO_2$, and normal PaO_2. The client's serum electrolyte levels also support metabolic acidosis, which include an elevated potassium level, normal to elevated chloride level, and normal calcium level. The client's anion gap of 30 mEq/L is high, also indicative of metabolic acidosis. This kind of metabolic acidosis occurs with diabetic ketoacidosis and other disorders.

Critical thinking strategy: Focus on the laboratory values and physiological changes associated with diabetic ketoacidosis.

Client needs category: Physiological integrity

Client needs subcategory: Physiological adaptation

Cognitive level: Analysis

Integrated process: Nursing process/analysis

Reference: Smeltzer, pages 335–336, 1412–1415

18. When reviewing the urinalysis report of a client with newly diagnosed diabetes mellitus, the nurse would expect which urine characteristics to be abnormal? Select all that apply.

☐ **1.** Amount

☐ **2.** Odor

☐ **3.** pH

☐ **4.** Specific gravity

☐ **5.** Glucose level

☐ **6.** Ketone bodies

Answer: 1, 3, 7, 8

Rationale: Diabetes mellitus is associated with increased amounts of urine, a sweet or fruity odor, and glucose and ketone bodies in the urine. It doesn't affect the urine's pH or specific gravity.

Critical thinking strategy: Focus on the pathophysiology and clinical manifestations of diabetes mellitus, and review laboratory values.

Client needs category: Physiological integrity

Client needs subcategory: Reduction of risk potential

Cognitive level: Comprehension

Integrated process: Nursing process/analysis

Reference: Smeltzer, pages 1382–1383

Integumentary disorders

1. A 30-year-old client presents at the physician's office with gray-brown burrows with epidermal curved ridges and follicular papules of the skin. The primary care provider diagnoses scabies. Which of the following teaching points should a nurse review with the client? Select all that apply.

☐ **1.** The disease is only actively contagious when the lesions are open.

☐ **2.** Scabies is transmitted by close person-to-person contact or contact with infected linens and clothing.

☐ **3.** The most commonly infected areas are the hands, feet, and neck.

☐ **4.** Severe itching of the affected areas, especially at night, is a common finding.

☐ **5.** Only the infected individual needs to use the prescribed medication.

☐ **6.** All of the client's linens and clothing should be washed immediately in hot water.

Answer: 2, 4, 6

Rationale: Scabies is a contagious disorder caused by a tiny mite that burrows under the skin; it's transmitted by close person-to-person contact or contact with infected linens or clothing. It causes severe itching, especially at night, in addition to the familiar papular rash. All of the client's linens and clothing should be washed promptly in hot water to reduce the risk of reinfestation. Scabies is transmissible from the time of infection to the time the burrows and papules appear, which may occur several weeks afterward. It remains transmissible until eradicated by a prescription cream or an oral medication. Scabies is most commonly seen in the finger webs, flexor surface of the wrists, and the antecubital fossae. When a family member is diagnosed, all members of the family must be treated with medication and their clothing and linens washed to prevent transmission and reinfestation.

Critical thinking strategy: Focus on the clinical manifestations of scabies, and review the recommended treatment and nursing interventions.

Client needs category: Health promotion and maintenance

Client needs subcategory: None

Cognitive level: Application

Integrated process: Teaching and learning

Reference: Smeltzer, pages 1963–1964

2. At an outpatient clinic, a medical assistant interviews a client and documents her findings. The staff nurse reads the progress notes below and begins planning client care based on which nursing diagnosis?

Progress notes	
2/9/09	Client very anxious because new black mole
0900	with shades of brown noted on upper outer
	right thigh. Asymmetrical in shape with an
	irregular border.————M. Rosenfeld, MA

☐ **1.** *Deficient knowledge related to potential diagnosis of basal cell carcinoma*

☐ **2.** *Fear related to potential diagnosis of malignant melanoma*

☐ **3.** *Risk for impaired skin integrity related to potential squamous cell carcinoma*

☐ **4.** *Readiness for enhanced knowledge of skin care precautions related to benign mole*

Answer: 2

Rationale: Documentation reveals that the client is anxious about her symptoms. These symptoms most closely resemble malignant melanoma. Therefore, *Fear related to potential diagnosis of malignant melanoma* is the most appropriate nursing diagnosis. The nursing note doesn't indicate that the client presently has deficient knowledge. The characteristics of the lesion aren't consistent with a basal or squamous cell carcinoma or a benign nevus (mole).

Critical thinking strategy: Focus on the nursing diagnosis that's most closely related to the client's statements, and review skin lesion assessment.

Client needs category: Physiological integrity

Client needs subcategory: Physiological adaptation

Cognitive level: Analysis

Integrated process: Communication and documentation

Reference: Smeltzer, pages 36–39

---

3. While assessing a client with a stage 2 pressure ulcer, the nurse would expect to note which of the following? Select all that apply.

☐ **1.** The skin is intact.

☐ **2.** Full-thickness skin loss is evident.

☐ **3.** Undermining is present.

☐ **4.** Sinus tracts have developed.

☐ **5.** The ulcer is superficial, like a blister.

☐ **6.** Partial-thickness skin loss of the epidermis is evident.

Answer: 5, 6

Rationale: A stage 2 pressure ulcer involves partial-thickness skin loss of the epidermis or dermis. The ulcer is superficial and presents clinically as an abrasion, blister, or shallow crater. Intact skin is characteristic of a stage 1 pressure ulcer. Full-thickness skin loss, undermining, and sinus tracts are characteristic of a stage 3 pressure ulcer.

Critical thinking strategy: Focus on the pathophysiology of pressure ulcers, and review pressure ulcer staging.

Client needs category: Physiological integrity

Client needs subcategory: Physiological adaptation

Cognitive level: Analysis

Integrated process: Nurisng process/analysis

Reference: Smeltzer, pages 208–211

4. Which of the following statements should the nurse include in the nursing care plan of a client with a pressure ulcer? Select all that apply.

☐ **1.** Use pressure reduction devices.

☐ **2.** Increase carbohydrates in the diet.

☐ **3.** Reposition the client every 1 to 2 hours.

☐ **4.** Teach the family members how to care for the wound.

☐ **5.** Clean the area around the ulcer with mild soap.

☐ **6.** Avoid the use of support-surface therapy.

Rationale: Using a pressure reduction device, repositioning the client every 1 to 2 hours, and cleaning the area around the wound with a mild soap will aid in healing or prevent further skin breakdown. Teaching family members how to care for the wound will assist with discharge planning. Protein, not carbohydrate, intake, should be increased to promote wound healing. Support-surface therapy is a major therapeutic modality for managing pressure, friction, and shearing forces on tissues such as ulcers.

Critical thinking strategy: Focus on nursing interventions for pressure ulcer care, and review pressure ulcer prevention guidelines.

Client needs category: Physiological integrity

Client needs subcategory: Basic care and comfort

Cognitive level: Analysis

Integrated process: Nursing process/planning

Reference: Smeltzer, pages 210–214

---

5. A triage nurse in the emergency department admits a 50-year-old male client with second-degree burns on the anterior and posterior portions of both legs. Based on the Rule of Nines, what percentage of the body is burned?

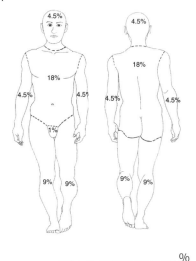

_____ %

Answer: 36

Rationale: The anterior and posterior portions of one leg amount to 18%. Because both legs are burned, the total is 36%.

Critical thinking strategy: Focus on the areas affected and the percentage of body surface area, and use simple math to add percentages together.

Client needs category: Physiological integrity

Client needs subcategory: Physiological adaptation

Cognitive level: Analysis

Integrated process: Nursing process/analysis

Reference: Smeltzer, pages 1997–1998

6. A client returns from the operating room with a partial-thickness skin graft on her left arm. The donor tissue was taken from her left hip. In planning her immediate postoperative care, which of the following interventions should the nurse include? Select all that apply.

☐ **1.** Change the dressing on the graft site every 8 hours.

☐ **2.** Elevate the left arm and provide complete rest of the grafted area.

☐ **3.** Administer pain medication every 4 hours as ordered for pain at the donor site.

☐ **4.** Perform range-of-motion (ROM) exercises to the left arm every 4 hours.

☐ **5.** Monitor the pulse in the left arm every 4 hours.

☐ **6.** Encourage the client to ambulate as desired on the first postoperative day.

Answer: 2, 3, 5

Rationale: The left arm should be elevated to reduce edema. Complete rest of the arm is needed to allow the graft to adhere. The donor site is usually more painful than the graft site, and the client will require pain medication to obtain relief. Because adequate circulation is needed for graft healing, it's important to monitor for presence of a pulse. Changing the dressing every 8 hours, performing ROM exercises every 4 hours, and ambulating on the first day are inappropriate because postoperative graft sites require immobilization for 3 to 5 days.

Critical thinking strategy: Focus on postoperative wound care and review skin grafts.

Client needs category: Physiological integrity

Client needs subcategory: Physiological adaptation

Cognitive level: Application

Integrated process: Nursing process/planning

Reference: Smeltzer, pages 1986–1987

---

7. A nurse is checking a client on bed rest with bathroom privledges who reported a rash when he awoke. The nurse assesses the client's skin and finds erythematous, slightly edematous areas on the client's back, posterior lower legs, and posterior elbows. The areas are quite itchy. The attending physician has diagnosed it as allergic contact dermatitis. Which of the following teaching points about contact dermatitis are correct? Select all that apply.

☐ **1.** The disorder is contagious.

☐ **2.** This is an allergic reaction.

☐ **3.** Based on the location of the rash, it's likely that detergents in the bed linens caused the rash.

☐ **4.** The skin is infected wherever the rash has developed.

☐ **5.** Oatmeal (Aveeno) baths are a good treatment for a rash of this type because of the large area involved.

☐ **6.** Washing with anti-bacterial soap will help the rash.

Answer: 2, 3, 5

Rationale: Contact dermatitis is classified as a reaction to an allergen and can appear when skin, especially if it's moist from perspiring or other reasons, remains in contact with an irritant for an extended time. It's a hypersensitivity reaction but usually requires extended contact. This client has a presentation often seen when clients remain in bed, perspiring on detergent-cleansed bed linens or gowns. This type of sensitivity to detergents may not have produced a reaction with a shorter time contact. The rash isn't contagious or infectious, although areas may become exudative and crusted. Treatment varies according to the intensity of the skin reaction and other factors, but oatmeal (Aveeno) baths are frequently prescribed.

Critical thinking strategy: Focus on the pathophysiology of contact dermatitis.

Client needs category: Physiological integrity

Client needs subcategory: Basic care and comfort

Cognitive level: Application

Integrated process: Teaching and learning

Reference: Smeltzer, pages 1964–1965

8. Which nursing interventions are effective in preventing pressure ulcers? Select all that apply.

☐ **1.** Clean the skin with warm water and a mild cleaning agent; then apply a moisturizer.

☐ **2.** When turning the client, slide him and avoid lifting him.

☐ **3.** Avoid raising the head of the bed more than 90 degrees.

☐ **4.** Turn and reposition the client every 1 to 2 hours unless contraindicated.

☐ **5.** If the client uses a wheelchair, seat him on a rubber or plastic doughnut.

☐ **6.** Use pillows to position the client and increase his comfort.

Answer: 1, 4, 6

Rationale: Nursing interventions that are effective in preventing pressure ulcers include cleaning the skin with warm water and a mild cleaning agent, and then applying a moisturizer; lifting—rather than sliding—the client when turning him to reduce friction and shear; avoiding raising the head of the bed more than 30 degrees, except for brief periods; repositioning and turning the client every 1 to 2 hours unless contraindicated; and using pillows to position the client and increase his comfort. If the client uses a wheelchair, the nurse should offer a pressure-relieving cushion as appropriate. She shouldn't seat him on a rubber or plastic doughnut because these devices can increase localized pressure at vulnerable points.

Critical thinking strategy: Focus on the causes of pressure ulcer development.

Nursing process step: Implementation

Client needs category: Safe, effective care environment

Client needs subcategory: Safety and infection control

Cognitive level: Application

Integrated process: Nursing process/planning

Reference: Taylor, page 1208

---

9. What terms would a nurse use to classify the lesion found on the feet of a client who presents with the one pictured below? Select all that apply.

☐ **1.** Linear

☐ **2.** Flat

☐ **3.** Fissure

☐ **4.** Crack

☐ **5.** Scale

☐ **6.** Ulcer

Answer: 1, 3

Rationale: It's important to use precise, descriptive terminology when documenting lesions to help aid diagnosis and track healing. The lesion depicted here is best described as a fissure, a linear crack in the skin. This type of lesion is commonly seen on clients with athlete's foot, usually between the toes.

Critical thinking strategy: Review types of skin lesions and focus on descriptors.

Client needs category: Physiological integrity

Client needs subcategory: Physiological adaptation

Cognitive level: Knowledge

Integrated process: Communication and documentation

Reference: Craven, pages 998–999

10. The nurse is caring for an 80-year-old male client who has been diagnosed with herpes zoster. The rash is located on his right lower back. Indicate the pathological development of herpes zoster in this client by placing the following signs and symptoms in chronological order, beginning with the earliest symptoms. Use all of the options.

1.	Crusted areas appearing in a linear pattern on the right lower back
2.	Burning sensation in the right lower back
3.	Localized itching in the right lower back
4.	Pain in the right lower back
5.	Stress for the past 2 months due to brother's severe illness
6.	Vesicles appearing in a linear pattern on right lower back

Answer: 5, 3, 2, 4, 6, 1

Rationale: Although herpes zoster can begin with any of the symptoms listed, and can skip items in the sequence, the typical course is one of symptoms preceded by psychosocial or physical stress. Symptoms typically progress from mild (often unrecognized by the client) to progressively worse. The area becomes painful, and then closed vesicles appear. These vesicles progress to crusted lesions, which then heal.

Critical thinking strategy: Focus on the pathophysiology of herpes zoster, and review early to late-stage signs and symptoms.

Client needs category: Physiological integrity

Client needs subcategory: Physiological adaptation

Cognitive level: Analysis

Integrated process: Nursing process/assessment

Reference: Smeltzer, pages 1958–1959

---

11. Which of the following integumentary system findings are a normal part of the aging process? Select all that apply.

☐ **1.** Less sebaceous gland activity

☐ **2.** Thinning of the epidermis

☐ **3.** Increased elasticity of skin

☐ **4.** Change in sensation to touch (may be decreased or increased)

☐ **5.** Decreased susceptibility to skin infections

☐ **6.** Delayed healing response

Answer: 1, 2, 4, 6

Rationale: Aging skin is drier and thinner due to loss of sebaceous gland activity as well as loss of subcutaneous tissue. The skin is also less elastic due to this loss of subcutaneous tissue. Aging sensory neurons and thinning skin can lead to decreased or increased skin sensation, which may vary at different body locations. Drying of the skin increases the susceptibility to infection and delays wound healing.

Critical thinking strategy: Focus on the physiological changes of aging skin.

Client needs category: Physiological integrity

Client needs subcategory: Physiological adaptation

Cognitive level: Knowledge

Integrated process: Nursing process/analysis

Reference: Smeltzer, page 233

Oncologic disorders

1. A client in the terminal stage of cancer is being transferred to hospice care. Which information regarding hospice care should the nurse include in the teaching plan? Select all that apply.

☐ **1.** The focus of care is on controlling symptoms and relieving pain.

☐ **2.** A multidisciplinary team provides care.

☐ **3.** Services are provided based on the ability to pay.

☐ **4.** Hospice care is provided only in hospice centers.

☐ **5.** Bereavement care is provided to the family.

☐ **6.** Care is provided in the home, independent of physicians.

Answer: 1, 2, 5

Rationale: Hospice care focuses on controlling symptoms and relieving pain at the end of life. A multidisciplinary team—consisting of nurses, physicians, chaplains, aides, and volunteers—provides the care. After the client's death, hospice provides bereavement care to the grieving family. Hospice services are provided based on need, not on the ability to pay. Hospice care may be provided in a variety of settings, such as freestanding hospice centers, the home, a hospital, or a long-term care facility. Care is provided under the direction of a physician, who's a key member of the hospice team.

Critical thinking strategy: Focus on the concepts and principles of hospice care

Client needs category: Physiological integrity

Client needs subcategory: Basic care and comfort

Cognitive level: Application

Integrated process: Teaching and learning

Reference: Smeltzer, pages 454–455

---

2. An adult client with Hodgkin's disease who weighs 143 lb is to receive vincristine (Oncovin) 25 mcg/kg I.V. What is the correct dose in micrograms that the client should receive? Record your answer as a whole number.

_____ micrograms

Answer: 1,625

Rationale: First, convert the client's weight from pounds to kilograms:

$$1 \text{ lb} = 2.2 \text{ kg}$$
$$143 \text{ lb} = X \text{ kg}$$
$$143 \text{ lb}/2.2 \text{ kg} = 65 \text{ kg}.$$

Next, multiply the weight in kilograms by the number of micrograms desired per kilogram:

$$65 \text{ kg} \times 25 \text{ mcg} = 1,625 \text{ mcg}$$

Critical thinking strategy: Focus on what the question is asking (the correct dose in micrograms based on the client's weight), and review common conversions.

Client needs category: Physiological integrity

Client needs subcategory: Pharmacological and parenteral therapies

Cognitive level: Application

Integrated process: Nursing process/planning

Reference: _Dosage Calculations Made Incredibly Easy,_ pages 111–112

3. A nurse has identified the nursing diagnosis *Situational low self-esteem related to hair loss and severe fatigue* for a client with cancer. Which of the following nursing interventions would be appropriate for this client's care? Select all that apply.

☐ **1.** Ask the client how the diagnosis and treatment are affecting her personal life and roles.

☐ **2.** Review any anticipated side effects of treatment with the client, stressing that some may not occur and others can be controlled.

☐ **3.** Teach the client how to resolve specific concerns related to the effects of treatment on her personal life.

☐ **4.** As a behavioral guide, describe the experiences of friends and other clients who have had this disease and treatment.

☐ **5.** Offer information on available counseling services and support groups, if desired, explaining that these techniques are helpful to many clients.

☐ **6.** Maintain eye contact with the client and use touch during interactions, if acceptable to the client.

Answer: 1, 2, 5, 6

Rationale: Discussing the client's feelings about her cancer diagnosis and treatment help to identify coping-related problems. Anticipating potential adverse effects can help the client begin to adapt and prepare to cope with these events. Referral to support groups or counseling services helps provide the client with validation and assistance with problem solving. Touch and eye contact can be therapeutic in affirming individuality and acceptance and can help build self-esteem. Instructing the client in how the nurse believes problems should be resolved isn't therapeutic. The nurse should help the client explore options for solving her problems in a manner consistent with the client's beliefs and values. Telling stories about others' experiences without their consent breaches confidentiality and may demonstrate a lack of listening and empathic interaction by the nurse. Validating the client's own personal story is beneficial to rebuilding self esteem.

Critical thinking strategy: Focus on the clinical manifestations and emotinal aspects of cancer, and review expected outcomes for clients with cancer.

Client needs category: Psychosocial integrity

Client needs subcategory: None

Cognitive level: Analysis

Integrated process: Caring

Reference: Smeltzer, page 413

---

4. A client with laryngeal cancer has undergone a laryngectomy and is now receiving radiation therapy to the head and neck. The nurse should monitor the client for which of the following adverse effects of external radiation? Select all that apply.

☐ **1.** Xerostomia

☐ **2.** Stomatitis

☐ **3.** Thrombocytopenia

☐ **4.** Cystitis

☐ **5.** Dysgeusia

☐ **6.** Leukopenia

Answer: 1, 2, 5

Rationale: Radiation of the head and neck often produces dry mouth (xerostomia), irritation of the oral mucous membranes (stomatitis), and diminished sense of taste (dysgeusia). Thrombocytopenia (reduced platelet count) and leukopenia (reduced white blood cell count) may occur with systemic radiation; cystitis may occur with radiation of the genitourinary system.

Critical thinking strategy: Focus on the specific area being irrradiated, and review localized adverse effects of radiation.

Client needs category: Physiological integrity

Client needs subcategory: Reduction of risk potential

Cognitive level: Application

Integrated process: Nursing process/planning

Reference: Smeltzer, pages 395–397

5. A nurse is teaching a community program on breast self-examination. She demonstrates the proper procedure for palpating each breast. In what sequence should the following actions be performed for proper self-examination? Use all the options.

1. Place the hand over the breast to be examined (use the right hand for the left breast and vice versa).
2. Lie down with one arm behind the head.
3. Palpate the breast in a perpendicular motion, going across the breast from side to side and top to bottom.
4. Use a circular motion to feel the breast tissue (with light, medium, and firm pressure).
5. Use the finger pads of the three middle fingers and touch the breast.

Rationale: Breast self-examination is a standard procedure described by national organizations designed to ensure palpation of all breast tissue. The exam also includes a visual inspection of the breasts while pressing the hands firmly against the hips and examining the underarms of each breast with the arms slightly raised.

Critical thinking stategy: Focus on the question being asked (the correct sequence for breast self-examination).

Client needs category: Health promotion and maintenance

Client needs subcategory: None

Cognitive level: Application

Integrated process: Teaching and learning

Reference: Smeltzer, page 1707

---

6. A client who is receiving chemotherapy for breast cancer develops myelosuppression. Which of the following instructions should the nurse include in the client's discharge teaching plan? Select all that apply.

☐ **1.** Avoid people who have recently received vaccines.

☐ **2.** Avoid activities that may cause bleeding.

☐ **3.** Wash hands frequently.

☐ **4.** Increase intake of fresh fruits and vegetables.

☐ **5.** Avoid crowded places such as shopping malls.

☐ **6.** Treat a sore throat with over-the-counter products.

Rationale: Chemotherapy can cause myelosuppression, which is a deceased number of red blood cells, white blood cells, and platelets. A client receiving chemotherapy needs to avoid people who have been vaccinated recently because an exaggerated reaction may occur. Because platelet counts are reduced, the client also needs to avoid activities that could cause trauma and bleeding. The client should wash her hands frequently because hand washing is the best way to prevent the spread of infection. A client receiving chemotherapy should avoid crowded places as well as people with colds during flu season because she has a reduced ability to fight infection. Fresh fruits and vegetables should be avoided because they can harbor bacteria that can't be removed easily by washing. Signs and symptoms of infection, such as a sore throat, fever, and a cough, should be reported immediately to the primary care provider.

Critical thinking strategy: Focus on the clinical manifestations of myelosuppression, and review leukopenia, thrombocytopenia, and anemia.

Client needs category: Physiological integrity

Client needs subcategory: Reduction of risk potential

Cognitive level: Application

Integrated process: Teaching and learning

Reference: Smeltzer, pages 400–401

7. A client with bladder cancer undergoes surgical removal of the bladder with construction of an ileal conduit. Which assessment findings indicate that the client is developing complications? Select all that apply.

☐ **1.** Urine output greater than 30 ml/hour

☐ **2.** Dusky appearance of the stoma

☐ **3.** Stoma protrusion from the skin

☐ **4.** Mucus shreds in the urine collection bag

☐ **5.** Edema of the stoma during the first 24 hours after surgery

☐ **6.** Sharp abdominal pain with rigidity

Answer: 2, 3, 6

Rationale: A dusky appearance of the stoma indicates decreased blood supply to the stoma; a healthy stoma should appear beefy-red. Protrusion indicates prolapse of the stoma, and sharp abdominal pain with rigidity suggests peritonitis. A urine output greater than 30 ml/hour is a sign of adequate renal perfusion and is a normal finding. Because mucous membranes are used to create the conduit, mucus in the urine is expected. Stomal edema is a normal finding during the first 24 hours after surgery.

Critical thinking strategy: Focus on the surgical procedure and potential complications.

Client needs category: Physiological integrity

Client needs subcategory: Reduction of risk potential

Cognitive level: Analysis

Integrated process: Nursing process/analysis

Reference: Smeltzer, pages 1598–1599

---

8. A client is ordered a dose of epoetin alfa (Aranesp) to treat anemia related to chemotherapy. The recommended dose is 150 units/kg. The client weighs 60 kg. The vial is labeled 10,000 units/ml. How many milliliters of epoetin alfa should the nurse administer? Record your answer using one decimal place.

_____ milliliters

Answer: 0.9

Rationale: First determine the number of units of epoetin alfa the client is to receive:

60 kg × 150 units = 9,000 units/kg.

Next, determine the number of milliliters required to deliver that dose:

10,000 units : 1 ml = 9,000 units : X

$$\frac{10,000 \text{ units} \times X}{10,000 \text{ units}} = \frac{9,000 \text{ units} \times 1 \text{ ml}}{10,000 \text{ units}}$$

X = 0.9 ml.

Critical thinking strategy: Focus on what the question is asking (the amount of milliliters to be administered), and review drug concentration calculations.

Client needs category: Physiological integrity

Client needs subcategory: Pharmacological and parenteral therapies

Cognitive level: Application

Integrated process: Nursing process/planning

Reference: *Dosage Calculations Made Incredibly Easy,* page 311

9. A client who is experiencing colon cancer is scheduled to undergo a colostomy. Which interventions would be appropriate to include in a preoperative teaching plan? Select all that apply.

☐ **1.** Demonstrate turning, coughing, deep breathing, splinting, and leg range-of-motion exercises, and provide rationales for each procedure.

☐ **2.** Encourage the client to rate his curent level of discomfort on 0-to-10 scale.

☐ **3.** Arrange for an enterostomal therapist to speak with the client about colostomy care.

☐ **4.** Explain the need for early postoperative ambulation.

☐ **5.** Instruct the client on signs and symptoms of intestinal obstruction.

☐ **6.** Encourage the client to express his feelings about changes in his body image.

Answer: 1, 3, 4, 6

Rationale: Preoperatively, the client will require instruction regarding the need for turning, coughing, deep breathing, splinting, and leg range-of-motion exercises. He'll also need to learn about colostomy care and the reason for early postoperative ambulation. Addressing feelings about body image changes is also appropriate at this time. Rating pain and discomfort and instructing the client about signs and symptoms of intestinal obstruction are part of the postoperative care.

Critical thinking strategy: Focus on preoperative interventions, and review colostomy surgery and care.

Client needs category: Physiological integrity

Client needs subcategory: Basic care and comfort

Cognitive level: Application

Integrated process: Teaching and learning

Reference: Taylor, pages 888–893, 898–904, 1581–1585

---

10. A client has been diagnosed with lung cancer and is scheduled to undergo a left pneumonectomy. He will have a chest tube inserted as part of the surgical procedure. Identify the area where the nurse will expect to see the chest tube inserted.

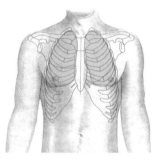

Answer:

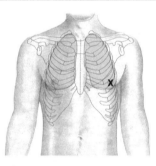

Rationale: A left pneumonectomy is surgical removal of the left lung. Therefore, a chest tube would be placed on the left side of the chest.

Critical thinking strategy: Focus on the clinical manifestations of pneumonectomy, and review the anatomical placement of a chest tube.

Client needs category: Health promotion and maintenance

Client needs subcategory: None

Cognitive level: Application

Integrated process: Nursing process/analysis

Reference: Smeltzer, pages 758–762

11. A client has been diagnosed with breast cancer and is scheduled to begin treatment with the antibiotic antineoplastic drug doxorubicin hydrochloride (Adriamycin). Which side effects should the nurse monitor for while the client is being treated with this medication? Select all that apply.

☐ **1.** Hair thinning

☐ **2.** Blue-green discoloration of urine

☐ **3.** Left ventricular failure

☐ **4.** Complete hair loss within 3-4 weeks

☐ **5.** Red discoloration of urine

Answer: 3, 4, 5

Rationale: Primary side effects of this drug include cardiac changes (including left ventricular failure and arrhythmias), complete hair loss within 3 to 4 weeks of receiving the drug, and red discoloration of the urine. Methotrexate rarely causes complete hair loss but may cause thinning or no hair loss. Methocarbamol (Robaxin), a muscle relaxant, causes the urine to turn a blue-green color.

Critical thinking strategy: Focus on common side effects of chemotherapeutic agents, and review doxurubicin hydrochloride (Adriamycin).

Client needs category: Physiological integrity

Client needs subcategory: Physiological adaptation

Cognitive level: Application

Integrated process: Nursing process/planning

Reference: Smeltzer, page 399

---

12. A client with pancreatic cancer has been prescribed fluorouracil (Adrucil) 12 mg/kg I.V. for 4 days. If no signs of toxicity occur, the client is to receive 6 mg/kg of the medication on days 6, 8, 10, and 12. The client weighs 198 lb. At the conclusion of day 12, how many total milligrams of fluorouracil will the client have received? Record your answer as a whole number.

_____ miligrams

Answer: 6,480

Rationale: The problem is calculated by initially converting 198 lb to kilograms:

$$1 \text{ lb} = 2.2 \text{ kg}$$
$$198 \text{ lb} = X \text{ kg}$$
$$198 \text{ lb} \div 2.2 \text{ kg} = 90 \text{ kg}$$

Next, multipy the weight in kilograms by the number of micrograms for each of the medication days:

$$12 \text{ mg} \times 90 = 1,080 \text{ mg}$$
$$(1,080 \text{ mg} \times 4 \text{ days} = 4,320 \text{ mg})$$
$$6 \text{ mg} \times 90 \text{ kg} = 540 \text{ mg}$$
$$(540 \text{ mg} \times 4 \text{ days} = 2,160 \text{ mg})$$

Then, add these amounts together:

$$4,320 \text{ mg} + 2,160 \text{ mg} = 6,480 \text{ mg}.$$

Critical thinking strategy: Focus on conversions and calculating dosage according to body weight.

Client needs category: Physiological integrity

Client needs subcategory: Pharmacological and parenteral therapies

Cognitive level: Application

Integrated process: Nursing process/planning

Reference: *Dosage Calculations Made Incredibly Easy,* pages 267–270

13. While undergoing treatment with a caustic chemotherapeutic agent, a client experiences extravasation. Indicate how the nurse should respond to extravasation by placing the following nursing interventions in chronological order. Use all the options.

1. Notify the physician.
2. Follow facility policy for dealing with extravasation.
3. Discontinue the intravenous infusion.
4. Implement physician's orders.
5. Document all signs and symptoms thoroughly.
6. Monitor the client throughout the shift, and give a detailed report to the oncoming shift.

Answer: 3, 2, 1, 4, 5, 6

Rationale: Initially, the intravenous infusion should be discontinued so that the client won't continue to receive more of the medication that caused the extravasation to occur. The facility will have a policy on how to deal with extravasation (usually the application of ice) that can be implemented while the physican is being notified. After the physician is notified, the specific orders will need to be implemented. All signs and symptoms that the client is experiencing should be documented thoroughly in preparation for the report to be given to the oncoming shift.

Critical thinking strategy: Focus on the clincal manifestations of extravasation and client safety, and review nursing interventions for extravasation.

Client needs category: Health promotion and maintenace

Client needs subcategory: None

Cognitive level: Analysis

Integrated process: Nursing process/implementation

Reference: Smeltzer, page 398

PART FOUR

Maternal-neonatal nursing

Antepartum period

1. During her first prenatal visit, a client asks a nurse what physiological changes she can expect during pregnancy. The nurse begins the discussion with the presumptive changes of pregnancy. Put the following presumptive changes in ascending chronological order according to when they occur. Use all of the options.

| **1.** Frequent urination |
| **2.** Breast changes |
| **3.** Quickening |
| **4.** Appearance of linea nigra, melasma, and striae gravidarum |
| **5.** Uterine enlargement in which the uterus can be palpated over the symphysis pubis |

Answer: 2, 1, 5, 3, 4

Rationale: Presumptive changes are subjective and can be caused by other medical conditions. Breast changes occur approximately 2 weeks after implantation of the embryo; frequent urination, at 3 weeks; fatigue and uterine enlargement over the symphysis pubis, at 18 weeks; quickening, between 18 and 20 weeks; and the appearance of linea nigra, melasma, and striae gravidarum, at 24 weeks.

Critical thinking strategy: Recall the physiologic changes of pregnancy and remember that presumptive changes are subjective.

Client needs category: Health promotion and maintenance

Client needs subcategory: None

Cognitive level: Application

Integrated process: Teaching and learning

Reference: Pillitteri, pages 222–225

2. A 30-year-old client comes to the office for a routine prenatal visit. After reading the chart entry below, the nurse should prepare the client for which of the following studies?

Progress notes

6/8/09 Pt. is 11 weeks pregnant; urine sample shows
1320   glycosuria. Pt. has a family history of
        diabetes. ——————— Chrissy Franks, RN

☐ **1.** Triple screen
☐ **2.** Indirect Coombs' test
☐ **3.** 1-hour glucose tolerance test
☐ **4.** Amniocentesis

Answer: 3

Rationale: A 1-hour glucose tolerance test is recommended to screen for gestational diabetes if the client is obese, has glycosuria or a family history of diabetes, or lost a fetus for unexplained reasons or gave birth to a large-for-gestational-age neonate. A triple screen tests for chromosomal abnormalities. The indirect Coombs' test screens maternal blood for red blood cell antibodies. Amniocentesis is used to detect fetal abnormalities.

Critical thinking strategy: Review laboratory studies and values for gestational diabetes as related to glucose.

Client needs category: Physiological integrity

Client needs subcategory: Reduction of risk potential

Cognitive level: Application

Integrated process: Teaching and learning

Reference: Pillitteri, pages 376–379

3. A nurse is preparing to teach a client about fetal growth and development during the first 3 months of pregnancy. Help prepare the teaching materials by putting the following milestones in order by month (month 1, month 2, month 3, and months 4 to 9). Use all of the options.

1. Teeth and bones begin to appear, the kidneys start to function and, at the end of the month, gender is distinguishable.

2. The embryo has a definite form; the head, trunk, and tiny buds for arms and legs develop; and the cardiovascular system begins to function.

3. Internal and external fetal growth continues at a rapid rate, and the fetus stores the fats and minerals it needs to live outside the womb.

4. The eyes, ears, nose, lips, tongue, and tooth buds develop; the umbilical cord has a definite form; and the external genitalia are present.

Answer: 2, 4, 1, 3

Rationale: Significant growth and development take place during the first 3 months. By the first month, the embryo has a definite form; the head, trunk, and tiny buds for arms and legs develop; and the cardiovascular system begins to function. By the second month, the eyes, ears, nose, lips, tongue, and tooth buds develop; the umbilical cord has a definite form; and the external genitalia are present. By the third month, teeth and bones begin to appear, the kidneys start to function and, at the end of the month, gender is distinguishable. By the fourth month, internal and external fetal growth begins accelerating at a more rapid rate; the fetus stores the fats and minerals it needs to live outside the womb, and growth continues until the fetus is full-term.

Critical thinking strategy: Recall fetal development by systems and weekly milestones.

Client needs category: Health promotion and maintenance

Client needs subcategory: None

Cognitive level: Application

Integrated process: Teaching and learning

Reference: Pillitteri, pages 189–197

---

4. A woman who is 15 weeks pregnant comes to the clinic for amniocentesis. The nurse knows that this test can be used to identify which of the following characteristics or problems? Select all that apply.

☐ **1.** Fetal lung maturity

☐ **2.** Gestational diabetes

☐ **3.** Chromosomal defects

☐ **4.** Neural tube defects

☐ **5.** Polyhydramnios

☐ **6.** Sex of the fetus

Answer: 3, 4, 6

Rationale: In early pregnancy, amniocentesis can be used to identify chromosomal and neural tube defects and to determine the sex of the fetus. It can also be used to evaluate fetal lung maturity during the last trimester of pregnancy. A blood test performed between 24 and 28 weeks' gestation is used to screen for gestational diabetes. Ultrasound is used to identify polyhydramnios; amniocentesis can be used to treat polyhydramnios by removing excess fluid.

Critical thinking strategy: Recall the fetal development at 15 weeks' gestation and relate this to an amniocentesis.

Client needs category: Physiological integrity

Client needs subcategory: Reduction of risk potential

Cognitive level: Application

Integrated process: Nursing process/planning

Reference: Pillitteri, pages 207–208

5. A client who is 41 weeks pregnant is about to undergo a biophysical profile (BPP) to evaluate her fetus's well-being. The nurse is aware that this test includes several components, some of which are listed below. Select all that apply.

☐ **1.** Fetal tone

☐ **2.** Fetal breathing

☐ **3.** Femur length

☐ **4.** Amniotic fluid volume

☐ **5.** Biparietal diameter

☐ **6.** Crown-rump length

Answer: 1, 2, 4

Rationale: A BPP is an ultrasound assessment of fetal well-being that includes the following components: nonstress test, fetal tone, fetal breathing, fetal motion, and volume of amniotic fluid. It's used to confirm the health of the fetus or identify abnormalities. Crown-rump length is used to assess gestational age during the first trimester. Biparietal diameter and femur length are also used to assess gestational age and are done in the second and third trimesters.

Critical thinking strategy: Focus on the five parameters of biophysical profile and relate them to fetal well-being.

Client needs category: Physiological integrity

Client needs subcategory: Reduction of risk potential

Cognitive level: Application

Integrated process: Nursing process/evaluation

Reference: Pillitteri, page 209

---

6. A nurse is performing a prenatal assessment on a client who is 32 weeks pregnant. She performs Leopold's maneuvers and determines that the fetus is in the cephalic position. Identify where the nurse should place the Doppler transducer to auscultate fetal heart tones.

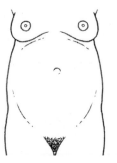

Answer:

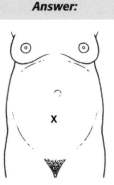

Rationale: When the fetus is in the cephalic position (head down), fetal heart tones are best auscultated midway between the symphysis pubis and the umbilicus. When the fetus is in the breech position, fetal heart tones are best heard at or above the level of the umbilicus.

Critical thinking strategy: Recall the fetal positions related to the fetal head placement and maternal anatomy.

Client needs category: Health promotion and maintenance

Client needs subcategory: None

Cognitive level: Analysis

Integrated process: Nursing process/assessment

Reference: Pillitteri, pages 225, 495

7. A nurse is palpating the uterus of a client who is 20 weeks pregnant to measure fundal height. Identify the area on the abdomen where the nurse should expect to feel the uterine fundus.

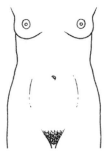

Answer:

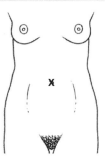

Rationale: At 20 weeks, the uterine fundus should be palpated approximately at the umbilicus. Fundal height should be measured from the symphysis pubis to the top of the uterus (McDonald's method). Serial measurements assess fetal growth over the course of the pregnancy. Between weeks 22 and 34, the number of centimeters measured correlate approximately with the week of gestation. However, if the client is very tall or short, fundal height will differ.

Critical thinking strategy: Recall the fundal height related to gestational age and fundal palpation technique.

Client needs category: Health promotion and maintenance

Client needs subcategory: None

Cognitive level: Application

Integrated process: Nursing process/assessment

Reference: Pillitteri, page 226

---

8. A client who is 32 weeks pregnant is being monitored in the antepartum unit for pregnancy-induced hypertension. She suddenly complains of continuous abdominal pain and vaginal bleeding. Which of the following nursing interventions should be included in the care of this client? Select all that apply.

☐ **1.** Evaluate maternal vital signs.

☐ **2.** Prepare for vaginal delivery.

☐ **3.** Reassure the client that she'll be able to continue the pregnancy.

☐ **4.** Auscultate fetal heart tones.

☐ **5.** Monitor the amount of vaginal bleeding.

☐ **6.** Monitor intake and output.

Answer: 1, 4, 5, 6

Rationale: The client's symptoms indicate that she's experiencing abruptio placentae. The nurse must immediately evaluate the mother's vital signs, auscultate fetal heart tones, monitor the amount of blood loss, and evaluate volume status by monitoring intake and output. After the severity of the abruption has been determined and blood and fluid have been replaced, a prompt cesarean (not vaginal) delivery is indicated if the fetus is in distress.

Critical thinking strategy: Focus on monitoring fetal and maternal well-being, and review pregnancy-induced hypertension.

Client needs category: Physiological integrity

Client needs subcategory: Physiological adaptation

Cognitive level: Analysis

Integrated process: Nursing process/implementation

Reference: Pillitteri, pages 415–417, 426–433

9. In early pregnancy, some clients complain of abdominal pain or pulling. Identify the area most commonly associated with this pain.

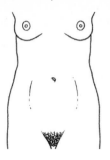

Rationale: As the uterus grows in early pregnancy, it deviates physically to the right. This shift, or dextrorotation, is due to the presence of the rectosigmoid colon in the left lower quadrant. As a result, many women complain of pain in the right lower quadrant.

Critical thinking strategy: Recall maternal anatomy, especially the enlarging uterus as it relates to the abdominal organs.

Client needs category: Health promotion and maintenance

Client needs subcategory: None

Cognitive level: Analysis

Integrated process: Nursing process/evaluation

Reference: Pillitteri, pages 283–284

---

10. During a prenatal visit, a physician decides to admit a client to the hospital. Based on the nurse's admission note below, which complication of pregnancy would the physician suspect?

Progress notes

2/2/09	30-year-old female admitted with nausea
1100	and vomiting. Pt. is 16 weeks pregnant and
	complains of thirst and vertigo. BP 120/70
	mm Hg, RR 20, P 104, Temp 100° F. Pt. has
	had nothing to eat or drink for 24 hours.
	———— S. Thomas, RN

☐ **1.** Iron-deficiency anemia

☐ **2.** Placenta previa

☐ **3.** Pregnancy-induced hypertension

☐ **4.** Hyperemesis gravidarum

Answer: 4

Rationale: Hyperemesis gravidarum is severe nausea and vomiting that persists after the first trimester. If untreated, it can lead to weight loss, starvation, dehydration, fluid and electrolyte imbalances, and acid-base disturbances. The client may report thirst, hiccups, oliguria, vertigo, and headache. A rapid pulse and elevated or subnormal temperature can also occur. Signs and symptoms of iron-deficiency anemia include fatigue, pallor, and exercise intolerance. Placenta previa causes painless, bright red, vaginal bleeding after 20 weeks of pregnancy. Pregnancy-induced hypertension usually develops after 20 weeks of pregnancy; the client reports sudden weight gain and presents with hypertension.

Critical thinking stategy: Review the assessment findings and relate them to complications of pregnancy.

Client needs category: Physiological integrity

Client needs subcategory: Physiological adaptation

Cognitive level: Application

Integrated process: Nursing process/assessment

Reference: Pillitteri, page 320

11. A pregnant client at 32 weeks' gestation has mild preeclampsia. She is discharged home with instructions to remain on bed rest. She should also be instructed to call her physician if she experiences which of the following symptoms? Select all that apply.

☐ **1.** Headache

☐ **2.** Increased urine output

☐ **3.** Blurred vision

☐ **4.** Difficulty sleeping

☐ **5.** Epigastric pain

☐ **6.** Severe nausea and vomiting

Answer: 1, 3, 5, 6

Rationale: Headache, blurred vision, epigastric pain, and severe nausea and vomiting can indicate worsening preeclampsia. Decreased, not increased, urine output is a concern because preeclampsia is associated with decreased renal perfusion, leading to a reduction in the glomerular filtration rate and decreased urine output. Difficulty sleeping, a common complaint during the third trimester, is only a concern if it's caused by any of the other symptoms.

Critical thinking strategy: Review the clinical manifestations of severe preeclampsia.

Client needs category: Physiological integrity

Client needs subcategory: Reduction of risk potential

Cognitive level: Application

Integrated process: Teaching and learning

Reference: Pillitteri, pages 427–429

---

12. A client who is 37 weeks pregnant comes to the office for a prenatal visit. A nurse performs Leopold's maneuvers to assess the position of the fetus. After performing the maneuvers, the nurse suspects that the physician will attempt external version. Where did the nurse palpate the head of the fetus?

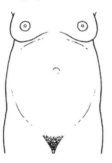

Answer:

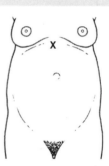

Rationale: If the fetal head is palpated at the top of the uterus, the fetus is in the breech position. That is, the head is not the presenting part and the physician may consider external version to convert the fetus to a vertex lie, or head-down position. This is accomplished by applying pressure on the maternal abdomen to turn the infant over, as in a somersault.

Critical thinking strategy: Recall the gestational age of the fetus and the expected fetal position as related to the maternal anatomy.

Client needs category: Physiological integrity

Client needs subcategory: Reduction of risk potential

Cognitive level: Analysis

Integrated process: Nursing process/planning

Reference: Pillitteri, pages 514–516

13. A nurse is teaching a course on the anatomy and physiology of reproduction. Identify the area where she should indicate that fertilization occurs.

Answer:

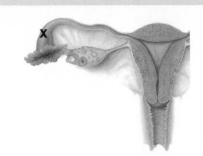

Rationale: After ejaculation, the sperm travel by flagellar movement through the cervical mucus into the fallopian tube to meet the descending ovum in the ampulla. Fertilization occurs in the ampulla (outer third) of the fallopian tube.

Critical thinking strategy: Review female anatomy and physiology as related to fertilization.

Client needs category: Health promotion and maintenance

Client needs subcategory: None

Cognitive level: Application

Integrated process: Teaching and learning

Reference: Pillitteri, pages 183–184

---

14. The nurse is giving prenatal instructions to a 32-year-old primagravida. Which nutritional instructions should the nurse review? Select all that apply.

☐ **1.** Caloric intake should be increased by 300 cal/day.

☐ **2.** Protein intake should be increased to more than 30 g/day.

☐ **3.** Vitamin intake shouldn't increase from prepregnancy requirements.

☐ **4.** Folic acid intake should be increased to 400 mg/day.

☐ **5.** Intake of all minerals, especially iron, should be increased.

Answer: 1, 2, 5

Rationale: A pregnant woman should increase her caloric intake by 300 cal/day. The protein requirements (76 g/day) of a pregnant woman exceed those of a nonpregnant woman by 30 g/day. All mineral requirements, especially iron, are increased in a pregnant woman. The woman should also increase her intake of all vitamins; a prenatal vitamin is usually recommended. Folic acid intake is particularly important to help prevent fetal anomalies such as neural tube defect. Intake should be increased from 400 to 800 mg/day.

Critical thinking strategy: Focus on the nutritional requirements of pregnancy including calorie, protein, vitamin, and mineral needs.

Client needs category: Physiological integrity

Client needs subcategory: Basic care and comfort

Cognitive level: Comprehension

Integrated process: Teaching and learning

Reference: Pillitteri, pages 303–306

15. A nurse is palpating the fundal height of a pregnant woman at 40 weeks' gestation. Identify the area on the abdomen where the nurse would expect to feel the uterine fundus.

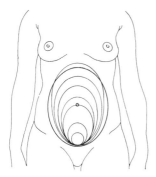

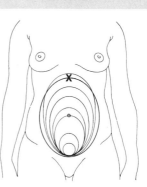

Rationale: Uterine height is measured from the top of the maternal symphsis pubis to the top of the uterine fundus. By the 36th week, the uterine fundus should touch the xiphoid process. About 2 weeks before term (the 38th week), the fetal head settles into the pelvis to prepare for birth and the uterus returns to the height it was at 36 weeks.

Critical thinking strategy: Recall the fundal height as related to the gestational age and fetal position.

Client needs category: Health promotion and maintenance

Client needs subcategory: None

Cognitive level: Application

Integrated process: Nursing process/assessment

Reference: Pillitteri, page 226

---

16. A 35-year-old client who is 28 weeks pregnant is admitted for testing. After reading the nursing notes below, which rationale best explains why a pregnant client should lie on her left side when resting or sleeping in the later stages of pregnancy?

Progress notes

5/12/09	Pt. admitted to short-term procedure unit
1430	for testing. States "I'm feeling a little
	faint." Skin slightly diaphoretic to touch. Pt.
	assisted to left side. VS stable. States "I'm
	feeling better now."
	————————————— S. Brown, RN

☐ **1.** To facilitate digestion

☐ **2.** To facilitate bladder empyting

☐ **3.** To prevent compression of the vena cava

☐ **4.** To prevent development of fetal anomalies

Rationale: The weight of the pregnant uterus is sufficiently heavy to compress the vena cava, which could impair blood flow to the uterus, possibly decreasing oxygen to the fetus. The client may experience supine hypotension syndrome (faintness, diaphoresis, and hypotension) from the pressure on the inferior vena cava. The side-lying position puts the weight of the fetus on the bed, not on the woman. The side-lying position hasn't been shown to prevent fetal anomalies, nor does it facilitate bladder emptying or digestion.

Critical thinking strategy: Review fetal positioning as related to maternal anatomy, particularly with respect to supine and side-lying positions.

Client needs category: Physiological integrity

Client needs subcategory: Reduction of risk potential

Cognitive level: Analysis

Integrated process: Nursing process/implementation

Reference: Pillitteri, page 276

17. A client is at risk for seizures due to pregnancy-induced hypertension. The physician orders 4 g magnesium sulfate in 250 ml D₅W to be infused at 1 g/hour following a loading dose. What is the flow rate in milliliters per hour? Round your answer to the nearest whole number.

_____ ml/hour

Rationale: To solve this, first set up a proportion and then solve for X:

$$4 \text{ g}/250 \text{ ml} = 1 \text{ g}/X \text{ ml}$$
$$4 \times X = 250$$
$$X = \frac{250 \text{ ml}}{4}$$
$$X = 62.5 \text{ ml}$$

Rounded off to a whole number, this is 63 ml/hour.

Critical thinking strategy: Focus on what the question is asking (the amount of milliliters to be infused in one hour), and set up a ratio and proportion using the known data.

Client needs category: Physiological integrity

Client needs subcategory: Pharmacological and parenteral therapies

Cognitive level: Application

Integrated process: Nursing process/planning

Reference: *Dosage Calculations Made Incredibly Easy*, pages 295–296

---

18. When teaching an antepartum client about the passage of the fetus through the birth canal during labor, the nurse describes the cardinal mechanisms of labor. Place these events in the proper sequence in which they occur. Use all of the options.

1. Flexion
2. External rotation
3. Descent
4. Expulsion
5. Internal rotation
6. Extension

Rationale: As the fetus moves through the birth canal, it goes through position changes to ensure that the smallest diameter of fetal head presents to the smallest diameter of the birth canal. Termed the cardinal mechanisms of labor, these position changes occur in the following sequence: descent, flexion, internal rotation, extension, external rotation, and expulsion.

Critical thinking strategy: Recall the relationship of the fetal head diameter to the diameter of the birth canal.

Client needs category: Health promotion and maintenance

Client needs subcategory: None

Cognitive level: Application

Integrated process: Teaching and learning

Reference: Pillitteri, pages 497–498

1. A nurse is evaluating a client who is 34 weeks pregnant for premature rupture of the membranes (PROM). Which findings indicate that PROM has occurred? Select all that apply.

☐ **1.** Fernlike pattern when vaginal fluid is placed on a glass slide and allowed to dry

☐ **2.** Acidic pH of fluid when tested with nitrazine paper

☐ **3.** Presence of amniotic fluid in the vagina

☐ **4.** Cervical dilation of 6 cm

☐ **5.** Alkaline pH of fluid when tested with nitrazine paper

☐ **6.** Contractions occurring every 5 minutes

Answer: 1, 3, 5

Rationale: The fernlike pattern that occurs when vaginal fluid is placed on a glass slide and allowed to dry, the presence of amniotic fluid in the vagina, and an alkaline pH of fluid are all signs of ruptured membranes. The fernlike pattern is a result of the high sodium and protein content of the amniotic fluid. The presence of amniotic fluid in the vagina results from the expulsion of the fluid from the amniotic sac. Amniotic fluid tests as an alkaline, not acidic, fluid. Cervical dilation and regular contractions are signs of progressing labor, but they don't indicate PROM.

Critical thinking strategy: Recall the clinical manifestations of PROM.

Client needs category: Physiological integrity

Client needs subcategory: Physiological adaptation

Cognitive level: Analysis

Integrated process: Nursing process/assessment

Reference: Pillitteri, page 425

2. A client in the first stage of labor is being monitored using an external fetal monitor. After the nurse reviews the monitoring strip from the client's chart (shown below), into which of the following positions should she assist the client?

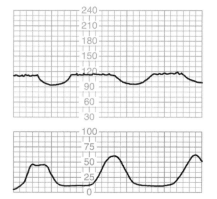

☐ **1.** Left lateral

☐ **2.** Right lateral

☐ **3.** Supine

☐ **4.** Prone

Answer: 1

Rationale: The fetal heart rate monitoring strip shows late decelerations, which indicate uteroplacental circulatory insufficiency and can lead to fetal hypoxia and acidosis if the underlying cause isn't corrected. The client should be turned onto her left side to increase placental perfusion and decrease contraction frequency. In addition, the I.V. fluid rate may be increased and oxygen administered. The right lateral, supine, and prone positions don't increase placental perfusion.

Critical thinking strategy: Remember that fetal heart rate patterns should mirror uterine contractions.

Client needs category: Physiological integrity

Client needs subcategory: Reduction of risk potential

Cognitive level: Analysis

Integrated process: Nursing process/implementation

Reference: Pillitteri, pages 524–527

3. On the waveform below, identify the area that indicates possible umbilical cord compression.

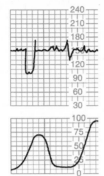

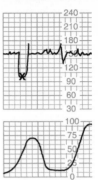

Rationale: Variable decelerations are decreases in fetal heart rate that aren't related to the timing of contractions. They're characteristic of umbilical cord compression, which reduces blood flow between the placenta and fetus. These decelerations generally occur as drops of 10 to 60 beats/minute below the baseline.

Critical thinking strategy: Recall that fetal oxygen depletion causes a decrease in fetal heart rate.

Client needs category: Physiological integrity

Client needs subcategory: Reduction of risk potential

Cognitive level: Analysis

Integrated process: Nursing process/analysis

Reference: Pillitteri, pages 525–527

---

4. A client who is 29 weeks pregnant comes to the labor and delivery unit. She states that she's having contractions every 8 minutes. The client is also 3 cm dilated. Which of the following can the nurse expect to administer? Select all that apply.

☐ **1.** Folic acid (Folvite)

☐ **2.** Terbutaline (Brethine)

☐ **3.** Betamethasone

☐ **4.** Rh₀(D) immune globulin (RhoGam)

☐ **5.** I.V. fluids

☐ **6.** Nalbuphine

Answer: 2, 3, 5

Rationale: The nurse can expect that terbutaline, a beta-2 agonist that relaxes smooth muscle, will be administered to halt contractions; that betamethasone, a corticosteroid, will be administered to decrease the risk of respiratory distress to the neonate if preterm delivery occurs; and that I.V. fluids will be given to expand the intravascular volume and decrease contractions if dehydration is the cause. Folic acid is a mineral recommended throughout pregnancy (especially in the first trimester) to decrease the risk of neural tube defects. RhoGam is given to Rh-negative clients who have been, or may have been, exposed to Rh-positive fetal blood. Nalbuphine is an opioid analgesic used during labor and delivery.

Critical thinking strategy: Focus on interventions to suppress preterm labor, and review medications used.

Client needs category: Physiological integrity

Client needs subcategory: Pharmacological and parenteral therapies

Cognitive level: Analysis

Integrated process: Nursing process/implementation

Reference: Pillitteri, pages 417–425

5. A nurse is monitoring a client who is receiving oxytocin (Pitocin) to induce labor. The nurse should observe for which of the following maternal adverse reactions? Select all that apply.

☐ **1.** Hypertension

☐ **2.** Jaundice

☐ **3.** Dehydration

☐ **4.** Fluid overload

☐ **5.** Uterine tetany

☐ **6.** Bradycardia

Answer: 1, 4, 5

Rationale: Adverse effects of oxytocin in the mother include hypertension, fluid overload, uterine tetany, and tachycardia, not bradycardia. The antidiuretic effect of oxytocin increases renal reabsorption of water, leading to fluid overload, not dehydration. Jaundice and bradycardia are adverse reactions that may occur in the neonate.

Critical thinking strategy: Recall the action and adverse effects of oxytocin.

Client needs category: Physiological integrity

Client needs subcategory: Pharmacological and parenteral therapies

Cognitive level: Application

Integrated process: Nursing process/assessment

Reference: Pillitteri, pages 609–610

---

6. A nurse is evaluating the external fetal monitoring strip (shown below) of a client who is in labor. Which of the following nursing interventions should the nurse implement?

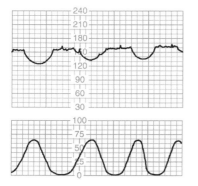

☐ **1.** Increase the I.V. fluid rate to boost intravascular volume.

☐ **2.** Reassure the client that the fetus isn't at risk, and continue to monitor the fetal heart rate.

☐ **3.** Elevate the client's legs.

☐ **4.** Administer supplemental oxygen.

Answer: 2

Rationale: The monitoring strip from this client's chart shows early decelerations. These can result from head compression during normal labor and don't indicate fetal distress. The nurse should reassure the client and continue to monitor the fetal heart rate. The other nursing interventions aren't appropriate.

Critical thinking strategy: Focus on the relationship between fetal heart rate patterns and uterine contraction patterns.

Client needs category: Health promotion and maintenance

Client needs subcategory: None

Cognitive level: Application

Integrated process: Nursing process/analysis

Reference: Pillitteri, pages 524–527

7. A client in labor is 8 cm dilated. The fetus, which is in vertex presentation, is 75% effaced and at 0 station. In the illustration below, identify the level of the fetus's head.

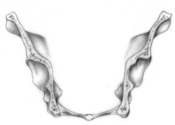

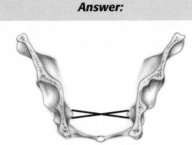

Rationale: Station refers to the level of the presenting part in relation to the pelvic inlet and the ischial spines. A 0 station indicates that the presenting part lies at the level of the ischial spines. Other stations are defined by their distance in centimeters above or below the ischial spines.

Critical thinking strategy: Recall maternal anatomy as it relates to fetal presentation and position.

Client needs category: Health promotion and maintenance

Client needs subcategory: None

Cognitive level: Application

Integrated process: Nursing process/assessment

Reference: Pillitteri, pages 493–494

---

8. A nurse is evaluating a fetal monitoring strip to time the contractions of a client in labor. Identify the beginning of the contraction in the illustration below.

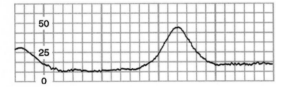

Answer:

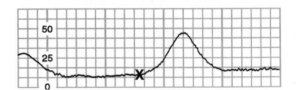

Rationale: The beginning of a contraction, identified by a rise in pressure in the uterus, is indicated on the monitoring strip by movement of the waveform away from the baseline.

Critical thinking strategy: Recall where to assess the starting point of uterine contraction on waveforms.

Client needs category: Health promotion and maintenance

Client needs subcategory: None

Cognitive level: Application

Integrated process: Nursing process/assessment

Reference: Pillitteri, pages 519–520

9. A nurse is caring for a client who's in the third stage of labor. The nurse knows that the client is likely to exhibit certain characteristic behaviors at this stage. Select all that apply.

☐ **1.** The client is excited about the process.

☐ **2.** The client is focused on the neonate's condition.

☐ **3.** The client is exhausted from the labor process.

☐ **4.** The client states she has discomfort from uterine contractions.

☐ **5.** The client is apprehensive about the process.

Answer: 2, 4

Rationale: In the third stage of labor, the client focuses on the neonate's condition. Before the placenta is expelled, she may also state that she is experiencing discomfort from uterine contractions. Excitement and apprehension are characteristic of the first stage of labor. Exhaustion is common in the second stage of labor.

Critical thinking strategy: Recall that the fetus is delivered during the second stage of labor.

Client needs category: Psychosocial integrity

Client needs subcategory: None

Cognitive level: Application

Integrated process: Caring

Reference: Pillitteri, pages 505–510, 538–539

---

10. The nurse is evaluating a client's external fetal monitoring strip (shown below). Identify the area on this strip that would cause concern about uteroplacental insufficiency.

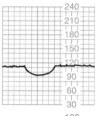

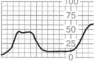

Answer:

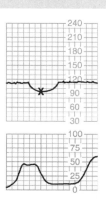

Rationale: This fetal monitoring strip illustrates a late deceleration. The decrease in fetal heart rate begins at the end of the contraction and doesn't return to baseline until the contraction is over. Late decelerations are caused by uteroplacental insufficiency resulting from decreased blood flow and oxygen transfer to the fetus through the intervillous spaces during uterine contractions.

Critical thinking strategy: Recall the relationship of fetal heart rate and uterine contraction patterns to fetal oxygenation.

Client needs category: Physiological integrity

Client needs subcategory: Reduction of risk potential

Cognitive level: Analysis

Integrated process: Nursing process/assessment

Reference: Pillitteri, pages 524–527

11. A client is being admitted to the labor and delivery unit. Her GTPAL classification is 5-2-1-1-2. Which statements are true about this client? Select all that apply.

☐ **1.** The client has had 4 previous pregnancies.

☐ **2.** The client has had 5 previous pregnancies.

☐ **3.** The client has had 1 full-term child, 1 abortion, and 1 premature child.

☐ **4.** The client has had 2 full-term children, 1 premature child, and 1 abortion.

☐ **5.** The client has 3 living children and is pregnant again.

☐ **6.** The client has 2 living children and is pregnant again.

Answer: 1, 4, 6

Rationale: Detailed information about a client's obstetric history is described using the GTPAL classification system. G represents gravida, or the number of times the client has been pregnant, including the current pregnancy. T is the number of full-term infants born (after 37 weeks), P is the number of preterm infants born (before 37 weeks), A is the number of induced or spontaneous abortions, and L is the number of living children.

Critical thinking strategy: Recall what each letter of the GTPAL pregnancy status classification system represents.

Client needs category: Health promotion and maintenance

Client needs subcategory: None

Cognitive level: Application

Integrated process: Communication and documentation

Reference: Pillitteri, pages 252–253

---

12. A nurse is assisting in the delivery room. The physician prepares to perform a midline episiotomy. On the illustration below, identify the area where the physican makes the incision.

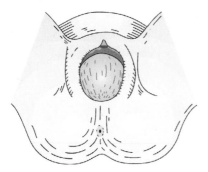

Answer:

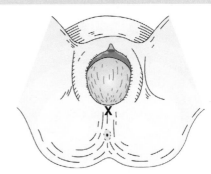

Rationale: An episiotomy is surgical enlargement of the vaginal opening that allows easier delivery of the fetus and prevents tearing of the perineum. The incision is made in the perineum and can be midline or right or left mediolateral.

Critical thinking strategy: Recall maternal anatomy and the purpose of an episiotomy.

Client needs category: Physiological integrity

Client needs subcategory: Reduction of risk potential

Cognitive level: Application

Integrated process: Nursing process/assessment

Reference: Pillitteri, pages 535–536

13. While caring for a client in labor, the nurse expresses concern after evaluating the external fetal monitoring strip below. What condition is the nurse most likely concerned about?

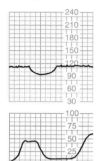

☐ **1.** Cephalopelvic disproportion

☐ **2.** Oligohydramnios

☐ **3.** Uteroplacental insufficiency

☐ **4.** Hydramnios

Rationale: This fetal monitoring strip illustrates a late deceleration. The decrease in fetal heart rate begins after the peak of the contraction and doesn't return to baseline until the contraction is over. Late decelerations are associated with uteroplacental insufficiency, shock, or fetal metabolic acidosis. Cephalopelvic disproportion may cause early, not late, decelerations early in labor. Oligohydramnios (less than normal amount of amniotic fluid) may be associated with variable decelerations. Hydramnios (excessive amniotic fluid) may be associated with uterine rupture.

Critical thinking strategy: Remember that fetal heart rate patterns occur in response to contractions.

Client needs category: Physiological integrity

Client needs subcategory: Reduction of risk potential

Cognitive level: Analysis

Integrated process: Nursing process/planning

Reference: Pillitteri, pages 524–526

14. A pregnant client in the first stage of labor has been ordered an oxytocin (Pitocin) drip. The order reads 1 ml (10 units) oxytocin in 1,000 ml NSS to infuse via infusion pump at 2 mU/ minute for 20 minutes. What is the flow rate needed to deliver 2 mU/ minute for 20 minutes? Record your answer using a whole number.

_____ milliliters

Answer: 4

Rationale: First, determine the concentration of the solution by setting up a proportion:

$$10 \text{ units}/1{,}000 \text{ ml} = X/1 \text{ ml}$$

Now, solve for X:

$$X \times 1{,}000 \text{ ml} = 10 \text{ units} \times 1 \text{ ml}$$
$$X = 10 \text{ units} \div 1{,}000$$
$$X = 0.01 \text{ unit/ml}$$

The amount 0.01 unit can be written in milliunits (mU):

1 mU is 1/1,000 of a unit; therefore $0.01 \times 1{,}000 = 10$ mU in 1 ml.

Next, determine the flow rate. If the prescribed dosage of oxytocin is 2 mU/minute for 20 minutes, the client receives a total of 40 mU (2 mU × 20 = 40 mU). To calculate the rate needed to provide that dose, set up a proportion with the known concentration in one proportion and the total oxytocin dose and unknown flow rate in the other:

$$10 \text{ mU}/1 \text{ ml} = 40 \text{ mU}/ X$$

Now, solve for X:

$$\frac{X \times 10 \text{ mU}}{10 \text{ mU}} = \frac{1 \text{ ml} \times 40 \text{ mU}}{10 \text{ mU}}$$
$$X = 4 \text{ ml}$$

The flow rate is 4 ml for 20 minutes.

Critical thinking strategy: Focus on solving the problem in stages, and review I.V. calculations.

Client needs category: Physiological integrity

Client needs subcategory: Pharmacological and parenteral therapies

Cognitive level: Application

Integrated process: Nursing process/planning

Reference: _Dosage Calculations Made Incredibly Easy,_ pages 293–294

15. Assessment of a client progressing through labor reveals the following findings. Order them in the sequence in which they would have occurred. Use all of the options.

| **1.** Uncontrollable urge to push |
| **2.** Cervical dilation of 7 cm |
| **3.** 100% cervical effacement |
| **4.** Strong Braxton Hicks contractions |
| **5.** Mild contractions lasting 20 to 40 seconds |

Rationale: Strong Braxton Hicks contractions typically occur prior to the onset of true labor and are considered a preliminary sign. During the latent phase of the first stage of labor, contractions are mild, lasting about 20 to 40 seconds. As the client progresses through labor, contractions increase in intensity and duration, and cervical dialation occurs. Cervical dialation of 7 cm indicates the client has entered the active phase of the first stage of labor. Cervical effacement also occurs, and effacement of 100% characterizes the transition phase of the first stage of labor. Progression into the second stage of labor is noted by the client's uncontrollable urge to push.

Critical thinking strategy: Recall the characteristics of the stages of labor.

Client needs category: Health promotion and maintenace

Client needs subcategory: None

Cognitive level: Application

Integrated process: Nursing process/assessment

Reference: Pillitteri, pages 489–490, 505–506

16. A nurse is monitoring the contractions of a client in the first stage of labor. Order the phases of a uterine contraction from the beginning of contraction to its conclusion. Use all of the options.

| **1.** Acme |
| **2.** Relaxation |
| **3.** Decrement |
| **4.** Increment |

Answer: 4, 1, 3, 2

Rationale: A contraction consists of three phases: the increment (when the intensity of the contraction increases), the acme (when the contraction is at its strongest), and the decrement (when the intensity decreases). Between contractions, the uterus relaxes. As labor progresses, the relaxation intervals decrease from 10 minutes early in labor to only 2 to 3 minutes later. The duration of contractions also changes, increasing from 20 to 30 seconds to a range of 60 to 90 seconds.

Critical thinking strategy: Focus on the definition of terms, and review the phases of contractions.

Client needs category: Health promotion and maintenance

Client needs subcategory: None

Cognitive level: Application

Integrated process: Nursing process/implementation

Reference: Pillitteri, page 502

Postpartum period

1. A client has received treatment for a warm, reddened, painful area in the breast as well as cracked and fissured nipples. The client expresses the desire to continue breast-feeding. Which instructions should the nurse include to prevent a recurrence of this condition? Select all that apply.

☐ **1.** Wash the nipples with soap and water.

☐ **2.** Change the breast pads frequently.

☐ **3.** Expose the nipples to air for part of each day.

☐ **4.** Wash hands before handling the breast and breast-feeding.

☐ **5.** Make sure that the baby grasps the nipple only.

☐ **6.** Release the baby's grasp on the nipple before removing the baby from the breast.

Answer: 2, 3, 4, 6

Rationale: To help prevent mastitis, an infection commonly associated with a break in the skin surface of the nipple, the nurse should suggest measures to prevent cracked and fissured nipples. Changing breast pads frequently and exposing the nipples to air for part of the day help keep the nipples dry and prevent irritation. Washing hands before handling the breast reduces the chance of accidentally introducing organisms into the breast. Releasing the baby's grasp on the nipple before removing the baby from the breast also reduces the chance of irritation. Nipples should be washed with water only; soap tends to remove the natural oils and increases the chance of cracking. The baby should grasp both the nipple and areola.

Critical thinking strategy: Review breast-feeding strategies and comfort measures.

Client needs category: Health promotion and maintenance

Client needs subcategory: None

Cognitive level: Comprehension

Integrated process: Teaching and learning

Reference: Pillitteri, page 670

---

2. A nurse is caring for a 1-day postpartum client. The progress note below informs the nurse that the client is in which phase of the postpartum period?

Progress notes	
5/24/09	Mother verbalizing labor and delivery
1715	experience. Doesn't appear confident about
	holding baby or changing diapers. Asking
	appropriate questions.——— J. Conners, RN

☐ **1.** Letting go

☐ **2.** Taking in

☐ **3.** Holding out

☐ **4.** Taking hold

Answer: 2

Rationale: The taking-in phase is normally the first postpartum phase. During this phase, the mother feels overwhelmed by the responsibilities of newborn care and is still fatigued from delivery. Taking hold is the next phase, when the client has rested and can learn mothering skills with confidence. Letting go is the final stage, when the client adapts to parenthood, her new role as a caregiver, and her new baby as a separate entity. Holding out isn't a valid phase.

Critical thinking strategy: Focus on the mother's behavior and review the postpartum phases.

Client needs category: Psychosocial integrity

Client needs subcategory: None

Cognitive level: Analysis

Integrated process: Caring

Reference: Pillitteri, pages 623–625

3. A nurse observes several interactions between a client and her neonate son. Which of the following behaviors by the mother would the nurse identify as evidence of mother-infant attachment? Select all that apply.

☐ **1.** Talks to and coos at her son

☐ **2.** Cuddles her son close to her

☐ **3.** Doesn't make eye contact with her son

☐ **4.** Requests that the nurse take the baby to the nursery for feedings

☐ **5.** Encourages the father to hold the baby

☐ **6.** Takes a nap when the baby is sleeping

Answer: 1, 2

Rationale: Talking to, cooing at, and cuddling with her son are positive signs that the client is adapting to her new role as a mother. Eye contact, touching, and speaking help establish attachment with a neonate. Avoiding eye contact is a nonbonding behavior. Feeding a neonate is an important role of a new mother and facilitates attachment. Encouraging the father to hold the neonate will facilitate attachment between the neonate and his father. Resting while the neonate is sleeping will conserve needed energy and allow the mother to be alert and awake when her infant is awake; however, it isn't evidence of bonding.

Critical thinking strategy: Focus on behaviors that relate to maternal-infant bonding.

Client needs category: Psychosocial integrity

Client needs subcategory: None

Cognitive level: Analysis

Integrated process: Caring

Reference: Pillitteri, pages 625–626

---

4. A nurse is caring for a postpartum client suspected of developing postpartum psychosis. Which of the following statements accurately characterize this disorder? Select all that apply.

☐ **1.** Symptoms start 2 days after delivery.

☐ **2.** The disorder is common in postpartum women.

☐ **3.** Symptoms include delusions and hallucinations.

☐ **4.** Suicide and infanticide are uncommon in this disorder.

☐ **5.** The disorder rarely occurs without a psychiatric history.

Answer: 3, 5

Rationale: A postpartum client should be suspected of psychosis if she exhibits delusions or hallucinations, generally starting within 4 weeks postpartum. Typically, the woman has a past history of a psychiatric disorder and treatment. A history of bipolar disorder is an important risk factor. The disorder occurs in less then 1% of postpartum mothers. It's considered a medical emergency. Suicide and infanticide are common.

Critical thinking strategy: Review the onset, symptoms, and etiology of postpartum psychosis and the differences with postpartal blues and depression.

Client needs category: Psychosocial integrity

Client needs subcategory: None

Cognitive level: Analysis

Integrated process: Caring

Reference: Pillitteri, pages 675–776

5. A mother with a history of varicose veins has just delivered her first baby. The nurse suspects that the mother has developed a pulmonary embolus. Which of the data below would lead to this nursing judgment? Select all that apply.

☐ **1.** Sudden dyspnea

☐ **2.** Chills, fever

☐ **3.** Diaphoresis

☐ **4.** Hypertension

☐ **5.** Confusion

Answer: *1, 3, 5*

Rationale: Sudden dyspnea with diaphoresis and confusion are classic signs and symptoms of a pulmonary embolus. In this disorder, a thrombus (stationary blood clot) dislodges from a varicose vein and becomes lodged in the pulmonary circulation. Chills and fever would indicate an infection. A client with an embolus could be hypotensive, not hypertensive.

Critical thinking strategy: Recall the pathophysiology and clinical manifestations of pulmonary embolism.

Client needs category: Physiological integrity

Client needs subcategory: Physiological adaptation

Cognitive level: Analysis

Integrated process: Nursing process/assessment

Reference: Pillitteri, pages 669–670

---

6. A nurse is palpating the uterine fundus of a client who delivered her neonate 8 hours ago. Identify the area where the nurse would expect to feel the fundus.

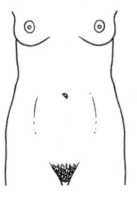

Answer:

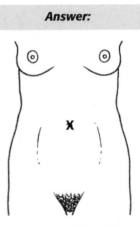

Rationale: The uterus should be felt at the level of the umbilicus from about 1 to 24 hours after birth.

Critical thinking strategy: Recall that the uterus decreases in size at a predictable rate following delivery.

Client needs category: Physiological integrity

Client needs subcategory: Reduction of risk potential

Cognitive level: Application

Integrated process: Nursing process/assessment

Reference: Pillitteri, pages 628–629

7. A nurse is caring for a client in the fourth stage of labor. Based on the nurse's note below, which postpartum complication has the client developed?

Progress notes

6/7/09	Pt.'s 24-hour blood loss is 600 ml. Uterus is
1745	soft and relaxed on palpation and pt. has
	a full bladder. Assisted pt. in emptying
	bladder and notified Dr. G. McMann of
	findings. Vital signs stable at present. See
	graphic sheet for ongoing assessments and
	perineal pad weights.————— S. Jones, RN

☐ **1.** Postpartum hemorrhage

☐ **2.** Puerperal infection

☐ **3.** Deep vein thrombosis

☐ **4.** Mastitis

Answer: 1

Rationale: Blood loss from the uterus that exceeds 500 ml in a 24-hour period is considered postpartum hemorrhage. If uterine atony is the cause, the uterus feels soft and relaxed. A full bladder can prevent the uterus from contracting completely, increasing the risk of hemorrhage. Puerperal infection is an infection of the uterus and structures above; its characteristic sign is fever. Two major types of deep vein thrombosis occur in the postpartum period: pelvic and femoral. Each has different signs and symptoms, but both occur later in the postpartum period (femoral, after 10 days postpartum; pelvic, after 14 days). Mastitis is an inflammation of the mammary glands that disrupts normal lactation and usually develops 1 to 4 weeks postpartum.

Critical thinking strategy: Identify the key assessment findings from the client's chart and relate them to the choices provided.

Client needs category: Physiological integrity

Client needs subcategory: Reduction of risk potential

Cognitive level: Analysis

Integrated process: Nursing process/evaluation

Reference: Pillitteri, pages 656–661

---

8. A nurse assesses a client's vaginal discharge on the first postpartum day and describes it in her progress note (shown below). Which of the following terms best describes the discharge?

Progress notes

3/30/09	Perineal pad changed two times this shift
1645	for moderate amount of red discharge.——
	————————————— J. Jones, RN

☐ **1.** Lochia alba

☐ **2.** Lochia

☐ **3.** Lochia serosa

☐ **4.** Lochia rubra

Answer: 4

Rationale: For the first 3 days after birth, the discharge is called lochia rubra. It consists almost entirely of blood, with only small particles of decidua and mucus. Lochia alba is a creamy white or colorless discharge that occurs 10 to 14 days postpartum. Lochia serosa is a pink or brownish discharge that occurs 4 to 14 days postpartum. The term *lochia* alone isn't a correct description of the discharge.

Critical thinking strategy: Focus on vaginal discharge, and relate it to the number of days postpartum.

Client needs category: Physiological integrity

Client needs subcategory: Physiological adaptation

Cognitive level: Application

Integrated process: Communication and documentation

Reference: Pillitteri, page 629

9. A home care lactation nurse has asked a client to keep a record of her intake, including calories, and output for 1 day. After reviewing the flow sheet that the client used to document the results (shown below), the nurse should make which of the following assessments?

Time period	Fluids (in ml)	Calories	Output (in ml)
7 a.m. to 11 a.m.	milk 240	breakfast 510	60
	orange juice 60		
11 a.m. to 3 p.m.	coffee 240	lunch 350	250
	orange juice 120	snack 80	200
	water 240		200
3 p.m. to 11 p.m.	water 240	dinner 500	100
	water 240	snack 350	230
	water 240		200
11 p.m. to 7 a.m.	water 240		300

☐ **1.** The client consumed an adequate amount of calories and fluids for breast-feeding.

☐ **2.** The client consumed an adequate amount of calories but not enough fluids for breast-feeding.

☐ **3.** The client consumed an adequate amount of fluids but not enough calories for breast-feeding.

☐ **4.** The client consumed an inadequate amount of fluids and calories for breast-feeding.

Answer: 4

Rationale: New mothers who are breast-feeding should consume 2 to 3 L of fluids and 2,300 to 2,700 calories daily.

Critical thinking strategy: Calculate the total calories and fluid intake and relate them to the nutritional needs of the lactating client.

Client needs category: Health promotion and maintenance

Client needs subcategory: None

Cognitive level: Analysis

Integrated process: Nursing process/evaluation

Reference: Pillitteri, pages 739–740

---

10. On examining a client who gave birth 3 hours ago, a nurse finds that the client has completely saturated a perineal pad within 15 minutes. Which actions should the nurse take? Select all that apply.

☐ **1.** Begin an I.V. infusion of lactated Ringer's solution.

☐ **2.** Assess the client's vital signs.

☐ **3.** Palpate the client's fundus.

☐ **4.** Place the client in high Fowler's position.

☐ **5.** Administer a pain medication.

Answer: 2, 3

Rationale: Checking vital signs provides information about the client's circulatory status and identifies significant changes that may need to be reported to the physician. By palpating the client's fundus, the nurse also gains valuable data. A boggy uterus may lead to excessive bleeding. Starting an I.V. infusion requires a physician's order. Placing the client in high Fowler's position may lower the blood pressure and be harmful to the client. Administration of a pain medication doesn't address the current problem.

Critical thinking strategy: Recall the nursing interventions related to excessive bleeding.

Client needs category: Physiological integrity

Client needs subcategory: Reduction of risk potential

Cognitive level: Application

Integrated process: Nursing process/implementation

Reference: Pillitteri, pages 656–660

11. A postpartum client is suspected of developing deep vein thrombosis. The nurse assesses the client for Homans' sign. Identify the area of the body below, where Homans' sign would be elicited.

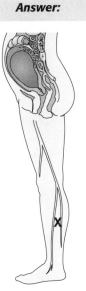

Answer:

Rationale: To elicit Homan's sign, the client dorsiflexes her ankle and then the nurse assesses for pain in the calf during that motion.

Critical thinking strategy: Recall the area where thrombophlebitis usually develops.

Client needs category: Physiological integrity

Client needs subcategory: Physiological adaptation

Cognitive level: Application

Integrated process: Nursing process/assessment

Reference: Pillitteri, page 645

---

12. The nurse is assessing a client who is 4 hours postpartum. Based on the findings documented by the nurse below, which action is most appropriate at this time?

Progress notes

06/11/09	Pt.'s vital signs stable at present. Perineal
1830	pad changed for moderate amount of red
	drainage. Uterus palpated at the level of
	the umbilicus and to the left side of the
	abdomen.———————N. Green, RN

☐ **1.** Ask the client to empty her bladder.

☐ **2.** Straight-catheterize the client immediately.

☐ **3.** Call the client's primary health care provider for direction.

☐ **4.** Straight-catheterize the client for half of her urine volume.

Answer: 1

Rationale: A full bladder may displace the uterine fundus to the left or right of the abdomen. A straight catheterization is unnecessarily invasive if the client can urinate on her own. Nursing interventions should be completed before notifying the primary health care provider in a nonemergency situation.

Critical thinking strategy: Focus on the assessment findings as they relate to the postpartal uterus.

Client needs category: Physiological integrity

Client needs subcategory: Physiological adaptation

Cognitive level: Application

Integrated process: Nursing process/implementation

Reference: Pillitteri, pages 670–673

13. A postpartum client has been ordered 500 mg of ampicillin oral suspension. The label reads *ampicillin 125 mg/5 ml.* How many milliliters should the client receive? Record your answer using a whole number.

_____ milliliters

Answer: 20

Rationale: To solve this problem, set up proportions as follows:

$$5 \text{ ml}/125 \text{ mg} = X \text{ ml}/500 \text{ mg}$$

$$X \times 125 \text{ mg} = 5 \text{ ml} \times 500 \text{ mg}$$

Solve for X by dividing both sides of the equation by 125 mg:

$$\frac{X \times 125 \text{ mg}}{125 \text{ mg}} = \frac{5 \text{ ml} \times 500 \text{ mg}}{125 \text{ mg}}$$

$$X = \frac{2,500 \text{ ml}}{125}$$

$$X = 20 \text{ ml}$$

Critical thinking strategy: Recall calculations using proportions and solving for X.

Client needs category: Physiological integrity

Client needs subcategory: Pharmacological and parenteral therapies

Cognitive level: Application

Integrated process: Nursing process/planning

Reference: *Dosage Calculations Made Incredibly Easy,* pages 176–178

---

14. The postpartum client transitions through phases while moving toward parenthood. Place the following phases in the order that they occur postpartally. Use all of the options.

| 1. Taking-hold phase |
| 2. Letting-go phase |
| 3. Taking-in phase |

Answer: 3, 1, 2

Rationale: The taking-in phase occurs in the first 24 hours after birth. The mother is concerned with her own needs and requires support from staff and relatives. The taking-hold phase occurs when the mother is ready to take responsibility for her care as well as her neonate's care. The letting-go phase begins several weeks later, when the mother incorporates the neonate into the family unit.

Critical thinking strategy: Focus on transitional maternal roles during the postpartum period.

Client needs category: Health promotion and maintenance

Client needs subcategory: None

Cognitive level: Analysis

Integrated process: Nursing process/evaluation

Reference: Pillitteri, pages 623–625

15. The nurse is preparing to perform a fundal massage on a client who is 2 hours postpartum. Order the sequence of events for performing this procedure. Use all of the options.

1.	Rotate the upper hand to massage the uterus until firm.
2.	Place the client in supine position.
3.	Gently press the fundus between the hands using slight downward pressure.
4.	Place one hand around the top of the fundus.
5.	Ask the client to void.
6.	Place one hand on the abdomen just above symphysis pubis.

Answer: 5, 2, 6, 4, 1, 3

Rationale: Fundal massage is performed to promote uterine tone and consistency and to minimize the risk of hemorrhage. First, have the client void to prevent displacement of the bladder and allow an accurate assessment of uterine tone. Then, place the client in proper supine positioning to allow for good visualization. To anchor the lower part of the uterus, place one hand on the abdomen just above the symphysis pubis and then place the other hand around the top of the fundus. Next, rotate the upper hand to massage the uterus until it's firm. Finally, when the uterus is firm, push gently on the fundus, using slight downward pressure against the lower hand.

Critical thinking strategy: Recall the fundal massage sequence and the reason for perfoming maneuvers.

Client needs category: Physiological integrity

Client needs subcategory: Reduction of risk potential

Cognitive level: Application

Integrated process: Nursing process/implementation

Reference: Pillitteri, pages 656–659

The neonate

1. A nurse is performing a neurologic assessment on a 1-day-old neonate in the nursery. Which of the following findings would indicate possible asphyxia in utero? Select all that apply.

- ☐ **1.** The neonate grasps the nurse's finger when she puts it in the palm of his hand.
- ☐ **2.** The neonate does stepping movements when held upright with the sole of his foot touching a surface.
- ☐ **3.** The neonate's toes don't curl downward when the soles of his feet are touched.
- ☐ **4.** The neonate doesn't respond when the nurse claps her hands above him.
- ☐ **5.** The neonate turns toward the nurse's finger when she touches his cheek.
- ☐ **6.** The neonate displays weak, ineffective sucking.

Answer: 3, 4, 6

Rationale: If the neonate's toes don't curl downward when the soles of his feet are touched and he doesn't respond to a loud sound, neurologic damage from asphyxia may have occurred. A normal neurologic response would be the downward curling of the toes when touched and extension of the arms and legs in response to a loud noise. Weak, ineffective sucking is another sign of neurologic damage. A neonate should grasp a person's finger when it's placed in the palm of his hand, do stepping movements when held upright with the sole of the foot touching a surface, and turn toward the nurse's finger when she touches his cheek.

Critical thinking strategy: Recall normal neurologic assessment findings.

Client needs category: Health promotion and maintenance

Client needs subcategory: None

Cognitive level: Application

Integrated process: Nursing process/assessment

Reference: Pillitteri, pages 686–689

2. What information should the nurse include when teaching postcircumcision care to the parents of a neonate prior to discharge from the hospital? Select all that apply.

☐ **1.** The infant must void before being discharged home.

☐ **2.** Petroleum jelly or antibiotic ointment should be applied to the glans of the penis with each diaper change.

☐ **3.** The infant can have tub baths while the circumcision heals.

☐ **4.** Any amount of blood noted on the front of the diaper should be reported.

☐ **5.** The circumcision will require care for 2 to 4 days after discharge.

Answer: 1, 2, 5

Rationale: The infant must void prior to discharge to ensure that the urethra isn't obstructed. A lubricating or antibiotic ointment should be applied with each diaper change. Typically, the penis heals within 2 to 4 days, and circumcision care is needed for that period only. To prevent infection, the infant shouldn't have tub baths until the circumcision is healed; sponge baths are appropriate. A small amount of bleeding is expected following a circumcision; parents should report only a large amount of bleeding.

Critical thinking strategy: Focus on teaching guidelines and actions that are unique to circumcision care.

Client needs category: Safe, effective care environment

Client needs subcategory: Management of care

Cognitive level: Application

Integrated process: Teaching and learning

Reference: Pillitteri, pages 715–716

---

3. A 14-day-old neonate is admitted for aspiration pneumonia. The results of a barium swallow confirm a diagnosis of gastroesophageal reflux with resulting aspiration pneumonia. Identify the area of the stomach associated with this diagnosis.

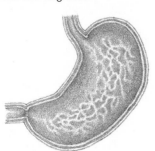

Answer:

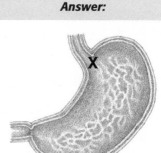

Rationale: Gastroesophageal reflux is a neuromotor disturbance in which the cardiac sphincter located between the stomach and the esophagus is weak. This allows easy regurgitation of gastric contents into the esophagus, causing possible aspiration into the lungs.

Critical thinking strategy: Recall the anatomy of the stomach and the pathophysiology of gastroesophageal reflux.

Client needs category: Physiological integrity

Client needs subcategory: Physiological adaptation

Cognitive level: Application

Integrated process: Nursing process/analysis

Reference: Pillitteri, page 1414

4. A nurse is demonstrating cord care to the mother of a neonate. Which actions would the nurse teach the mother to perform? Select all that apply.

☐ **1.** Keep the diaper below the cord.

☐ **2.** Tug gently on the cord as it begins to dry.

☐ **3.** Apply antibiotic ointment to the cord twice daily.

☐ **4.** Only sponge-bathe the infant until the cord falls off.

☐ **5.** Clean the length of the cord with alcohol several times daily.

☐ **6.** Wash the cord with mild soap and water.

Rationale: The diaper should be positioned below the cord to allow it to air-dry and to prevent urine from getting on the cord. The nurse should instruct the parents to sponge-bathe the infant until the cord falls off. Soap and water shouldn't be used as a part of cord care. The entire cord should be cleaned with alcohol, using a cotton swab or another appropriate method, several times a day. Parents should also be instructed to never pull on the cord, but to allow it to fall off naturally. Antibiotic ointments are contraindicated unless there are signs of infection.

Critical thinking strategy: Focus on teaching guidelines and actions that are unique to cord care.

Client needs category: Safe and effective care environment

Client needs subcategory: Management of care

Cognitive level: Application

Integrated process: Teaching and learning

Reference: Pillitteri, pages 711–712

---

5. At 5 minutes of age, a neonate is pink with acrocyanosis; has flexed knees, clenched fists, a whimpering cry, and a heart rate of 128 beats/minute; and withdraws his foot when slapped on the sole. What 5-minute Apgar score would the nurse record for this neonate?

Sign	Apgar Score		
	0	**1**	**2**
Heart rate	Absent	Less than 100 beats/minute (slow)	More than 100 beats/minute
Respiratory effort	Absent	Slow, irregular	Good cry
Muscle tone	Flaccid	Some flexion and resistance to extension of extremities	Active motion
Reflex irritability	No response	Grimace or weak cry	Vigorous cry
Color	Pallor, cyanosis	Pink body, blue Extremities	Completely pink

☐ **1.** 5

☐ **2.** 7

☐ **3.** 8

☐ **4.** 10

Rationale: The Apgar score provides an assessment of a neonate's health immediately after birth and at 5 minutes of age. Criteria assessed include heart rate, respiratory effort, muscle tone, reflex irritability, and color, each receiving a score from zero (poor) to 2 (normal). This neonate has a heart rate above 100 beats/minute (score of 2); a weak cry (score of 1); good flexion (score of 2); a good response to a slap on the sole (score of 2); and pink color with acrocyanosis (score of 1). Thus, his total Apgar score is 8.

Critical thinking strategy: Review the Apgar scale and focus on the data given in the question.

Client needs category: Physiological integrity

Client needs subcategory: Physiological adaptation

Cognitive level: Analysis

Integrated process: Communication and documentation

Reference: Pillitteri, pages 700–701

6. A nurse is administering vitamin K (AquaMEPHY-TON) to a neonate following delivery. The medication comes in a concentration of 2 mg/ml, and the ordered dose is 0.5 mg to be given subcutaneously. How many milliliters should the nurse administer? Record your answer using two decimal places.

_____ milliliters

Rationale: Use the following formula to calculate drug dosages:

Dose on hand/Quantity on hand = Dose desired/X

2 mg/ml = 0.5 mg/X

X = 0.25 ml.

Critical thinking strategy: Recall dosage calculations using ratio and proportion and solving for X.

Client needs category: Physiological integrity

Client needs subcategory: Pharmacological and parenteral therapies

Cognitive level: Analysis

Integrated process: Nursing process/planning

Reference: *Dosage Calculations Made Incredibly Easy,* pages 58–60

---

7. A nurse is eliciting reflexes in a neonate during a physical examination. Identify the area that the nurse would touch to elicit a plantar grasp reflex.

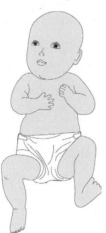

Answer:

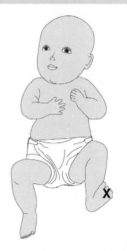

Rationale: To elicit a plantar grasp reflex, the nurse should touch the sole of the foot near the base of the digits, causing flexion or grasping. This reflex disappears at around age 9 months.

Critical thinking strategy: Recall the definition of *plantar,* and review neonatal reflexes.

Client needs category: Health promotion and maintenance

Client needs subcategory: None

Cognitive level: Application

Integrated process: Nursing process/implementation

Reference: Pillitteri, pages 686–689

8. A nurse is providing care to a neonate. Place the following steps in the order that the nurse should implement them to properly perform ophthalmia neonatorum prophylaxis. Use all of the options.

1. Close and manipulate the eyelids to spread the medication over the eye.

2. Shield the neonate's eyes from direct light, and tilt his head slightly to the side that will receive the treatment.

3. Repeat the procedure for the other eye.

4. Wash hands and put on gloves.

5. Instill the ointment in the lower conjunctival sac.

6. Gently raise the neonate's upper eyelid with the index finger, and pull the lower eyelid down with the thumb.

Answer: 4, 2, 6, 5, 1, 3

Rationale: Ophthalmia neonatorum prophylaxis involves the instillation of 0.5% erythromycin or 1% tetracycline ointment into a neonate's eyes. This procedure is performed to prevent gonorrheal and chlamydial conjunctivitis. All 50 states mandate that this treatment be given within 1 hour after delivery to decrease the risk of permanent eye damage and blindness.

Critical thinking strategy: Focus on assessment and prevention of maternal-neonatal infections, and review the ophthalmia neonatorum prophylaxis procedure.

Client needs category: Physiological integrity

Client needs subcategory: Physiological adaptation

Cognitive level: Application

Integrated process: Nursing process/implementation

Reference: Pillitteri, page 790

---

9. A nurse would expect to observe which of the following signs in the neonate with developmental dysplasia of the hip (DDH)? Select all that apply.

☐ **1.** Negative Ortolani test

☐ **2.** Positive Barlow test

☐ **3.** Asymmetrical leg skin folds.

☐ **4.** Limitation in adduction of the affected leg.

☐ **5.** Lengthening of the affected leg.

Answer: 2, 3

Rationale: A neonate with DDH will have a positive Ortolani test, a positive Barlow test, and asymmetrical skin folds in the thigh. The affected leg has limited abduction and appears shorter than the unaffected leg in a neonate with DDH.

Critical thinking strategy: Recall the clinical findings of DDH.

Client needs category: Physiological integrity

Client needs subcategory: Physiological adaptation

Cognitive level: Application

Integrated process: Nursing process/assessment

Reference: Pillitteri, pages 1214–1218

10. Following the admission assessment of a neonate born at 42 weeks' gestation, the nurse identifies which of the following findings as normal? Select all that apply.

☐ **1.** A three-vessel umbilical cord

☐ **2.** Peeling skin on the feet

☐ **3.** Absence of sole creases

☐ **4.** Absence of vernix caseosa

☐ **5.** Cyanosis of the hands and feet

☐ **6.** Large amounts of frothy oral secretions

Answer: 1, 2, 3, 4, 5

Rationale: All of the answers are expected findings in a healthy infant at 42 weeks' gestation except for large amounts of frothy oral secretions. This is indicative of tracheoesophageal fistula; it's an abnormal finding in any neonate, regardless of gestational age at the time of birth.

Critical thinking strategy: Focus on normal assessment findings for full-term neonates.

Client needs category: Health promotion and maintenance

Client needs subcategory: None

Cognitive level: Application

Integrated process: Nursing process/evaluation

Reference: Pillitteri, pages 705–707

---

11. A neonate has been placed on cardiac and apnea monitoring in the neonatal nursery. The nurse notes that apnea alarm repeatedly triggers. Place the following actions in the order in which they should be completed by the nurse. Use all of the options.

1. Silence the alarm to decrease environmental stimuli.
2. Perform a focused assessment on the neonate.
3. Count the respiratory rate for 60 seconds.
4. Document the assessment findings, interventions, and neonate's response.

Answer: 2, 3, 1, 4

Rationale: The priority action is to perform a focused assessment on the neonate. Afterward, the nurse should evaluate the respiratory rate by counting respirations for 60 seconds. Afterward, the nurse should silence the alarm and, finally, document the information. Remember to "nurse the client," not the equipment.

Critical thinking strategy: Recall the ABCs (airway, breathing, circulation) of care when prioritizing actions.

Client needs category: Physiological integrity

Client needs subcategory: Physiological adaptation

Cognitive level: Application

Integrated process: Nursing process/implementation

Reference: Pillitteri, page 783

12. A 2-week-old neonate is admitted to the hospital with a diagnosis of possible sepsis. The neonate weighs 3.2 kg. The physican writes the following orders for the neonate and signs the order sheet. Which order should the nurse question?

Order sheet

05/12/09	Acetaminophen (Tylenol) 10 mg/kg per
1000	rectum, Q4–6 hours prn pain
	Ampicillin 200 mg/kg IV Q6 hrs
	D₅½ Normal saline IV @ 125 ml/hr
	Mom may breastfeed ad lib.
	Draw blood cultures x 3 in A.M.
	Send Urine C & S in A. M.
	————————————R. Richard, M.D.

☐ **1.** Acetaminophen (Tylenol) 10 mg/kg per rectum, q 4-6 hrs. prn pain

☐ **2.** Ampicillin 200 mg/kg IV q 6hrs

☐ **3.** Mom may breastfeed ad lib

☐ **4.** Draw blood cultures 3 3 in A. M.

Answer: 4

Rationale: After the adminstration of ampicillin, the neonate's blood cultures will be invalid; the cultures should be obtained prior to the administration of the antibiotics. It's the nurse's responsibility to notify the physician and seek further clarification before carrying out this order. All of the other physican orders are appropriate as written.

Critical thinking strategy: Recall the timing of blood cultures and administration of antibiotics.

Client needs category: Physiological integrity

Client needs subcategory: Pharmacologic and parenteral therapies

Cognitive level: Analysis

Integrated process: Nursing process/analysis

Reference: Pillitteri, pages 1120–1121

---

13. The nurse is caring for a neonate who has a suspected neonatal sepsis. The physician's order is for ampicillin 100 mg/kg/day to be given in 4 divided doses. The client weighs 7 lb, 8 ounces. How many milligrams should the nurse give with each dose? Record your answer using a whole number.

_____ milligrams/dose

Answer: 85

Rationale: First, convert the weight to kilograms:

$$7 \text{ lb, 8 oz} = 7.5 \text{ lb}$$
$$1 \text{ lb} = 2.2 \text{ kg}$$
$$7.5 \text{ lb} \div 2.2 \text{ kg} = 3.4 \text{ kg}$$

Then, multiply the kilograms of body weight by 100 mg (dose given):

$$3.4 \text{ kg} \times 100 \text{ mg} = 340 \text{ mg/kg}$$

Next, divide 340 mg/kg by 4 doses per day:

$$340 \div 4 = 85 \text{ mg per dose.}$$

Critical thinking strategy: Focus on what the question is asking (the milligrams to give with each dose), and review conversions and dosage calculations based on body weight.

Client needs category: Physiological integrity

Client needs subcategory: Pharmacological and parenteral therapies

Cognitive level: Application

Integrated process: Nursing process/planning

Reference: *Dosage Calculations Made Incredibly Easy,* pages 267–270

14. The nurse is preparing to perform a heelstick procedure to obtain blood from a neonate. Identify the area where the nurse would perform this procedure.

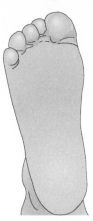

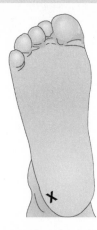

Rationale: The correct location is in the lower left outer aspect of the heel. The capillary blood supply is rich here, and the specimen can be obtained most easily form this area. It shouldn't be taken from the center part of the heel because of the potential for nerve injury.

Critical thinking strategy: Recall the vascular anatomy of the heel area, and review specimen collection techniques.

Client needs category: Physiological integrity

Client needs subcategory: Basic care and comfort

Cognitive level: Analysis

Integrated process: Nursing process

Reference: Pillitteri, page 1122

PART FIVE

Pediatric nursing

The infant

1. A physician orders an I.V. infusion of dextrose 5% in quarter-normal saline solution to be infused at 7 ml/kg/hr for a 10-month-old infant. The infant weighs 22 lb. How many milligrams of the ordered solution should the nurse infuse each hour? Record your answer using a whole number.

_____ milliliters/hour

Answer: 70

Rationale: To perform this calculation, the nurse should first convert the infant's weight to kilograms:

$$2.2 \text{ lb/kg} = 22 \text{ lb}/X \text{ kg}$$
$$X = 22 \times 2.2$$
$$X = 10 \text{ kg}.$$

Next, she should multiply the infant's weight by the ordered rate:

$$10 \text{ kg} \times 7 \text{ ml/kg/hour} = 70 \text{ ml/hour}.$$

Critical thinking strategy: Recall conversions, and calculate the answer based on the infant's weight.

Client needs category: Physiological integrity

Client needs subcategory: Pharmacological and parenteral therapies

Cognitive level: Application

Integrated process: Nursing process/implementation

Reference: _Dosage Calculations Made Incredibly Easy,_ pages 267–270, 279–280

---

2. A nurse is teaching the parents of a 6-month-old infant about normal growth and development. Which of the following statements regarding infant development are true? Select all that apply.

☐ **1.** A 6-month-old infant has difficulty holding objects.

☐ **2.** A 6-month-old infant can usually roll from prone to supine and supine to prone positions.

☐ **3.** A teething ring is appropriate for a 6-month-old infant.

☐ **4.** Stranger anxiety usually peaks at age 12 to 18 months.

☐ **5.** Head lag is commonly noted in infants at age 6 months.

☐ **6.** Lack of visual coordination usually resolves by age 6 months.

Answer: 2, 3, 6

Rationale: Gross motor skills of the 6-month-old infant include rolling from front to back and back to front. Teething usually begins around age 6 months and, therefore, a teething ring is appropriate. Visual coordination is usually resolved by age 6 months. At age 6 months, fine motor skills include purposeful grasping and releasing of objects and transferring objects from one hand to another. Stranger anxiety normally peaks at 8 months. The 6-month-old infant also should have good head control and no longer display head lag when pulled up to a sitting position.

Critical thinking strategy: Recall infant developmental milestones.

Client needs category: Health promotion and maintenance

Client needs subcategory: None

Cognitive level: Application

Integrated process: Teaching and learning

Reference: Pillitteri, pages 829–833

3. An infant who weighs 8 kg is to receive ampicillin (Omnipen) 25 mg/kg I.V. every 6 hours. How many milligrams should a nurse administer per dose? Record the answer as a whole number.

_____ mg/dose

Answer: 200

Rationale: The nurse should calculate the correct dose by multiplying the infant's weight by the ordered rate:

$$8 \text{ kg} \times 25 \text{ mg/kg} = 200 \text{ mg.}$$

Critical thinking strategy: Remember to use the drop-down calculator during the NCLEX and, even if the math seems easy, double-check figures.

Client needs category: Physiological integrity

Client needs subcategory: Pharmacological and parenteral therapies

Cognitive level: Application

Integrated process: Nursing process/planning

Reference: *Dosage Calculations Made Incredibly Easy,* pages 267–270

---

4. A nurse is conducting a physical examination on an infant. Identify the anatomic landmark she should use to measure chest circumference.

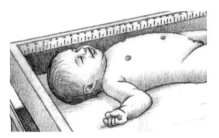

Answer:

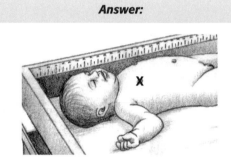

Rationale: Chest circumference is most accurately measured by placing the measuring tape around the infant's nipples. Measuring above or below the nipples will yield a false measurement. The measurement should be taken after exhalation.

Critical thinking strategy: Review assessment techniques for infant body measurements.

Client needs category: Health promotion and maintenance

Client needs subcategory: None

Cognitive level: Application

Integrated process: Nursing process/implementation

Reference: Pillitteri, page 994

5. A healthy 2-month-old infant is being seen in the local clinic for a well-child checkup and his initial immunizations. Which immunizations should the nurse anticipate administering at this appointment? Select all that apply.

☐ **1.** DTaP (diphtheria, tetanus, and acellular pertussis)

☐ **2.** MMR (measles, mumps, and rubella)

☐ **3.** OPV (oral polio vaccine)

☐ **4.** HBV (hepatitis B vaccine)

☐ **5.** Varicella zoster (chickenpox) vaccine

☐ **6.** HIB (*Haemophilus influenzae* vaccine)

☐ **7.** Pneumococcal vaccine

Answer: 1, 4, 6, 7

Rationale: At age 2 months, the American Academy of Pediatrics recommends the administration of DTaP, IPV (inactivated polio vaccine), HBV, HIB, and pneumococcal vaccine. The MMR immunization should be administered at 12 to 15 months. The IPV—not the OPV—is currently used to minimize spread of the disease. The varicella zoster vaccine may be given any time after the child's first birthday.

Critical thinking strategy: Recall the recommended childhood immunization schedule.

Client needs category: Health promotion and maintenance

Client needs subcategory: None

Cognitive level: Application

Integrated process: Nursing process/planning

Reference: Pillitteri, pages 1026–1029

---

6. When assessing an infant for changes in intracranial pressure (ICP), it's important to palpate the fontanels. Identify the area where a nurse should palpate to assess the anterior fontanel.

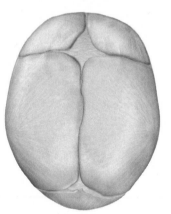

Answer:

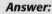
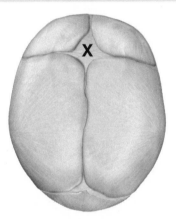

Rationale: The anterior fontanel is formed by the junction of the sagittal, frontal, and coronal sutures. It's shaped like a diamond and normally measures 4 to 5 cm at its widest point. A widened, bulging fontanel is a sign of increased ICP.

Critical thinking strategy: Review the configuration of the anterior and posterior fontanels in infants.

Client needs category: Health promotion and maintenance

Client needs subcategory: None

Cognitive level: Application

Integrated process: Nursing process/assessment

Reference: Pillitteri, page 694

7. A parent is planning to enroll her 9-month-old infant in a day-care facility. The parent asks a nurse what to look for as indicators that the facility is adhering to good infection control measures. How should the nurse reply? Select all that apply.

☐ **1.** The facility keeps boxes of gloves in the director's office.

☐ **2.** Soiled diapers are discarded in covered receptacles.

☐ **3.** Toys are kept on the floor for the children to share.

☐ **4.** Disposable papers are used on the diaper-changing surfaces.

☐ **5.** Facilities for handwashing are located in every classroom.

☐ **6.** Soiled clothing and cloth diapers are sent home in labeled paper bags.

Answer: 2, 4, 5

Rationale: A parent can assess infection control measures by appraising steps taken by the facility to prevent the spread of disease. Placing soiled diapers in covered receptacles, covering the diaper-changing surfaces with disposable papers, and ensuring that sinks are available for personnel to wash their hands after activities are all indicators that infection control measures are being followed. Gloves should be readily available to personnel and, therefore, should be kept in every room—not in an office. Toys typically are shared by numerous children; however, this contributes to the spread of germs and infections. All soiled clothing and cloth diapers should be placed in a sealed plastic bag before being sent home.

Critical thinking strategy: Focus on the location of care, and recall standard precautions for infection control.

Client needs category: Safe, effective care environment

Client needs subcategory: Safety and infection control

Cognitive level: Application

Integrated process: Teaching and learning

Reference: Pillitteri, pages 902–905

---

8. A nurse is performing cardiopulmonary resuscitation (CPR) on an infant. Identify the area where the nurse should assess for a pulse.

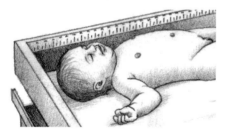

Answer:

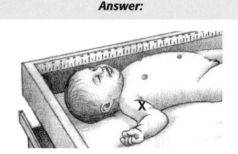

Rationale: The brachial pulse is the pulse to assess when performing infant CPR. The carotid pulse, which is used in children and adults, is extremely difficult to locate in an infant because of his short neck.

Critical thinking strategy: Focus on cardiovascular system anatomy, and review infant CPR.

Client needs category: Physiological adaptation

Client needs subcategory: Physiological integrity

Cognitive level: Application

Integrated process: Nursing process/assessment

Reference: Pillitteri, pages 1316–1318

9. A nurse is assessing a 10-month-old infant during a checkup. Which developmental milestones would the nurse expect the infant to display? Select all that apply.

☐ **1.** Holding the head erect

☐ **2.** Self-feeding

☐ **3.** Demonstrating good bowel and bladder control

☐ **4.** Sitting on a firm surface without support

☐ **5.** Bearing the majority of weight on legs

☐ **6.** Walking alone

Answer: 1, 4, 5

Rationale: By age 4 months, an infant should be able to hold his head erect. By age 9 months, the infant should be able to sit on a firm surface without support and bear the majority of weight on his legs (for example, walking while holding onto furniture). Self-feeding and bowel and bladder control are developmental milestones of toddlers. By age 12 months, the infant should be able to stand on his own and may take his first steps.

Critical thinking strategy: Recall the developmental milestones (especially motor skills) of infants and toddlers.

Client needs category: Health promotion and maintenance

Client needs subcategory: None

Cognitive level: Application

Integrated process: Nursing process/evaluation

Reference: Pillitteri, pages 833–834

---

10. A nurse is conducting an infant nutrition class for parents. Which of the following foods should the nurse tell parents that they may introduce during the first year of life? Select all that apply.

☐ **1.** Sliced beef

☐ **2.** Pureed fruits

☐ **3.** Whole milk

☐ **4.** Rice cereal

☐ **5.** Strained vegetables

☐ **6.** Fruit juice

Answer: 2, 4, 5

Rationale: The first food provided to a neonate is breast milk or formula. Between ages 4 and 6 months, rice cereal can be introduced, followed by pureed or strained fruits and vegetables, then strained or ground meat. Meats must be chopped or ground before they're fed to an infant to prevent choking. Infants shouldn't be given whole milk until they're at least 1-year old. Fruit drinks provide no nutritional benefit and shouldn't be encouraged.

Critical thinking strategy: Review infant feeding schedules, including timing and type of solid foods introduced in the first year of life.

Client needs category: Health promotion and maintenance

Client needs subcategory: None

Cognitive level: Application

Integrated process: Teaching and learning

Reference: Pillitteri, pages 845–847

11. A nurse is teaching parents about the developmental milestones of an infant. Place the following developmental activities for an infant in order of occurrence by age from earliest to latest. Use all the options.

1. Crawling on hands and knees
2. Sitting alone
3. Turning self from supine to prone
4. Turning self from prone to supine
5. Effectively using pincer grasp

Rationale: Infants turn first from prone to supine, and then supine to prone by age 3 to 4 months. Sitting alone usually occurs at about age 6 months. Crawling occurs at around age 7 to 8 months. The use of pincer grasp usually occurs at around 9 to 10 months.

Critical thinking strategy: Recall infant developmental milestones, focusing on gross motor skills.

Client needs category: Health promotion and maintenance

Client needs subcategory: None

Cognitive level: Analysis

Integrated process: Teaching and learning

Reference: Pillitteri, pages 833–834

---

12. The nurse is teaching an infant's parents about introducing foods to their infant's diet. Identify the correct sequence in which the following foods are introduced into the infant's diet during the first year of life. Use all of the options.

1. Strained vegetables
2. Honey
3. Strained chicken
4. Rice cereal
5. Whole milk
6. Breast milk or formula

Rationale: From birth through the first birthday or longer if desired, the infant is given breast milk or formula. Cereals are commonly introduced to the diet at 4 to 6 months of age. At 6 to 7 months, strained vegetables may be started. Strained meats, including chicken, can be started at 9 months. Whole milk shouldn't be given until at least 12 months, and honey not until after 12 months. Introduction of solids can be delayed because an infant gains his primary nutrition, including protein for growth, from breast milk or formula.

Critical thinking strategy: Focus on the principles and practice of introducing foods into the infant's diet, and review allergy risks.

Client needs category: Health promotion and maintenance

Client needs subcategory: None

Cognitive level: Analysis

Integrated process: Teaching and learning

Reference: Pillitteri, pages 845–847

1. A nurse is preparing a dose of amoxicillin for a 3-year-old with acute otitis media. The child weighs 33 lb. The dosage prescribed is 50 mg/kg/day in divided doses every 8 hours. The concentration of the drug is 250 mg/5 ml. How many milliliters should the nurse administer? Record your answer using a whole number.

_____ milliliters

Answer: 5

Rationale: To calculate the child's weight in kilograms, the nurse should use the following formula:

$$2.2 \text{ lb}/1 \text{ kg} = 33 \text{ lb}/X \text{ kg}$$
$$X = 33 \div 2.2$$
$$X = 15 \text{ kg}.$$

Next, the nurse should calculate the daily dosage for the child:

$$50 \text{ mg/kg/day} \times 15 \text{ kg} = 750 \text{ mg/day}.$$

To determine divided daily dosage, the nurse should know that "every 8 hours" means 3 times per day. So, she should perform that calculation in this way:

$$\text{Total daily dosage} \div 3 \text{ times per day} = \text{Divided daily dosage}$$
$$750 \text{ mg/day} \div 3 = 250 \text{ mg}.$$

The drug's concentration is 250 mg/5 ml, so the nurse should administer 5 ml.

Critical thinking strategy: Focus on whether this amount is a reasonable volume of oral medication to give to a toddler in a single dose, and review math skills.

Client needs category: Physiological integrity

Client needs subcategory: Pharmacological and parenteral therapies

Cognitive level: Application

Integrated process: Nursing process/implementation

Reference: _Dosage Calculations Made Incredibly Easy,_ pages 267–270

2. A 3-year-old is to receive 500 ml of dextrose 5% in normal saline solution over 8 hours. At what rate (in milliliters per hour) should a nurse set the infusion pump? Round your answer to a whole number.

_____ ml/hr

Answer: 63

Rationale: To calculate the rate per hour for the infusion, the nurse should divide 500 ml by 8 hours:

$$500 \text{ ml} \div 8 \text{ hours} = 62.5 \text{ ml/hour } (63 \text{ ml/hr}).$$

Critical thinking strategy: Recall dosage calculations for hourly flow rates, and double-check the math.

Client needs category: Physiological integrity

Client needs subcategory: Pharmacological and parenteral therapies

Cognitive level: Application

Integrated process: Nursing process/implementation

Reference: _Dosage Calculations Made Incredibly Easy,_ pages 235–236

3. A 2-year-old is being treated for pneumonia. After reviewing the respiratory section of the client care flow sheet (shown below), the nurse concludes that she should place the child in which position to maximize oxygenation?

Flow sheet

Date: 4/2/09	2300–0700	0700–1500	1500–2300
Breath sounds	Diminished BS LLL	Diminished BS LLL	Crackles LLL
Treatment/results	-----------	CPT & postural drainage	CPT & postural drainage
Cough/results	Nonproductive	Nonproductive	Yellow sputum
Oxygen therapy	Humidifier	Humidifier	Humidifier

☐ **1.** Left side-lying

☐ **2.** Right side-lying

☐ **3.** Supine

☐ **4.** Supine with the head of the bed elevated 30 degrees

Answer: 2

Rationale: The client should be positioned on his right side. Gravity will help mobilize secretions from the affected (left) lung, thereby allowing for improved blood flow and oxygenation.

Critical thinking strategy: Focus on the pathophysiology of pneumonia and related nursing interventions.

Client needs category: Physiological integrity

Client needs subcategory: Physiological adaptation

Cognitive level: Analysis

Integrated process: Nursing process/implementation

Reference: Pillitteri, pages 1264–1265

---

4. A 15-month-old has just received his routine immunizations, including diphtheria, tetanus, and acellular pertussis (DTaP); inactivated polio vaccine (IPV); and measles, mumps, and rubella (MMR). What information should the nurse give to the parents before they leave the office? Select all that apply.

☐ **1.** Minor symptoms can be treated with acetaminophen (Tylenol).

☐ **2.** Minor symptoms can be treated with aspirin.

☐ **3.** Call the office if the toddler develops a fever above 103° F (39.4° C), seizures, or difficulty breathing.

☐ **4.** Soreness at the immunization site and mild fever are common.

☐ **5.** The immunizations prevent the toddler from contracting their associated diseases.

☐ **6.** The toddler should restrict his activity for the remainder of the day.

Answer: 1, 3, 4

Rationale: Minor symptoms, such as soreness at the immunization site and mild fever, can be treated with acetaminophen or ibuprofen. Aspirin should be avoided in children because of its association with Reye's syndrome. The parents should notify the clinic if serious complications (such as a fever above 103° F, seizures, or difficulty breathing) occur. Minor discomforts, such as soreness and mild fever, are common after immunizations. Immunizing the child decreases the health risks associated with contracting certain diseases; it doesn't prevent the toddler from acquiring them. Although the child may prefer to rest after immunizations, it isn't necessary to restrict his activity.

Critical thinking strategy: Review nursing care and parent instructions related to childhood immunizations.

Client needs category: Health promotion and maintenance

Client needs subcategory: None

Cognitive level: Application

Integrated process: Teaching and learning

Reference: Pillitteri, pages 1031–1032

5. A nurse is feeling the apical impulse of a 28-month-old child. Identify the area where the nurse should assess the apical impulse.

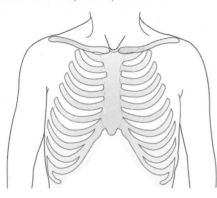

Answer:

Answer:

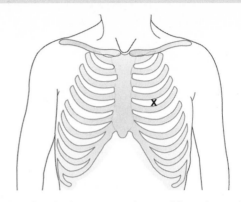

Rationale: The heart's apex for a toddler is located at the fourth intercostal space, immediately to the left of the midclavicular line. It's one or two intercostal spaces above what's considered normal for an adult because the heart's position in a child of this age is more horizontal and larger in diameter than that of an adult.

Critical thinking strategy: Identify the point of maximal impulse, then count the number of ribs to identify the intercostal spaces.

Client needs category: Health promotion and maintenance

Client needs subcategory: None

Cognitive level: Application

Integrated process: Nursing process/assessment

Reference: Craven, page 453

---

6. A nurse is caring for a 3-year-old with viral meningitis. Which signs and symptoms would the nurse expect to find during the initial assessment? Select all that apply.

☐ **1.** Bulging anterior fontanel

☐ **2.** Fever

☐ **3.** Nuchal rigidity

☐ **4.** Petechiae

☐ **5.** Irritability

☐ **6.** Photophobia

☐ **7.** Hypothermia

Answer: 2, 3, 5, 6

Rationale: Common signs and symptoms of viral meningitis include fever, nuchal rigidity, irritability, and photophobia. A bulging anterior fontanel is a sign of hydrocephalus, which isn't likely to occur in a toddler because the anterior fontanel typically closes by age 24 months. A petechial, purpuric rash may be seen with bacterial meningitis. Hypothermia is a common sign of bacterial meningitis in an infant younger than age 3 months.

Critical thinking strategy: Focus on the child's age, and review clinical findings in viral meningitis.

Client needs category: Physiological integrity

Client needs subcategory: Physiological adaptation

Cognitive level: Application

Integrated process: Nursing process/evaluation

Reference: Pillitteri, pages 1558–1560

7. A 3-year-old is being treated for severe status asthmaticus. After reviewing the progress notes below, a nurse should determine that this client is being treated for which of the following conditions?

Progress notes

4/5/09	Pt. was acutely restless, diaphoretic, and with
0600	SOB at 0530. Dr. T. Smith notified and
	ordered ABG analysis. ABG drawn from R
	radial artery. Stat results as follows: pH
	7.28, PacO₂ 55 mm Hg, HCO₃⁻ 26 mEq/L. Dr.
	Smith with pt. now. ———— J. Collins, RN.

- ☐ **1.** Metabolic acidosis
- ☐ **2.** Respiratory alkalosis
- ☐ **3.** Respiratory acidosis
- ☐ **4.** Metabolic alkalosis

Answer: 3

Rationale: A pH less than 7.35 and a partial pressure of arterial carbon dioxide ($PaCO_2$) greater than 45 mm Hg indicate respiratory acidosis. Status asthmaticus is a medical emergency characterized by respiratory distress. At first, the client hyperventilates; then respiratory alkalosis occurs, followed by metabolic acidosis. If treatment is ineffective or hasn't started, symptoms can progress to hypoventilation and respiratory acidosis, both of which are life-threatening. A client with respiratory alkalosis would have a pH greater than 7.45 and a $PaCO_2$ less than 35 mm Hg. Metabolic acidosis is characterized by a pH less than 7.35 and a bicarbonate (HCO_3^-) level less than 22 mEq/L. Metabolic alkalosis is characterized by a pH greater than 7.45 and HCO_3^- above 26 mEq/L.

Critical thinking strategy: Recall the normal range for each of the blood gas values, and then analyze the ABG values provided.

Client needs subcategory: Physiological integrity

Client needs subcategory: Physiological adaptation

Cognitive level: Analysis

Integrated process: Nursing process/analysis

Reference: Pillitteri, pages 1229–1230

---

8. A 30-month-old toddler is being evaluated for a ventricular septal defect (VSD). Identify the area where a VSD occurs.

Answer:

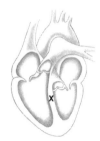

Rationale: A VSD is a small hole between the right and left ventricles that allows blood to shunt between them, causing right ventricular hypertrophy and, if left untreated, biventricular heart failure. It's a common congenital heart defect and accounts for 20% to 30% of all heart lesions.

Critical thinking strategy: Review congenital heart defects and how blood flow is altered by each defect.

Client needs category: Physiological integrity

Client needs subcategory: Physiological adaptation

Cognitive level: Application

Integrated process: Nursing process/analysis

Reference: Pillitteri, page 1297

9. A child weighing 44 lb is to receive 45 mg/kg/day of penicillin V potassium oral suspension in four divided doses every 6 hours. The suspension that's available is penicillin V potassium 125 mg/5 ml. How many milliliters should the nurse administer for each dose? Record your answer using a whole number.

_____ milliliters

Answer: 9

Rationale: First convert the child's weight to kilograms:

$$44 \text{ lb} \div 2.2 \text{ kg/lb} = 20 \text{ kg}.$$

Next, determine the daily dose:

$$45 \text{ mg}: 1 \text{ kg} = X \text{ mg} : 20 \text{ kg}$$
$$45 \times 20 = 1 \times X$$
$$900 = X.$$

Then determine the dose to administer every 6 hours (4 doses):

$$900 \text{ mg} \div 4 = 225 \text{ mg}.$$

Finally, determine the volume to be given at each dose:

$$225 \text{ mg} : X = 125 \text{ mg} : 5 \text{ ml}$$
$$1,125 \text{ mg/ml} = 125 \text{ mg}/X$$
$$9 \text{ ml} = X.$$

Critical thinking strategy: Recall conversion of pounds to kilograms, and don't confuse milligrams (dosage) with milliliters (volume to be given).

Client needs category: Physiological integrity

Client needs subcategory: Pharmacological and parenteral therapies

Cognitive level: Application

Integrated process: Nursing process/planning

Reference: _Dosage Calculations Made Incredibly Easy,_ pages 267–270

10. A 34-month-old is hospitalized for a lengthy illness. Which of the following behaviors are examples of expected developmental regression for the child's age-group. Select all that apply.

☐ **1.** Enuresis

☐ **2.** Encopresis

☐ **3.** Immature speech patterns

☐ **4.** Altered gait

☐ **5.** Loss of fine motor skills

Answer: 1, 2, 3

Rationale: Enuresis (uncontrolled voiding) and encopresis (uncontrolled stooling) are often seen in toddlers who were previously toilet trained and return to diapers during hospitalization. Language regression ("baby talk") is often observed during hospitalization. Altered gait and loss of fine motor skills aren't typical regressive behaviors; when seen in a child, they may indicate musculoskeletal or neurological problems.

Critical thinking strategy: Recall the developmental milestones of toddlers, and focus on how hospitalization might lead to regressive behaviors.

Client needs category: Health promotion and maintenance

Client needs subcategory: None

Cognitive level: Application

Integrated process: Nursing process/analysis

Reference: Pillitteri, pages 1072–1073, 1085–1088

11. Which of the following clients require contact precautions? Select all that apply.

☐ **1.** A toddler with scabies

☐ **2.** A toddler with mumps

☐ **3.** A toddler with streptococcal pharyngitis

☐ **4.** A toddler with pulmonary tuberculosis

☐ **5.** A toddler with a multidrug-resistant organism

Answer: 1, 5

Rationale: Scabies is a skin infection and requires contact precautions. Multidrug-resistant infection also requires contact precautions because of potential contamination. A toddler with mumps or streptococcal pharyngitis requires droplet precautions. Pulmonary tuberculosis requires airborne precautions.

Critical thinking strategy: Review the pathophysiology of the listed diseases and transmission-based precautions.

Client needs category: Safe and effective care environment

Client needs subcategory: Safety and infection control

Cognitive level: Application

Integrated process: Nursing process/implementation

Reference: Craven, page 473

---

12. Maslow's hierarchy of needs is often used as a framework for prioritization of client needs. Prioritize the following nursing care activities for a toddler according to Maslow's framework. Use all of the options.

| **1.** Progressing the diet after surgery |
| **2.** Clearing the airway of secretions |
| **3.** Changing a soiled diaper |
| **4.** Administering antipyretics for an axillary temperature of 104° F |
| **5.** Notifying the practitioner about suspected compartment syndrome |

Answer: 2, 5, 3, 4, 1

Rationale: According to Maslow's framework, the five categories, or hierarchy of needs in order of priority, are as follows: physiologic needs, safety, love, esteem, and self-actualization. Within the physiologic needs category are the essentials for existence air, nutrition, water, elimination, sleep and rest, thermoregulation, and sex. Therefore, maintaining a patent airway is the first priority, followed by notifying the practitioner of suspected compartment syndrome because of the risk of loss of limb. Changing a soiled diaper would be next because this is necessary to prevent skin breakdown. Administering antipyretics for fever primarily provides comfort to the child. The lowest priority, although important, is progressing the child's diet following surgery.

Critical thinking strategy: Review Maslow's hierachy of needs

Client needs category: Safe and effective care environment

Client needs subcategory: Management of care

Cognitive level: Application

Integrated process: Nursing process/implementation

Reference: Craven, pages 52–54

13. The nurse is preparing to insert an intravenous catheter into an anxious toddler. Place the following steps in the order the nurse should follow. Use all of the options.

1. Wash hands and gather supplies.
2. Prepare the equipment.
3. Inform the toddler of the procedure.
4. Inform the parents of the procedure.
5. Select and prep the appropriate site.
6. Insert the I.V. catheter and secure it appropriately.

Answer: 4, 1, 2, 3, 5, 6

Rationale: It's important to inform the parents and gain their support for the procedure first, especially if the child is anxious. A toddler doesn't understand the concept of time, so the nurse shouldn't inform him until very shortly before the I.V. insertion. Next, the nurse should wash her hands and prepare the supplies and equipment, keeping them out of the child's sight to decrease anxiety. Finally, the nurse to inform the toddler what's about to happen, then perform the procedure by selecting and prepping the site, inserting the I.V. catheter, and securing it.

Critical thinking strategy: Recall that the child is anxious, and prioritize the nursing interventions accordingly.

Client needs category: Physiological integrity

Client needs subcategory: Basic care and comfort

Cognitive level: Application

Integrated process: Nursing process/planning

Reference: Pillitteri, pages 1150–1155

The preschooler

1. A 4½-year-old is ordered to receive 25 ml/hour of I.V. solution. The nurse is using a pediatric microdrip chamber to administer the medication. For how many drops per minute should the microdrip chamber be set? Record your answer using a whole number.

_____ drops/minute

Answer: 25

Rationale: When using a pediatric microdrip chamber, the number of milliliters per hour equals the number of drops per minute. If 25 ml/hour is ordered, the I.V. solution should infuse at 25 drops/minute.

Critical thinking strategy: Recall the formula for using the pediatric doses in a microdrip chamber; remember that the number of milliliters per hour equals the number of drops per minute.

Client needs category: Physiological integrity

Client needs subcategory: Pharmacological and parenteral therapies

Cognitive level: Application

Integrated process: Nursing process/planning

Reference: _Dosage Calculations Made Incredibly Easy,_ pages 236–237

2. A 44-lb preschooler is being treated for inflammation. The physician orders 0.2 mg/kg/day of dexamethasone by mouth to be administered every 6 hours. The elixir comes in a strength of 0.5 mg/5 ml. How many milliliters of dexamethasone should the nurse give the child at each dose? Record your answer using a whole number.

_____ milliliters/dose

Answer: 10

Rationale: To perform this dosage calculation, the nurse should first convert the child's weight from pounds to kilograms:

$$44 \text{ lb} \div 2.2 \text{ lb/kg} = 20 \text{ kg.}$$

Then she should calculate the total daily dose for the child:

$$20 \text{ kg} \times 0.2 \text{ mg/kg/day} = 4 \text{ mg.}$$

Next, the nurse should calculate the amount to be given at each dose:

$$4 \text{ mg} \div 4 \text{ doses} = 1 \text{ mg/dose.}$$

The available elixir contains 0.5 mg of drug per 5 ml. Determine how much to give for a 1-mg dose:

$$0.5 \text{ mg}: 5 \text{ ml} = 1 \text{ mg} : X \text{ ml}$$
$$0.5 \text{ mg} \times X = 5 \text{ ml} \times 1 \text{ mg}$$
$$X = 5 \div 0.5$$
$$X = 10 \text{ ml}$$

Therefore, to give 1 mg of the drug, the nurse should administer 10 ml to the child at each dose.

Critical thinking strategy: Remember to calculate the total daily dose, then divide the total daily dose into the amount given at each individual dose.

Client needs category: Physiological integrity

Client needs subcategory: Pharmacological and parenteral therapies

Cognitive level: Analysis

Integrated process: Nursing process/planning

Reference: *Dosage Calculations Made Incredibly Easy,* pages 266–270

---

3. A nurse is performing a Denver Developmental Screening Test II on a 4½-year-old child. What behaviors should the nurse expect the child to demonstrate? Select all that apply.

☐ **1.** He balances on each foot for at least 6 seconds.

☐ **2.** He copies a square that has straight lines and square corners.

☐ **3.** He prepares his own cereal without help.

☐ **4.** He copies a circle that's closed or very nearly closed.

☐ **5.** He speaks clearly.

☐ **6.** He draws a person with at least three body parts.

Answer: 3, 4, 5, 6

Rationale: By age 4½, a child should be able to prepare a bowl of cereal without help, copy a circle, speak clearly, and draw a person with at least three body parts. The majority of children don't achieve balancing on each foot for 6 seconds until about age 5½. Less than 25% of all children are able to correctly copy a square by age 4.

Critical thinking strategy: Recall that cognitive growth is substantial during these years, and each year during this period marks a major step forward in gross motor, fine motor, and language development.

Client needs category: Health promotion and maintenance

Client needs subcategory: None

Cognitive level: Analysis

Integrated process: Nursing process/analysis

Reference: Pillitteri, pages 1020–1023, 1815–1816

4. A 4-year-old child has recently been diagnosed with acute lymphocytic leukemia (ALL). What information about ALL should the nurse provide when educating the child's parents? Select all that apply.

☐ **1.** ALL is a rare form of childhood leukemia.

☐ **2.** ALL affects all blood-forming organs and systems throughout the body.

☐ **3.** Because of the increased risk of bleeding, the child shouldn't brush his teeth.

☐ **4.** Adverse effects of chemotherapy include sleepiness, alopecia, and stomatitis.

☐ **5.** There's a 95% chance of obtaining a first remission with treatment.

☐ **6.** The child shouldn't be disciplined during this difficult time.

Answer: 2, 4, 5

Rationale: In ALL, immature white blood cells (WBCs) crowd out healthy WBCs, red blood cells, and platelets in the bone marrow. These abnormal WBCs affect all blood-forming organs and systems. Common adverse effects of chemotherapy and radiation include nausea, vomiting, diarrhea, sleepiness, alopecia, anemia, stomatitis, pain, and increased susceptibility to infection. A first remission occurs in about 95% of cases. Brushing teeth doesn't result in increased or abnormal bleeding. A child with leukemia still needs appropriate discipline and limits because a lack of consistent parenting may lead to negative behaviors and fear.

Critical thinking strategy: Review the pathophysiology of ALL, and focus on parent teaching guidelines.

Client needs category: Physiological integrity

Client needs subcategory: Reduction of risk potential

Cognitive level: Application

Integrated process: Teaching and learning

Reference: Pillitteri, pages 1696–1701

---

5. A critically ill 4-year-old is in the pediatric intensive care unit. Telemetry monitoring reveals junctional tachycardia. Identify where this arrhythmia originates.

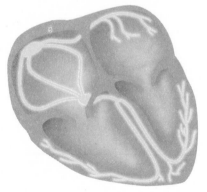

Answer:

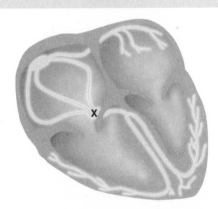

Rationale: In junctional tachycardia, the atrioventricular node fires rapidly. The atria are depolarized by retrograde conduction; however, conduction through the ventricles remains normal.

Critical thinking strategy: Recall the heart's anatomy, physiology, and conduction system.

Client needs category: Physiological integrity

Client needs subcategory: Physiological adaptation

Cognitive level: Analysis

Integrated process: Nursing process/assessment

Reference: Smeltzer, pages 824, 834

6. A school nurse is gathering registration data for a child entering first grade. Which of the following immunizations should the school nurse verify that the child has had? Select all that apply.

☐ **1.** Hepatitis B series

☐ **2.** Diphtheria-tetanus-pertussis series

☐ **3.** *Haemophilus influenzae* type b series

☐ **4.** Varicella zoster vaccine

☐ **5.** Pneumonia vaccine

☐ **6.** Oral polio series

Answer: 1, 2, 3

Rationale: Hepatitis B series, diphtheria-tetanus-pertussis series, *Haemophilus influenzae* type b series, and inactivated (not oral) polio series are the immunizations that the child should receive before entering first grade. The oral polio vaccine was discontinued; the safer inactivated polio vaccine is now used. The varicella zoster vaccine is administered only if the child hasn't had chickenpox. Some states require proof of vaccination if the child hasn't had chickenpox, but it isn't required in all states. Pneumonia vaccine isn't required or routinely given to children.

Critical thinking strategy: Review immunization and infection control recommendations provided by the American Academy of Pediatrics and the Centers for Disease Control and Prevention.

Client needs category: Physiological integrity

Client needs subcategory: Physiological adaptation

Cognitive level: Analysis

Integrated process: Nursing process/analysis

Reference: Pillitteri, pages 1026–1027

---

7. A 4-year-old child is brought to the emergency department in cardiac arrest. The staff performs cardiopulmonary resuscitation (CPR). Identify the area where the child's pulse should be checked.

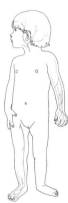

Answer:

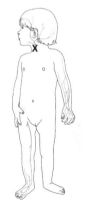

Rationale: The carotid artery should be used to check for a pulse when performing CPR on children and adults. The brachial pulse should be used when performing CPR on an infant.

Critical thinking strategy: Recall the recommendations for CPR in children and the differences in CPR for infants and adults.

Client needs category: Physiological integrity

Client needs subcategory: Physiological adaptation

Cognitive level: Application

Integrated process: Nursing process/assessment

Reference: Pillitteri, pages 1316–1318

8. A preschooler is scheduled to have a Wilms' tumor removed. Identify the area of the urinary system where this tumor is located.

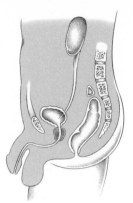

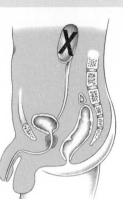

Answer:

Rationale: Wilms' tumor, also known as a nephroblastoma, is located on the kidney. The most common intra-abdominal tumor in children, Wilms' tumor usually affects children ages 6 months to 4 years and favors the left kidney.

Critical thinking strategy: Recall the anatomy of the urinary system and the pathophysiology of Wilms' tumor.

Client needs category: Physiological integrity

Client needs subcategory: Physiological adaptation

Cognitive level: Application

Integrated process: Nursing process/analysis

Reference: Pillitteri, page 1711

---

9. A nurse is caring for a 5-year-old child who is in the terminal stages of cancer. Which statements about the child's impending death are most likely to be true? Select all that apply.

☐ **1.** The parents may be at different stages of grief in dealing with the child's impending death.

☐ **2.** The child is thinking about the future and knows he may not be able to participate.

☐ **3.** The dying child may become clingy and act like a toddler.

☐ **4.** Whispering in the child's room will help the child to cope.

☐ **5.** The death of a child may have long-term disruptive effects on the family.

☐ **6.** The child doesn't fully understand the concept of death.

Answer: 1, 3, 5, 6

Rationale: When dealing with a dying child, parents may be at different stages of grief at different times. The child may regress in his behaviors. The stress of a child's death commonly results in divorce and behavioral problems in siblings. Preschoolers see illness and death as a form of punishment. They fear separation from parents and might worry about who will provide care for them. Preschoolers have only a rudimentary concept of time; thinking about the future is typical of an adolescent facing death, not a preschooler. Whispering in front of the child only increases his fear of death.

Critical thinking strategy: Recall the stages of the grief process and review the developmental stage of preschoolers.

Client needs category: Psychosocial integrity

Client needs subcategory: None

Cognitive level: Analysis

Integrated process: Caring

Reference: Pillitteri, Pages 1771–1776

---

10. A 3-year-old boy has arrived in the emergency room. The nurse documents the following assessment findings in the client's chart, knowing that they're consistent with which disease process?

Progress notes

5/15/09	Pt. admitted to ER with T. 103.6° F, HR
1100	100, RR 24. Respirations are shallow, and
	breath sounds are decreased, with rales
	auscultated bilaterally. Pt. has a harsh cough
	and mother states he has had a discolored
	productive cough at home.—S. Jones, RN

☐ **1.** Bronchiolitis

☐ **2.** Pneumonia

☐ **3.** Asthma

☐ **4.** Cystic fibrosis

Answer: 2

Rationale: The elevated fever, shallow respirations, decreased breath sounds, rales, harsh cough, and productive mucus are findings associated with pneumonia. Typically, there's no fever with asthma and cystic fibrosis, and bronchiolitis presents with a low-grade fever. Wheezing is associated with asthma and bronchiolitis; however, this wasn't found upon physical examination of this client. Bronchiolitis produces a dry cough, and pneumonia causes a productive, harsh cough. The client with cystic fibrosis typically presents with wheezing, rhonchi, and thick, tenacious mucus.

Critical thinking strategy: Focus on the clinical findings as they related to pneumonia, and review disorders of the lower respiratory tract.

Client needs category: Physiological integrity

Client needs subcategory: Physiological adaptation

Cognitive level: Analysis

Integrated process: Nursing process/analysis

Reference: Pillitteri, pages 1259–1271

---

11. A 4-year-old postoperative child is found unresponsive and in cardiopulmonary arrest. Place the following actions in the correct sequence to perform cardiopulmonary resuscitation (CPR) after the child has been assessed for responsiveness and help has been called. Use all of the options.

1. Perform abdominal thrusts.
2. Feel for the carotid pulse.
3. Put the child on his back.
4. Perform 30 compressions and 2 ventilations, and repeat the procedure.
5. Place the child's head in a neutral position, and open his mouth.
6. Provide 2 rescue breaths.

Answer: 3, 5, 6, 1, 2, 4

Rationale: The first step in resuscitation is to assess if the child is responsive to shaking and calling his name. If he is unresponsive, then call for help. Next, place the child on his back. Place the child's head in a neutral position and open his mouth to allow for a patent airway. Next, administer 2 breaths at a rate of 1 per second—either by an Ambu bag, when available, or mouth-to mouth, pinching the child's nose slightly. Observe the child's chest with each breath to see if it rises. If it doesn't rise, this indicates an airway obstruction. Perform abdominal thrusts to relieve the obstruction. Once the airway is patent, administer two ventilations. Next, feel for a carotid pulse for 10 seconds. If it's absent, perform chest compressions and pause after 30 compressions in order to give 2 ventilations.

Critical thinking strategy: Focus on the CPR steps and checking the ABCs (aiway, breathing, and circulation).

Client needs category: Physiological integrity

Client needs subcategory: Physiological adaptation

Cognitive level: Application

Integrated process: Nursing process/implementation

Reference: Pillitteri, pages 1316–1318

12. A nurse is caring for a 4-year-old child who developed acute renal failure after a traumatic injury and hemorrhaging. Place the following events in the order in which they most likely occurred during progression of his severe renal deterioration. Use all of the options.

| **1.** Acidosis |
| **2.** Severe hypocalcemia |
| **3.** Azotemia |
| **4.** Oliguria |

Answer: 4, 3, 1, 2

Rationale: The first symptom of acute renal failure is oliguria (urine output less than 1 ml per kilogram of the child's body weight per hour). The inability to produce urine causes azotemia, an accumulation of nitrogen waste in the bloodstream, which leads to rising blood urea nitrogen (BUN) levels. This leads to acidosis because of the body's inability to excrete $H+$ ions. The acidotic state results in hyperphosphatemia (high phosphorus levels), which in turn causes hypocalcemia (low calcium levels). When hypocalcemia is severe, muscle twitching and tetany can occur.

Critical thinking strategy: Recall the pathophysiology of acute renal failure.

Client needs category: Physiological integrity

Client needs subcategory: Physiological adaptation

Cognitive level: Application

Integrated process: Nursing process/implementation

Reference: Pillitteri, page 1476

The school-age child

1. A 7-year-old child is admitted to the hospital for a course of I.V. antibiotics. What actions should the nurse take before inserting the peripheral I.V. catheter? Select all that apply.

- ☐ **1.** Explain the procedure to the child immediately before the procedure.
- ☐ **2.** Apply a topical anesthetic to the I.V. site before the procedure.
- ☐ **3.** Ask the child which hand he uses for drawing.
- ☐ **4.** Explain the procedure to the child using abstract terms.
- ☐ **5.** Don't let the child see the equipment to be used in the procedure.
- ☐ **6.** Tell the child that the procedure won't hurt.

Answer: 2, 3

Rationale: Topical anesthetics reduce the pain of a venipuncture. The cream should be applied about 1 hour before the procedure and requires a physician's order. The I.V. should be inserted into the hand opposite the one the child indentifies as his drawing hand. The procedure should be explained to the child in simple, concrete words well before it takes place so that he has time to ask questions. Unfamiliar terms should be defined. To help ease his anxiety, the child should be shown the equipment that will be used for the procedure. Although the topical anesthetic will relieve some pain, there's usually some pain or discomfort involved in venipuncture, so the child shouldn't be told otherwise.

Critical thinking strategy: Recall that the cognitive development of a school-age child is concrete operational thinking, and review the nursing process for administration of I.V. fluids.

Client needs category: Health promotion and maintenance

Client needs subcategory: None

Cognitive level: Application

Integrated process: Nursing process/implementation

Reference: Pillitteri, pages 919–920

2. A mother brings her child to the pediatrician's office for evaluation of chronic stomach pain. The mother states that the pain seems to go away when she tells the child that he can stay home from school. The physician diagnoses school phobia. Which other behaviors or symptoms may the child exhibit? Select all that apply.

☐ **1.** Nausea

☐ **2.** Headaches

☐ **3.** Weight loss

☐ **4.** Dizziness

☐ **5.** Fever

Answer: 1, 2, 4

Rationale: Children with school phobia commonly complain of vague symptoms, such as stomachaches, nausea, headaches, and dizziness, to avoid going to school. These symptoms typically don't occur on weekends. A careful history must be taken to identify a pattern of school avoidance. Weight loss and fever are more likely to have a physiological cause and are uncommon in children with school phobia.

Critical thinking strategy: Recall that fears manifest with acute episodes of symptoms (such as GI problems).

Client needs category: Psychosocial integrity

Client needs subcategory: None

Cognitive level: Analysis

Integrated process: Caring

Reference: Pillitteri, page 932

---

3. A child with sickle cell anemia is being discharged after treatment for a crisis. Which instructions for avoiding future crises should the nurse provide to the child and his family? Select all that apply.

☐ **1.** Avoid foods high in folic acid.

☐ **2.** Drink plenty of fluids.

☐ **3.** Use cold packs to relieve joint pain.

☐ **4.** Report a sore throat to an adult immediately.

☐ **5.** Restrict activity to quiet board games.

☐ **6.** Wash hands before meals and after playing.

Answer: 2, 4, 6

Rationale: Fluids should be encouraged to prevent stasis in the bloodstream, which can lead to sickling. Sore throats and all other cold symptoms should be reported promptly because they may indicate an infection, which can precipitate a crisis (red blood cells sickle and obstruct blood flow to tissues). Children with sickle cell anemia should learn appropriate measures to prevent infection, such as proper hand-washing techniques and good nutrition. Folic acid intake should be encouraged to help support new cell growth; new cells replace fragile sickled cells. Warm packs should be applied to promote comfort and relieve pain; cold packs cause vasoconstriction. The child should maintain an active, normal life but should avoid excessive exercise, which can precipitate an attack. When the child experiences a crisis, he'll typically limit his own activity according to his pain level.

Critical thinking strategy: Recall the events that may trigger a sickle cell crisis, such as dehydration or infection.

Client needs category: Physiological integrity

Client needs subcategory: Reduction of risk potential

Cognitive level: Application

Integrated process: Teaching and learning

Reference: Pillitteri, pages 1396–1397

4. A nurse is preparing to administer I.V. methylprednisolone sodium succinate (Solu-Medrol) to a child who weighs 42 lb. The order is for 0.03 mg/kg I.V. daily. How many milligrams should the nurse prepare? Record your answer using one decimal place.

_____ milligrams

Answer: 0.6

Rationale: To perform this dosage calculation, the nurse should first convert the child's weight to kilograms:

$$44 \text{ lb} \div 2.2 \text{ kg/lb} = 20 \text{ kg.}$$

Then she should use this formula to determine the dose:

$$20 \text{ kg} \times 0.03 \text{ mg/kg} = X \text{ mg}$$
$$X = 0.6 \text{ mg.}$$

Critical thinking strategy: Remember that most drugs are based on the child's weight in kilograms. Recall that dosage calculations should be calculated per day, and then divided into the amount given at each dose.

Client needs category: Physiological integrity

Client needs subcategory: Pharmacological and parenteral therapies

Cognitive level: Application

Integrated process: Nursing process/planning

Reference: *Dosage Calculations Made Incredibly Easy,* pages 267–270

---

5. An 8-year-old child has just returned from the operating room after having a tonsillectomy. The nurse preparing to perform a postoperative assessment should be alert for which signs and symptoms of bleeding? Select all that apply.

☐ **1.** Frequent clearing of the throat

☐ **2.** Breathing through the mouth

☐ **3.** Frequent swallowing

☐ **4.** Sleeping for long intervals

☐ **5.** Pulse rate of 98 beats/minute

☐ **6.** Blood-red vomitus

Answer: 1, 3, 6

Rationale: A classic sign of bleeding after tonsillectomy is frequent swallowing; this occurs because blood drips down the back of the throat, tickling it. Other signs include frequent clearing of the throat and vomiting of bright red blood. Vomiting of dark blood may occur if the child swallowed blood during surgery, but this doesn't indicate postoperative bleeding. Breathing through the mouth is common because of dried secretions in the nares. Sleeping for long intervals is normal after receiving sedation and anesthesia. A pulse rate of 98 beats/minute is in the normal range for this age-group.

Critical thinking strategy: Review the postoperative management of a child after a tonsillectomy and the signs and symptoms of complications, which may be subtle.

Client needs category: Physiological integrity

Client needs subcategory: Reduction of risk potential

Cognitive level: Application

Integrated process: Nursing process/assessment

Reference: Pillitteri, pages 1248–1249

6. A 6-year-old child with complaints of fever, malaise, and anorexia is diagnosed with varicella (chickenpox). The nurse explains to the mother how skin lesions will develop. Place the following descriptions in the order that they will occur as the disease progresses. Use all of the options.

1. As initial lesions progress through stages, new lesions form on the trunk and extremities.

2. Papules develop into clear vesicles on an erythematous base.

3. Itchy red macules on the face, scalp, and trunk progress to papules.

4. Vesicles become cloudy and break easily.

5. Scabs form.

Rationale: Fever, malaise, and anorexia occur 24 to 48 hours before a rash develops. The rash begins as itchy red macules on the face, scalp, and trunk. These macules progress to papules, which develop into clear vesicles on an erythematous base. The vesicles become cloudy and break, forming scabs. New lesions continue to form on the trunk and extremities.

Critical thinking strategy: Focus on the pathophysiology of varicella, and review the stages and characteristics of lesions.

Client needs category: Physiological integrity

Client needs subcategory: Basic care and comfort

Cognitive level: Analysis

Integrated process: Teaching and learning

Reference: Pillitteri, pages 1359–1360

---

7. A nurse is teaching bicycle safety to a child and his parents. Indicate the part of the body that's most important to protect while riding a bicycle.

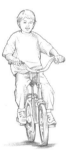

Answer:

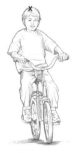

Rationale: Unprotected, the head is vulnerable to skull and brain injuries in the event of a bicycle accident. A well-fitting helmet can protect the head and is the most important safety feature for the nurse to stress to children and parents. According to the American Academy of Pediatrics, wearing a helmet correctly can prevent or lessen the severity of brain injuries resulting from bicycle crashes.

Critical thinking strategy: Focus on the types of bicycle-related head injuries, including skull fractures and brain damage from inertial force.

Client needs category: Safe and effective care environment

Client needs subcategory: Safety and infection control

Cognitive level: Application

Integrated process: Teaching and learning

Reference: Pillitteri, pages 892–893

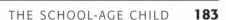

8. A 10-year-old child visits the pediatrician's office for his annual physical examination. When a nurse asks how he's doing, he becomes quiet and states that his grandmother died last week. Which statements by the child show that he understands the concept of death? Select all that apply.

☐ **1.** "Death is final."

☐ **2.** "All people must die."

☐ **3.** "My grandmother's death has been hard to understand."

☐ **4.** "My grandmother died because she was sick and nothing could make her better."

☐ **5.** "My grandmother is dead, but she'll come back."

☐ **6.** "My grandmother died because someone in the family did something bad."

Answer: 1, 3, 4

Rationale: By age 10, most children know that death is irreversible and final. However, a child may still have difficulty understanding the death of a specific loved one or understanding that children can die. School-age children should be able to identify cause-and-effect relationships, such as when a terminal illness causes someone to die. Adolescents, not school-age children, understand that death is a universal process. Preschoolers see death as temporary and may think of it as a punishment.

Critical thinking strategy: Focus on the cognitive stages of development for a school-age child, particularly with regard to coping with death.

Client needs category: Psychosocial integrity

Client needs subcategory: None

Cognitive level: Analysis

Integrated process: Caring

Reference: Pillitteri, pages 1776–1777

---

9. A child with sickle cell anemia is being treated for sickle cell crisis. The physician orders morphine sulfate (Duramorph) 2 mg I.V. The concentration of the vial is 10 mg/1 ml of solution. How many milliliters of solution should the nurse administer? Record your answer using one decimal place.

_____ milliliters

Answer: 0.2

Rationale: The nurse should calculate the volume to be given using this equation:

$$2 \text{ mg}/X \text{ ml} = 10 \text{ mg}/1 \text{ ml}$$

$$\frac{10 \text{ mg} \times X}{10 \text{ mg}} = \frac{2 \text{ mg} \times 1 \text{ ml}}{10 \text{ mg}}$$

$$X = 0.2 \text{ ml.}$$

Critical thinking strategy: Review the unit doses for medications and how to calculate fractional doses.

Client needs category: Physiological integrity

Client needs subcategory: Pharmacological and parenteral therapies

Cognitive level: Application/planning

Integrated process: Nursing process/planning

Reference: *Dosage Calculations Made Incredibly Easy,* pages 208–211

10. A 6-year-old boy arrives at the hospital for treatment of a medullablastoma. Indicate below where this tumor originated in his brain.

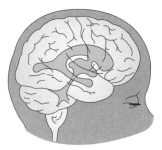

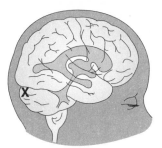

Rationale: A medullablastoma is a fast-growing, malignant tumor that originates in the cerebellum. It rarely spreads to other parts of the body but, when it does, it metastasizes to other parts of the brain or spinal cord. It's found more commonly in children than adults (peak age is 3 to 5 years), and it's more prevalent in boys than girls. The first symptoms are related to increased intracranial pressure (ICP) and include vomiting, visual disturbances, headaches, irritability, behavioral changes, fatigue, ataxia, muscle weakness, nystagmus, and speech problems. If the tumor blocks the ventricles, the increased ICP can lead to hydrocephalus, necessitating surgical placement of a shunt to drain excess cerebrospinal fluid. The treatment for medullabastoma includes surgery to remove the tumor, radiation, and/or chemotherapy.

Critical thinking strategy: Review the anatomy and physiology of the brain, focusing on the cerebellum.

Client needs category: Physiological integrity

Client needs subcategory: Physiological adaptation

Cognitive level: Application

Integrated process: Nursing process/analysis

Reference: Pillitteri, page 1704–1707

11. An 11-year-old girl comes into the physician's office complaining of dysuria. The nurse suspects a urinary tract infection. Which of the following findings on the laboratory report is consistent with a urinary tract infection?

Laboratory results

Test: Urinalysis
Date: 07/16/09   **Time collected:** 0700

Parameter	Results
Color	Pale yellow
Turbidity	Clear
pH	7.8
Specific gravity	1.015
Protein	Negative
Glucose	Positive
Ketones	Positive
Red blood cells	Less than 1 per high-power field
White blood cells	20 per high-power field
Casts	None

☐ **1.** White blood cells: 20 per high-power field

☐ **2.** pH 7.8

☐ **3.** Ketones: positive

☐ **4.** Glucose: positive

Answer: 1

Rationale: A normal urinalysis would show less than 5 white blood cells per high-power field. An elevated white blood cell count of 20 is an indication of bacteria and urinary tract infection. The normal range of urinary pH is 4.6 to 8.0. The presence of glucose or ketones in the urine doesn't indicate a urinary tract infection, but may indicate diabetes mellitus.

Critical thinking strategy: Recall the normal findings for a urinalysis.

Client needs category: Physiological integrity

Client needs subcategory: Reduction of risk potential

Cognitive level: Analysis

Integrated process: Nursing process/analysis

Reference: Craven, page 1084

---

12. A 10-year-old child has been admitted to the hospital with Reye's syndrome. Place the following findings in chronological order to show the clinical stages of Reye's syndrome. Use all of the options.

1. Flaccid paralysis
2. Coma
3. Vomiting
4. Presence of a viral infection
5. Deepened coma
6. Disorientation

Answer: 4, 3, 6, 2, 5, 1

Rationale: Reye's syndrome is an acute multisystem disorder that causes encephalopathy and predominately affects school-age children. Symptoms develop within a few days to weeks after a viral infection, beginning with vomiting, sleepiness, and liver dysfunction. About 24 to 48 hours after onset of symptoms, the child's condition rapidly deteriorates, causing disorientation, hallucinations, and sometimes a coma with decorticate posturing. The coma may progress to a deepened coma with decerebrate posturing and, eventually, flaccid paralysis. The majority of children who survive the acute stage of illness completely recover.

Critical thinking strategy: Review the clinical findings and deteriorating stages of Reye's syndrome.

Client needs category: Physiological integrity

Client needs subcategory: Reduction of risk potential

Cognitive level: Analysis

Integrated process: Nursing process/analysis

Reference: Pillitteri, page 1561

The adolescent

1. A nurse is caring for an adolescent girl who was admitted to the hospital's medical unit after attempting suicide by ingesting acetaminophen (Tylenol). Which interventions should the nurse incorporate into the client's care plan? Select all that apply.

☐ **1.** Limit care until the client initiates a conversation.

☐ **2.** Ask the client's parents if they keep firearms in their home.

☐ **3.** Ask the client if she's currently having suicidal thoughts.

☐ **4.** Assist the client with bathing and grooming as needed.

☐ **5.** Inspect the client's mouth after giving oral medications.

☐ **6.** Assure the client that anything she says will be held in strict confidence.

Answer: 2, 3, 4, 5

Rationale: Safety is the primary consideration when caring for suicidal clients. Because firearms are the most common method used in suicides, the client's parents should be taught to lock firearms and ammunition in separate locations and not give the client access to the keys. Safety also includes assessing for current suicidal ideation. Many suicidal people are depressed and don't have the energy to care for themselves, so the client may need assistance with bathing and grooming. Because depressed and suicidal clients may hide pills in their cheeks, the nurse should inspect the client's mouth after giving oral medications. Rather than limit care, the nurse should try to establish a trusting relationship through nursing interventions and therapeutic communication. The client can't be guaranteed confidentiality when self-destructive behavior is an issue.

Critical thinking strategy: Focus on the nursing care of the suicidal adolescent, remembering that safety is the priority.

Client needs category: Physiological integrity

Client needs subcategory: Reduction of risk potential

Cognitive level: Application

Integrated process: Caring

Reference: Pillitteri, pages 968–970

---

2. A nurse is teaching a 16-year-old female client with inflammatory bowel disease about her corticosteroid treatment. Which adverse effects are likely to be concerns for this client? Select all that apply.

☐ **1.** Acne

☐ **2.** Hirsutism

☐ **3.** Mood swings

☐ **4.** Osteoporosis

☐ **5.** Growth spurts

☐ **6.** Adrenal suppression

Answer: 1, 2, 3, 4, 6

Rationale: Adverse effects of corticosteroids include acne, hirsutism, mood swings, osteoporosis, and adrenal suppression. Steroid use in children and adolescents may cause delayed growth, not growth spurts.

Critical thinking strategy: Review the pharmacology of corticosteroids and how the adverse effects of corticosteroids relate to adolescents.

Client needs category: Physiological integrity

Client needs subcategory: Pharmacological and parenteral therapies

Cognitive level: Application

Integrated process: Teaching and learning

Reference: Smeltzer, pages 1484–1486

3. A nurse is caring for a 17-year-old female client with cystic fibrosis who has been admitted to the hospital for administration of I.V. antibiotics and respiratory treatment for exacerbation of a lung infection. The client has a number of questions about her future and the consequences of the disease. Which statements about the course of cystic fibrosis are true? Select all that apply.

☐ **1.** Breast development is commonly delayed.

☐ **2.** The client is at risk for developing diabetes.

☐ **3.** Pregnancy and childbearing aren't affected.

☐ **4.** Normal sexual relationships can be expected.

☐ **5.** Only males carry the gene for the disease.

☐ **6.** By age 20, the client should be able to decrease the frequency of respiratory treatment.

Answer: 1, 2, 4

Rationale: Cystic fibrosis delays growth and the onset of puberty. Children with cystic fibrosis tend to be smaller than average size and develop secondary sex characteristics later in life. In addition, they're at risk for developing diabetes mellitus because the pancreatic duct becomes obstructed as pancreatic tissues are destroyed. Clients with cystic fibrosis can expect to have normal sexual relationships, but thick secretions that obstruct the cervix and block sperm entry may impair fertility. Males and females carry the gene for cystic fibrosis. Pulmonary disease commonly progresses as the client ages, requiring additional respiratory treatment, not less.

Critical thinking strategy: Recall the pathophysiology of cystic fibrosis and its effect on the exocrine glands.

Client needs category: Physiological integrity

Client needs subcategory: Physiological adaptation

Cognitive level: Analysis

Integrated process: Teaching and learning

Reference: Pillitteri, pages 1269–1273

---

4. A nurse is preparing to administer the first dose of tobramycin (Nebcin) to an adolescent with cystic fibrosis. The order is for 3 mg/kg I.V. daily in three divided doses. The client weighs 99 lb. How many milligrams should the nurse administer per dose? Record your answer using a whole number.

_____ milliliters

Answer: 45

Rationale: To perform this dosage calculation, the nurse should first convert the client's weight to kilograms using this formula:

$$1 \text{ kg}/2.2 \text{ lb} = X \text{ kg}/99 \text{ lb}$$

$$\frac{2.2 \text{ lb} \times X}{2.2 \text{ lb}} = \frac{99 \text{ lb} \times 1 \text{ kg}}{2.2 \text{ lb}}$$

$$X = 45 \text{ kg.}$$

Then she should calculate the client's daily dose using this formula:

$$45 \text{ kg} \times 3 \text{ mg/kg} = 135 \text{ mg.}$$

Finally, the nurse should calculate the divided dose:

$$135 \text{ mg} \div 3 \text{ doses} = 45 \text{ mg/dose.}$$

Critical thinking strategy: Recall conversions based on body weight, and remember to calculate the dosage per day and then the dosage per each dose.

Client needs category: Physiological integrity

Client needs subcategory: Pharmacological and parenteral therapies

Cognitive level: Application

Integrated process: Nursing process/planning

Reference: *Dosage Calculations Made Incredibly Easy,* pages 267–270

---

5. A 14-year-old boy arrives in the emergency room complaining of abdominal pain with nausea and vomiting for the past 24 hours. The suspected diagnosis is appendicitis. Indicate below where the nurse would anticipate the area of sharpest pain would be during the assessment.

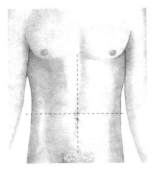

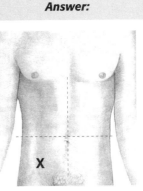

Rationale: Appendicitis typically begins with anorexia, nausea, and vomiting for the first 12 to 24 hours. Abdominal pain, a late sign, is usually diffuse at first and gradually localizes to the right lower quadrant. The sharpest pain should be noted at McBurney's point, which is one-third of the way between the anterior and superior iliac crest and the umbilicus.

Critical thinking strategy: Recall the anatomy of the gastrointestinal system and the organs within each of the abdominal quadrants.

Client needs category: Physiological integrity

Client needs subcategory: Reduction of risk potential

Cognitive level: Application

Integrated process: Nursing process/assessment

Reference: Pillitteri, page 1435

---

6. A 15-year-old boy with a history of asthma and chronic bronchitis is admitted to the hospital. The nurse documents the following assessment findings in the chart below. Which of the following conditions is the client most likely experiencing?

Progress notes

5/17/09	15-year-old male admitted with productive
1430	cough, hypoventilation, and limited chest
	expansion. Pt. is confused as to time and
	place with difficulty reorienting, and
	appears lethargic. VS: T. 103.4° F, P 88, RR
	16, BP 98/56. ABG results pH 7.1, PaCO₂ 50
	mm Hg, HCO₃⁻ 29 mEq/L. Dr. Lewis with Pt.
	now————————M. Burns, RN

- ☐ **1.** Metabolic acidosis
- ☐ **2.** Respiratory alkalosis
- ☐ **3.** Respiratory acidosis
- ☐ **4.** Metabolic alkalosis

Answer: 3

Rationale: Arterial blood gas analysis can determine the effectiveness of ventilation, information about oxygenation of the blood, and acid-base status. A pH less than 7.35, a partial pressure of arterial carbon dioxide ($PaCO_2$) greater than 45 mm Hg, and a bicarbonate (HCO_3^-) level of greater than 26 mEq/L indicate respiratory acidosis. A client with respiratory alkalosis would have a pH greater than 7.45 and a $PaCO_2$ less than 35 mm Hg. Metabolic acisdosis is characterized by a pH less than 7.35 and an HCO_3^- less than 22 mEq/L. Metabolic alkalosis is characterized by a pH greater than 7.45 and an HCO_3^- above 26 mEq/L.

Critical thinking strategy: Recall the normal findings of arterial blood gas levels.

Client needs category: Physiological integrity

Client needs subcategory: Physiological adaptation

Cognitive level: Analysis

Integrated process: Nursing process/analysis

Reference: Pillitteri, pages 1229–1230

7. The nurse knows that sexual maturation in adolescent boys normally follows a predictable timeline, with some individual variation. Place the following milestones in chronological order according to the development or appearance of secondary sex characteristics. Use all of the options.

| 1. Penile growth |
| 2. Voice changes |
| 3. Increase in height |
| 4. Spermatogenesis |
| 5. Growth of testes |
| 6. Growth of face, axillary, and pubic hair |

Rationale: Adolescence is the physiologic period that starts at the beginning of puberty and ends with the cessation of bodily growth. Development of secondary sex characteristics coincides with the growth and maturation of reproductive organs, which typically occurs at about age 12 to 14 in boys. The testosterone level is low in boys until puberty, at which time it increases to influence sexual maturation. The first signs are usually an increase in weight followed by testicular growth. This is followed by growth of pubic, axillary, and facial hair, accompanied by laryngeal enlargement and voice changes. The next stage is penile growth, then an increase in height, and finally sperm production.

Critical thinking strategy: Review the timeline of the development of male secondary sex changes.

Client needs category: Health promotion and maintenance

Client needs subcategory: None

Cognitive level: Application

Integrated process: Nursing process/analysis

Reference: Pillitteri, page 944

8. The nurse performs a physical examination on a 16-year-old male client and notes that he is short and underweight for his age. His history reveals that he's had type I diabetes mellitus since age 5. Place the following events in chronological order to describe the progression of disease that ultimately lead to his short stature and low weight. Use all of the options.

| 1. Breakdown of protein and fat |
| 2. Hyperglycemia |
| 3. Short stature, underweight |
| 4. Lack of insulin |
| 5. Glycosuria, electrolyte depletion |
| 6. Severe acidosis |

Rationale: Type I diabetes mellitus results from the inability of pancreatic islet cells to produce insulin. The body's cells need glucose to function and, when glucose can't enter the cells because of a lack of insulin, the glucose level builds up in the bloodstream (hyperglycemia). The kidneys then attempt to lower the level by excreting the excess glucose into the urine (glycosuria). The body also excretes large amounts of fluids (polyuria) while excreting the glucose. Potassium and phosphate pass from the body's cells into the bloodstream, causing electrolyte depletion. When the body can't use the gluocse for energy, the body resorts to breaking down protein and fat, resulting in an accumulation of ketone bodies, the acidic end products of fat breakdown. This leads to severe acidosis. Due to the large amounts of fat and protein used for energy, children generally remain short in stature and underweight.

Critical thinking strategy: Focus on the pathophysiology of diabetes mellitus and the consequences of lack of insulin.

Client needs category: Physiological integrity

Client needs subcategory: Physiological adaptation

Cognitive level: Analysis

Integrated process: Nursing process/analysis

Reference: Pillitteri, pages 1520–1521

PART SIX

Psychiatric and mental health nursing

Foundations of psychiatric nursing

1. A hospitalized client becomes angry and belligerent toward a nurse after speaking on the phone with his mother. The nurse learns that the mother can't visit as expected. Which interventions might the nurse use to help the client deal with his displaced anger? Select all that apply.

☐ **1.** Explore the client's unmet needs.

☐ **2.** Avoid the client until he apologizes.

☐ **3.** Suggest that the client direct his anger at his mother.

☐ **4.** Invite the client to a quiet place to talk.

☐ **5.** Assist the client in identifying alternate ways of approaching the problem.

Answer: 1, 4, 5

Rationale: Feelings of displacement or directing his anger toward the nurse need to be identified and understood by the client before the nurse can help guide him to choose appropriate actions. Avoiding the client or having him direct anger at another person is inappropriate. Approaching the client in a calm manner and offering to assist in the problem-solving process allows the client to identify needs that aren't being met and explore constructive ways of dealing with his anger.

Critical thinking strategy: Focus on the optimal therapeutic approach and effective anger management techniques.

Client needs category: Psychosocial integrity

Client needs subcategory: None

Cognitive level: Application

Integrated process: Caring

Reference: Boyd, pages 144–152

---

2. Electroconvulsive therapy (ECT) is an effective treatment for severe depression when which of the following conditions are present? Select all that apply.

☐ **1.** The client also has dementia.

☐ **2.** The client can't tolerate tricyclic antidepressants.

☐ **3.** The client lives in a long-term care facility.

☐ **4.** The client is undergoing a stressful life change.

☐ **5.** The client is having acute suicidal thoughts.

Answer: 2, 5

Rationale: ECT is used to treat acute depressive illnesses in an attempt to rapidly reverse a life-threatening situation, such as disturbing delusions, agitation, or attempted suicide. It's also used when the client can't tolerate tricyclic antidepressants, since other medication regimens for depression can take weeks to become effective. ECT usually isn't indicated for situational depression caused by intense stress. Clients with dementia aren't given ECT because ECT may further exacerbate cognitive impairment. The decision to use ECT isn't based on where the client lives.

Critical thinking strategy: Recall the major symptoms of depression and environmental factors that influence treatment for depression

Client needs category: Psychosocial integrity

Client needs subcategory: None

Cognitive level: Application

Integrated process: Nursing process/implementation

Reference: Boyd, page 361

3. A nurse knows that her initial approach to a rape victim should aim to decrease the client's anxiety. Which of the following interventions would be appropriate? Select all that apply.

☐ **1.** Admit the client to the treatment area right away.

☐ **2.** Encourage the client to undergo an examination immediately in order to get it behind her.

☐ **3.** Assure the client that she's safe in the examination room.

☐ **4.** Touch the client early on so that she knows the nurse is supportive.

☐ **5.** Allow a third party to be present if the client requests it.

☐ **6.** Ask "what" questions to determine the type of assault.

Answer: 1, 3, 5, 6

Rationale: Immediately admitting a rape victim to the treatment area may help her feel cared for and safe. Allowing a third party to remain with her, if requested, also increases her feeling of safety. "What" questions help to clarify events in a nonjudgmental way. At a time of great distress, the nurse should pace the interview and examination according to the client's level of comfort. Touching a client who has recently been assaulted may increase her anxiety. The nurse should wait for the client to initiate contact or ask permission prior to initiating physical contact.

Critical thinking strategy: Remember the client's physical and emotional needs after experiencing rape.

Client needs category: Psychosocial integrity

Client needs subcategory: None

Cognitive level: Application

Integrated process: Caring

Reference: Boyd, pages 844–846

---

4. A nurse is engaging in a therapeutic relationship with a client. Which of the following nursing actions are appropriate with this type of relationship? Select all that apply.

☐ **1.** Identify and meet the needs and specific desires of the client.

☐ **2.** Help the client explore different problem-solving techniques.

☐ **3.** Encourage the practice of new coping skills.

☐ **4.** Give advice to the client.

☐ **5.** Exchange personal information with the client.

☐ **6.** Discuss the client's feelings with her family members.

Answer: 2, 3

Rationale: The goal of a therapeutic relationship is to enhance the personal growth of the client. This is achieved by helping clients explore problem-solving techniques and develop coping skills. Giving advice, exchanging personal information, and striving to meet the personal needs and special desires of the client are characteristic of social relationships. Discussing the client's feelings with family members is a breach of confidentiality, unless previously approved by the client.

Critical thinking strategy: Focus on how the nurse assists the client to meet basic needs, and review therapeutic communication.

Client needs category: Psychosocial integrity

Client needs subcategory: None

Cognitive level: Analysis

Integrated process: Caring

Reference: Boyd, pages 137–142

5. A nurse is explaining the Bill of Rights for psychiatric patients to a client who has voluntarily sought admission to an inpatient psychiatric facility. Which of the following rights should the nurse include in the discussion? Select all that apply.

- ☐ **1.** Right to select health care team members
- ☐ **2.** Right to refuse treatment
- ☐ **3.** Right to a written treatment plan
- ☐ **4.** Right to obtain disability benefits
- ☐ **5.** Right to confidentiality
- ☐ **6.** Right to personal mail

Answer: 2, 3, 5, 6

Rationale: An inpatient client usually receives a copy of the Bill of Rights for psychiatric patients, which includes the right to refuse treatment, to have a written treatment plan, to have all her medical information kept confidential, and to receive mail. A client in an inpatient setting doesn't have the right to select health care team members. Although the client may apply for disability benefits as a result of a chronic or incapacitating illness, obtaining disability compensation isn't a patient right and members of a psychiatric institution don't decide who should receive it.

Critical thinking strategy: Review the rights of clients in hospitalized settings and the responsibilities of health care providers.

Client needs category: Psychosocial integrity

Client needs subcategory: None

Cognitive level: Application

Integrated process: Teaching and learning

Reference: Boyd, pages 21–26

---

6. In the emergency department, a client reveals to the nurse a lethal plan for committing suicide and agrees to a voluntary admission to the psychiatric unit. Which information should the nurse discuss with the client to answer the question "How long do I have to stay here?" Select all that apply.

- ☐ **1.** "You may leave the hospital at any time unless you're suicidal or homicidal or unable to meet your basic needs."
- ☐ **2.** "Let's talk more after the health care team has assessed you."
- ☐ **3.** "Once you've signed the papers, you have no say."
- ☐ **4.** "Because you could hurt yourself, you must be safe before being discharged."
- ☐ **5.** "You need a lawyer to help you make that decision."
- ☐ **6.** "There must be a court hearing before you can leave the hospital."

Answer: 1, 2, 4

Rationale: A person who is admitted to a psychiatric hospital may voluntarily sign out of the hospital unless the health care team determines that the person is harmful to himself or others. The health care team evaluates the client's condition before discharge. If there's reason to believe that the client may be harmful to himself or others, a hearing can be held to determine if the admission status should be changed from voluntary to involuntary. The client still has rights after committing himself to a psychiatric unit. The client doesn't need a lawyer to leave the hospital. A court hearing is held only if the client may pose a threat to himself or others and requires further treatment.

Critical thinking strategy: Focus on the factors that determine the length of stay.

Client needs category: Psychosocial integrity

Client needs subcategory: None

Cognitive level: Application

Integrated process: Teaching and learning

Reference: Boyd, pages 33–34

7. A nurse has developed a relationship with a client who has an addiction problem. Which actions would indicate that the therapeutic interaction is in the working phase? Select all that apply.

☐ **1.** The client discusses how the addiction has contributed to family distress.

☐ **2.** The client reluctantly shares the family history of addiction.

☐ **3.** The client verbalizes difficulty identifying personal strengths.

☐ **4.** The client discusses the financial problems related to the addiction.

☐ **5.** The client expresses uncertainty about what topic to discuss.

☐ **6.** The client acknowledges the addiction's effects on his children.

Answer: 1, 3, 4, 6

Rationale: Acknowledging the addiction's effects on the family and discussing its financial impact will help the client to identify personal strengths in dealing with addiction and strengthen the therapeutic relationship in the process. Discussing the family history of addiction and expressing uncertainty about what topics to address with the nurse typically happen during the introductory phase of a nurse-client relationship.

Critical thinking strategy: Focus on the dynamics occuring in the introductory phase of a therapeutic relationship.

Client needs category: Psychosocial integrity

Client needs subcategory: None

Cognitive level: Application

Integrated process: Caring

Reference: Boyd, pages 564–566

---

8. When psychiatric nurses intitiate therapeutic relationships with clients, they must be aware of client testing behaviors. Which of the following situations demonstrate testing behaviors from a client? Select all that apply.

☐ **1.** Placing the nurse in the role of parent

☐ **2.** Dressing in a flamboyant or seductive manner

☐ **3.** Requesting personal information from the nurse

☐ **4.** Following the contract established between the nurse and client

☐ **5.** Stating information to try to shock the nurse

☐ **6.** Violating the nurse's personal space

Answer: 1, 3, 5, 6

Rationale: A client will test the nurse-client relationship by acting in ways to control the relationship or to elicit an emotional response from the nurse. Examples of the testing behavior include speaking about things that will shock the nurse, violating personal space, requesting personal information, and placing the nurse in the role of parent. Dressing in a flamboyant or seductive manner demonstrates a lack of rules or expected behaviors; this is a violation of boundary setting. A contract is used to develop or negotiate an agreement between the nurse and the client to achieve a mutual goal.

Critical thinking strategy: Focus on what behaviors test the nurse's professional demeanor.

Client needs category: Psychosocial integrity

Client needs subcategory: None

Cognitive level: Analysis

Integrated process: Nursing process/analysis

Reference: Boyd, pages 148–151

Anxiety disorders

1. A nurse is caring for a client with agoraphobia. Which of the following signs and symptoms would the nurse expect to find in this client? Select all that apply.

☐ **1.** Hallucinations

☐ **2.** Panic attacks

☐ **3.** Inability to leave home

☐ **4.** Eating disorders

☐ **5.** Alcohol consumption

☐ **6.** Tobacco use

Answer: 2, 3

Rationale: Agoraphobia is characterized by extreme anxiety and a fear of being in open places. Panic attacks and an inability to leave home are symptoms associated with the disorder. No correlation exists between fear of open spaces and hallucinations, eating disorders, alcohol consumption, or tobacco use.

Critical thinking strategy: Focus on conditions that commonly occur with phobias or unrealistic fears.

Client needs category: Psychosocial integrity

Client needs subcategory: None

Cognitive level: Analysis

Integrated process: Nursing process/assessment

Reference: Boyd, pages 395–396

---

2. A client is being seen in the clinic after returning from military service abroad. The nurse is aware that posttraumatic stress disorder (PTSD) can be acute or chronic. Which of the following statements about PTSD are accurate? Select all that apply.

☐ **1.** PTSD is a syndrome that affects only those who have experienced traumatic episodes during war.

☐ **2.** PTSD is characterized by nightmares and flashbacks.

☐ **3.** Hypervigilance is characteristic of clients with PTSD.

☐ **4.** Substance abuse is a common coping mechanism used by clients with PTSD.

☐ **5.** Psychotic episodes can occur in clients with PTSD.

☐ **6.** Clients with PTSD may complain of feeling empty inside.

Answer: 2, 3, 4, 5, 6

Rationale: Although PTSD is commonly associated with combat, it can manifest itself after any kind of trauma. If symptoms occur within 6 months of the traumatic event, the disorder is considered acute. If symptoms occur more than 6 months after the traumatic event, PTSD is considered delayed or chronic. PTSD is characterized by nightmares or flashbacks. Clients are hypervigilant but typically describe themselves as "empty inside." Sometimes, the events can present as a psychotic episode. Substance abuse is a common "symptom" used for coping.

Critical thinking strategy: Recall the defining characteristics and clinical manifestions of PTSD.

Client needs category: Psychosocial integrity

Client needs subcategory: None

Cognitive level: Analysis

Integrated process: Nursing process/assessment

Reference: Boyd, pages 428–429

3. An 8-year-old child diagnosed with obsessive-compulsive disorder is admitted to a psychiatric facility. Which behaviors would a nurse assessing the client characterize as compulsions? Select all that apply.

☐ **1.** Checking and rechecking that the television is turned off before going to school

☐ **2.** Repeatedly washing the hands

☐ **3.** Brushing teeth three times per day

☐ **4.** Routinely climbing up and down a flight of stairs three times before leaving the house

☐ **5.** Feeding the dog the same meal every day

☐ **6.** Wanting to play the same video game each night

Answer: 1, 2, 4

Rationale: Compulsions involve symbolic rituals that relieve anxiety when they're performed. The disorder is caused by anxiety from obsessive thoughts, and acts are seen as irrational. Examples include repeatedly checking the television set, washing hands, or climbing stairs. An activity such as playing the same video game each night may be indicative of normal development for a school-age child. Frequent brushing of the teeth and feeding the dog a consistent meal aren't abnormal.

Critical thinking strategy: Focus on activities that are defined as compulsions.

Client needs category: Psychosocial integrity

Client needs subcategory: None

Cognitive level: Analysis

Integrated process: Nursing process/assessment

Reference: Boyd, pages 471–473

---

4. A client with the nursing diagnosis of *Fear related to being embarrassed in the presence of others* exhibits symptoms of social phobia. What nursing outcomes should the nurse establish for this client? Select all that apply.

☐ **1.** The client manages her fear in group situations.

☐ **2.** The client develops a plan to avoid situations that may cause stress.

☐ **3.** The client verbalizes feelings that occur in stressful situations.

☐ **4.** The client develops a plan for responding to stressful situations.

☐ **5.** The client denies feelings that may contribute to irrational fears.

☐ **6.** The client uses suppression to deal with underlying fears.

Answer: 1, 3, 4

Rationale: Improving stress management skills, verbalizing feelings, and anticipating and planning for stressful situations are adaptive responses to stress. Avoidance, denial, and suppression are maladaptive defense mechanisms.

Critical thinking strategy: Focus on actions that help the client cope with fear.

Client needs category: Psychosocial integrity

Client needs subcategory: None

Cognitive level: Application

Integrated process: Nursing process/planning

Reference: Boyd, page 428

5. A nurse recognizes improvement in a client with the nursing diagnosis of *Ineffective role performance related to the need to perform rituals.* Which of the following behaviors indicates improvement? Select all that apply.

☐ **1.** The client refrains from performing rituals during stress.

☐ **2.** The client says that he uses "thought stopping" when obsessive thoughts occur.

☐ **3.** The client verbalizes the relationship between stress and ritualistic behaviors.

☐ **4.** The client avoids stressful situations.

☐ **5.** The client rationalizes ritualistic behavior.

☐ **6.** The client performs ritualistic behaviors in private.

Answer: 1, 2, 3

Rationale: Refraining from performing rituals demonstrates that the client manages stress appropriately. Using "thought stopping" demonstrates the client's ability to employ appropriate interventions for obsessive thoughts. Verbalizing the relationship between stress and behaviors indicates that the client understands the disease process. Avoiding stressful situations and rationalizing or hiding ritualistic behaviors are maladaptive methods of managing stress and anxiety.

Critical thinking strategy: Focus on options that promote healthy behaviors.

Client needs category: Psychosocial integrity

Client needs subcategory: None

Cognitive level: Analysis

Integrated process: Nursing process/evaluation

Reference: Boyd, pages 471–472

---

6. A recent diagnosis of cancer has caused a client severe anxiety. Which of the following interventions should the nurse include in the care plan? Select all that apply.

☐ **1.** Maintain a calm, nonthreatening environment.

☐ **2.** Explain relevant aspects of chemotherapy.

☐ **3.** Encourage the client to verbalize her concerns regarding the diagnosis.

☐ **4.** Encourage the client to use deep-breathing exercises and other relaxation techniques during periods of increased stress.

☐ **5.** Provide distractions for the client during periods of stress.

☐ **6.** Teach the stages of grieving to the client.

Answer: 1, 3, 4

Rationale: During periods of acute stress, interventions that help the client regain control will help her to master this new threat. Providing a calm, nonthreatening environment and encouraging verbalization of concerns will help the client face the unknown. Relaxation techniques have a physiologic and psychological effect in calming the client, which in turn allows further exploration of thoughts and feelings as well as problem solving. The ability to learn is limited during extreme stress, so teaching the client about grief and chemotherapy wouldn't be effective at this stage. Providing distractions would be ineffective at this point in the grief process.

Critical thinking strategy: Focus on interventions that attempt to relieve stress and promote relaxation.

Client needs category: Psychosocial integrity

Client needs subcategory: None

Cognitive level: Application

Integrated process: Nursing process/implementation

Reference: Boyd, pages 222–234

7. The nurse is teaching a client diagnosed with a generalized anxiety disorder how to effectively cope with severe distress. Which interventions would the nurse use to promote effective coping with anxiety? Select all that apply.

- ☐ **1.** Discuss previous methods that were effective in handling stress.

- ☐ **2.** Encourage the client to limit the time spent worrying to only 15 minutes per day.

- ☐ **3.** Help the client to establish a goal and develop a plan to meet the goal.

- ☐ **4.** Teach the client how to label his feelings and how to express them.

- ☐ **5.** Examine ways to differentiate between realistic and unrealistic thoughts.

- ☐ **6.** Assist the client to acknowledge the major consequences of blaming others.

Answer: 1, 2, 3, 4

Rationale: To promote effective skills, the nurse should focus on having the client identify successful coping skills used in the past and on building on the client's knowledge of his disorder. Setting a limit on the amount of time spent worrying gives him boundaries and acknowledges his concerns. Establishing a goal and plan to meet the goal allows the client to engage in problem solving and exercise control over the stressful situation. Labeling and expressing feelings is a healthy way to acknowledge feelings. Clients with schizophrenia, not generalized anxiety disorder, require help with focusing on reality-based behaviors. Clients who demonstrate oppositional behavior tend to blame others instead of taking responsibility for their inappropriate behavior.

Critical thinking strategy: Focus on the defining characteristics and clinical manifestations of generalized anxiety disorder, and review coping skills.

Client needs category: Psychosocial integrity

Client needs subcategory: None

Cognitive level: Application

Integrated process: Teaching and learning

Reference: Boyd, pages 423–427

Mood, adjustment, and dementia disorders

1. A nurse is conducting a group session for children and adolescents who have been diagnosed with depression. Which of the following behaviors would a nurse expect to see in this group? Select all that apply.

- ☐ **1.** Delusions

- ☐ **2.** Anxiety

- ☐ **3.** Sadness

- ☐ **4.** Irritability

- ☐ **5.** Somatic symptoms, such as headache or stomachache

- ☐ **6.** Suicidal thoughts

Answer: 2, 4, 5, 6

Rationale: Children and adolescents with depression commonly experience anxiety and irritability (rather than sadness) as well as somatic symptoms. Suicide is a serious risk in these age-groups. These age-groups seldom experience psychotic symptoms. If psychotic symptoms do occur, they are more likely to be auditory hallucinations, not delusions.

Critical thinking strategy: Focus on the symptoms of child and adolescent depression.

Client needs category: Psychosocial integrity

Client needs subcategory: None

Cognitive level: Analysis

Integrated process: Nursing process/assessment

Reference: Boyd, pages 660–661

2. A nurse is caring for a client diagnosed with dysthymia. Which of the following defining characteristics are associated with this disorder? Select all that apply.

☐ **1.** Insomnia or hypersomnia

☐ **2.** Delusions or hallucinations

☐ **3.** Suicidal thoughts

☐ **4.** Onset of symptoms within a 2-week period

☐ **5.** Symptoms that occur in the winter and resolve in spring

☐ **6.** Appetite disturbance

Answer: 1, 3, 6

Rationale: Sleep and appetite disturbances and suicidal thoughts can appear in clients with dysthymia or major depressive disorders. Onset of symptoms are gradual and may appear over weeks or months. Delusions and other psychotic symptoms may occur in major depression but don't occur in dysthymia, a milder and more chronic mood disorder. Episodes of depression occurring solely in the winter are indicative of seasonal affective disorder.

Critical thinking strategy: Review the defining characteristics of dysthymia.

Client needs category: Psychosocial integrity

Client needs subcategory: None

Cognitive level: Analysis

Integrated process: Nursing process/assessment

Reference: Boyd, pages 349–350

---

3. A nurse is developing a care plan for a client with acute mania. Place the following behaviors according to the order in which they progress in a client with acute mania. Use all of the options.

1. Has delusions of grandeur
2. Uses relevant, calm speech patterns
3. Shows high productivity and competitive attitude in work and leisure activities
4. Becomes easily irritated
5. Demonstrates poor judgement and impulse control

Answer: 2, 3, 4, 5, 1

Rationale: Relevant and calm speech patterns are indicative of normal behavior. An early sign of dysphoria at the beginning of a manic episode is the client's lack of sleep. Since sleep isn't a priority, the client soon begins displaying a high level of productivity and competitiveness in work and leisure activities. As the mania increases, the client becomes more easily irritated and requires medication. The client demonstrates poor judgement and impulse control; therefore, client safety becomes a major concern. Lastly, the client becomes psychotic and has grandiose ideas that evolve into delusions of grandeur.

Critical thinking strategy: Recall the progression of behaviors of mania from mild to major.

Client needs category: Psychosocial integrity

Client needs subcategory: None

Cognitive level: Analysis

Integrated process: Nursing process/assessment

Reference: Boyd, pages 366–372

4. A physician prescribes lithium for a client diagnosed with bipolar disorder. Which of the following topics should a nurse cover when teaching the client? Select all that apply.

☐ **1.** Potential for addiction

☐ **2.** Signs and symptoms of drug toxicity

☐ **3.** Potential for tardive dyskinesia

☐ **4.** Importance of a low-tyramine diet

☐ **5.** Need to consistently monitor blood levels

☐ **6.** Amount of time that may be needed for mood changes to occur

Answer: 2, 5, 6

Rationale: Client education should cover the signs and symptoms of drug toxicity, the need to report them to the physician, and the need for regular monitoring of drug blood levels. The nurse should also inform the client that mood changes may not be apparent for 7 to 21 days after treatment is initiated. Lithium doesn't have addictive properties and doesn't cause tardive dyskinesia. Tyramine is a potential concern to clients who are also taking monoamine-oxidase inhibitors.

Critical thinking strategy: Remember that increased blood levels are related to increased side effects.

Client needs category: Physiological integrity

Client needs subcategory: Pharmacological and parenteral therapies

Cognitive level: Application

Integrated process: Teaching and learning

Reference: Boyd, pages 116–117, 372–375

---

5. After interviewing a client diagnosed with recurrent depression, a nurse determines the client's potential to commit suicide. Which of the factors listed below might contribute to the client's risk for suicide? Select all that apply.

☐ **1.** Psychomotor retardation

☐ **2.** Impulsive behaviors

☐ **3.** Overwhelming feelings of guilt

☐ **4.** Chronic, debilitating illness

☐ **5.** Decreased physical activity

☐ **6.** Repression of anger

Answer: 2, 3, 4, 6

Rationale: Impulsive behavior, overwhelming guilt, chronic illness, and repressed anger are factors that contribute to suicide potential. Psychomotor retardation and decreased physical activity are symptoms of depression, but they don't typically lead to suicide because the client doesn't have the energy and cognitive abilities to harm himself.

Critical thinking strategy: Recall the risk factors for suicide.

Client needs category: Psychosocial integrity

Client needs subcategory: None

Cognitive level: Analysis

Integrated process: Nursing process/analysis

Reference: Boyd, pages 349, 362

6. A nurse is assessing a client who talks freely about feeling depressed. During the interaction, the nurse hears the client state, "Things will never change." What other indications of hopelessness should the nurse look for? Select all that apply.

☐ **1.** Bouts of anger

☐ **2.** Periods of irritability

☐ **3.** Preoccupation with delusions

☐ **4.** Feelings of worthlessness

☐ **5.** Self-destructive behaviors

☐ **6.** Auditory hallucinations

Answer: 1, 2, 4, 5

Rationale: Clients who are depressed and feeling hopeless are often irritable and express inappropriate anger, feelings of worthlessness, and suicidal thoughts. In addition, they may demonstrate self-destructive behaviors. Preoccupation with delusions and auditory hallucinations is generally seen in clients with schizophrenia or other psychotic disorders rather than in those expressing hopelessness.

Critical thinking strategy: Focus on behaviors associated with hopelessness and depression.

Client needs category: Psychosocial integrity

Client needs subcategory: None

Cognitive level: Analysis

Integrated process: Nursing process/assessment

Reference: Boyd, page 262

---

7. A nurse interviews the family of a client hospitalized with severe depression and suicidal ideation. What family assessment information is essential to know when formulating an effective plan of care? Select all that apply.

☐ **1.** Physical pain

☐ **2.** Personal responsibilities

☐ **3.** Employment skills

☐ **4.** Communication patterns

☐ **5.** Role expectations

☐ **6.** Current family stressors

Answer: 4, 5, 6

Rationale: When working with the family of a depressed client, it's helpful for the nurse to be aware of the family's communication style, role expectations, and current family stressors. This information can help to identify family difficulties and teaching points that could benefit the client and the family. Information concerning physical pain, personal responsibilities, and employment skills wouldn't be helpful because these areas aren't directly related to their experience of having a depressed family member.

Critical thinking strategy: Focus on the family assessment, not assessment of the client.

Client needs category: Psychosocial integrity

Client needs subcategory: None

Cognitive level: Analysis

Integrated process: Nursing process/planning

Reference: Boyd, pages 364–365

8. A client is prescribed sertraline (Zoloft), a selective serotonin reuptake inhibitor. Which adverse effects would the nurse cover when creating a medication teaching plan? Select all that apply.

☐ **1.** Agitation

☐ **2.** Agranulocytosis

☐ **3.** Sleep disturbance

☐ **4.** Intermittent tachycardia

☐ **5.** Dry mouth

☐ **6.** Seizures

Answer: 1, 3, 5

Rationale: Common adverse effects of sertraline are agitation, sleep disturbance, and dry mouth. Agranulocytosis, intermittent tachycardia, and seizures are adverse effects of clozapine (Clozaril).

Critical thinking strategy: Review the side effects of serotonin reuptake inhibitors.

Client needs category: Physiological integrity

Client needs subcategory: Pharmacological and parenteral therapies

Cognitive level: Application

Integrated process: Teaching and learning

Reference: Boyd, page 120

---

9. A nurse is assessing a client for dementia. What history findings would the nurse expect to learn while talking with the client and her family? Select all that apply.

☐ **1.** The progression of symptoms has been slow.

☐ **2.** The client admits to feelings of sadness.

☐ **3.** The client acts apathetic and pessimistic.

☐ **4.** The family can't determine when the symptoms first appeared.

☐ **5.** The client has been exhibiting basic personality changes.

☐ **6.** The client has great difficulty paying attention to others.

Answer: 1, 4, 5, 6

Rationale: Dementia is characterized by a slow onset of symptoms, which makes it difficult to determine when symptoms first occurred. It progresses to noticeable changes in the individual's personality and impaired ability to pay attention to other people. Sadness, apathy, and pessimism are symptoms of depression.

Critical thinking strategy: Focus on the clinical manifestations of dementia and differentiate them from depression.

Client needs category: Health promotion and maintenance

Client needs subcategory: None

Cognitive level: Analysis

Integrated process: Nursing process/assessment

Reference: Boyd, pages 707–711

10. A client has been diagnosed with an adjustment disorder with mixed anxiety and depression. What are the primary nursing diagnoses the nurse would associate with this type of adjustment disorder? Select all that apply.

☐ **1.** Activity intolerance

☐ **2.** Impaired social interaction

☐ **3.** Risk for situational low self-esteem

☐ **4.** Disturbed personal identity

☐ **5.** Acute confusion

☐ **6.** Impaired memory

Answer: 2, 3

Rationale: A client with an adjustment disorder is likely to exhibit *Impaired social interaction* and *Risk for situational low self-esteem.* The other diagnoses listed aren't applicable to adjustment disorder.

Critical thinking strategy: Recall the defining characteristics of adjustment disorder, and focus on the client's anxiety and depression.

Client needs category: Psychosocial integrity

Client needs subcategory: None

Cognitive level: Analysis

Integrated process: Nursing process/analysis

Reference: Boyd, pages 393, 353–354

---

11. A nurse is preparing discharge instructions for a client with resistant depression who was prescribed a new medication regimen that includes phenelzine (Nardil). If the teaching was successful, which of the following foods should the client state he needs to avoid? Select all that apply.

☐ **1.** Aged cheese

☐ **2.** Cottage cheese

☐ **3.** Milk

☐ **4.** Wine

☐ **5.** Salami

☐ **6.** Fruit

Answer: 1, 4, 5

Rationale: Phenelzine is a monoamine oxidase inhibitor, which requires being on a tyramine-free diet to avoid hypertensive crisis. Aged cheese, salami, and wine will cause vasoconstriction and a rise in blood pressure. Cottage cheese, milk, and fruit are allowed on a tyramine-free diet.

Critical thinking strategy: Review the pharmacologic effects of monoamine oxidase inhibitors.

Client needs category: Physiological integrity

Client needs subcategory: Pharmacological and parenteral therapies

Cognitive level: Application

Integrated process: Teaching and learning

Reference: Boyd, pages 122–123

Psychotic disorders

1. A nurse is assessing a new client and notices clang associations in his speech pattern. This symptom is commonly seen in clients with which of the following disorders? Select all that apply.

☐ **1.** Dissociative identity disorder

☐ **2.** Schizophrenia

☐ **3.** Narcolepsy

☐ **4.** Mania

☐ **5.** Organic disorders

☐ **6.** Intermittent explosive disorder

Answer: 2, 4, 5

Rationale: This speech pattern, characterized by meaningless rhymes, is found most commonly in clients with schizophrenia but may also be present in those with bipolar disorder (during the manic phase) and organic disorders. It isn't characteristic of dissociative identity disorders, narcolepsy, or explosive disorders.

Critical thinking strategy: Focus on defining the term *clang associations.*

Client needs category: Psychosocial integrity

Client needs subcategory: None

Cognitive level: Analysis

Integrated process: Nursing process/assessment

Reference: Boyd, page 280

---

2. A nurse is monitoring a client who appears to be hallucinating. The client is gesturing at a figure on the television. He appears agitated and his speech contains paranoid content. Which nursing interventions are appropriate at this time? Select all that apply.

☐ **1.** In a firm voice, instruct the client to stop the behavior.

☐ **2.** Reassure the client that he's not in any danger.

☐ **3.** Acknowledge the presence of the hallucinations.

☐ **4.** Instruct other team members to ignore the client's behavior.

☐ **5.** Immediately implement physical restraints.

☐ **6.** Give simple commands in a calm voice.

Answer: 2, 3, 6

Rationale: Using a calm voice and giving simple commands, the nurse should reassure the client that he is safe. She shouldn't challenge the client; rather, she should acknowledge his hallucinatory experience. It isn't appropriate to ask the client to stop the behavior. Ignoring behavior won't reduce the client's agitation. Implementing restraints isn't warranted at this time. Although the client is agitated, he doesn't appear to be at risk for harming himself or others.

Critical thinking strategy: Focus on client safety and providing reassurance to the client.

Client needs category: Psychosocial integrity

Client needs subcategory: None

Cognitive level: Application

Integrated process: Nursing process/implementation

Reference: Boyd, page 724

3. A client with schizophrenia is taking the atypical antipsychotic medication clozapine (Clozaril). Which of the following signs and symptoms suggest that the client may be experiencing an adverse effect associated with this medication? Select all that apply.

☐ **1.** Sore throat

☐ **2.** Pill-rolling movements

☐ **3.** Polyuria

☐ **4.** Fever

☐ **5.** Polydipsia

☐ **6.** Orthostatic hypotension

Answer: 1, 4, 6

Rationale: Sore throat, fever, and the sudden onset of other flulike symptoms are signs of agranulocytosis, an adverse effect of clozapine. The condition is caused by a deficiency of granulocytes (a type of white blood cell), which causes the individual to be susceptible to infection. The client's white blood cell count should be monitored at least weekly during clozapine treatment. Orthostatic hypotension may occur with initial use of the drug. Dizziness upon standing with or without fainting can also occur during clozapine treatment. Extrapyramidal effects (such as pill-rolling) either don't occur or occur at a much lesser rate with the atypical antipsychotic medications. Polydipsia (excessive thirst) and polyuria (increased urination) are common adverse effects of lithium.

Critical thinking strategy: Review the adverse effects of antipsychotic medications.

Client needs category: Physiological integrity

Client needs subcategory: Pharmacological and parenteral therapies

Cognitive level: Application

Integrated process: Nursing process/evaluation

Reference: Boyd, pages 301–302

---

4. A delusional client says to a nurse "I am the Easter bunny," and insists that the nurse refer to him as such. The belief appears to be fixed and unchanging. Which of the following nursing interventions should the nurse implement when working with this client? Select all that apply.

☐ **1.** Consistently use the client's name in interactions.

☐ **2.** Smile at the humor of the situation.

☐ **3.** Agree that the client is the Easter bunny.

☐ **4.** Logically point out why the client couldn't be the Easter bunny.

☐ **5.** Provide an as-needed medication.

☐ **6.** Provide the client with structured activities.

Answer: 1, 6

Rationale: This client needs continuous reality-based orientation, so the nurse should use the client's name in all interactions. Structured activities can help the client refocus and resolve his delusion. The nurse shouldn't contribute to the delusion by smiling at the comment or agreeing with the client. Logical arguments and an as-needed medication aren't likely to change the client's beliefs.

Critical thinking strategy: Review communication methods and focus on delusional thinking.

Client needs category: Psychosocial integrity

Client needs subcategory: None

Cognitive level: Application

Integrated process: Nursing process/implementation

Reference: Boyd, pages 340–341

5. A physician starts a client on the antipsychotic medication haloperidol (Haldol). The nurse is aware that this medication produces extrapyramidal adverse effects. Which measures should the nurse take while the client is receiving this drug? Select all that apply.

- ☐ **1.** Review subcutaneous injection technique.
- ☐ **2.** Closely monitor vital signs, especially temperature.
- ☐ **3.** Observe for increased pacing and restlessness.
- ☐ **4.** Monitor blood glucose levels.
- ☐ **5.** Provide the client with hard candy.
- ☐ **6.** Monitor for signs and symptoms of urticaria.

Rationale: Neuroleptic malignant syndrome is a life-threatening extrapyramidal adverse effect of antipsychotic medications such as haloperidol. It's associated with a rapid increase in temperature. The most common extrapyramidal adverse effect, akathisia, is a form of psychomotor restlessness that's often exhibited as pacing. Haloperidol and the anticholinergic medications that are provided to alleviate its extrapyramidal effects can result in dry mouth. Providing the client with hard candy to suck on can help alleviate this problem. Haloperidol isn't given subcutaneously and doesn't affect blood glucose levels. Urticaria isn't usually associated with haloperidol administration.

Critical thinking strategy: Recall that extrapyramidal effects are associated with abnormal motor movement.

Client needs category: Physiological integrity

Client needs subcategory: Pharmacological and parenteral therapies

Cognitive level: Analysis

Integrated process: Nursing process/planning

Reference: Boyd, pages 113–115

---

6. When teaching a group of students in a psychiatric assistant class about the use of antipsychotic medications, the nurse advises them that certain symptoms can occur within the first few weeks of treatment. Which symptoms are likely to occur? Select all that apply.

- ☐ **1.** Acute dystonic reactions
- ☐ **2.** Akathisia
- ☐ **3.** Tardive dyskinesia
- ☐ **4.** Neuroleptic malignant syndrome
- ☐ **5.** Hearing loss
- ☐ **6.** Orthostatic hypotension

Rationale: Acute dystonia, akathisia, neuroleptic malignant syndrome, and orthostatic hypotension can occur during the first few weeks of treatment with antipsychotic drugs. Tardive dyskinesia doesn't typically occur until at least 6 months after starting treatment. Hearing loss isn't an adverse effect of antipsychotic drugs.

Critical thinking strategy: Review the adverse effects of the different classes of antipsychotic medications.

Client needs category: Psychosocial integrity

Client needs subcategory: None

Cognitive level: Analysis

Integrated process: Teaching and learning

Reference: Boyd, pages 111–116

7. A nurse is working with a schizophrenic client who suddenly begins experiencing auditory hallucinations. Place the following interventions in the order that best prevents exacerbation of the client's anxiety. Use all of the options.

1. Ask the client, "What are you experiencing right now?"

2. Encourage the client to relate the history of his hallucinations.

3. Tell the client, "I'd like to spend time with you to discuss your hallucinations. Is that okay with you?"

4. Ask the client if he has recently taken any drugs or alcohol.

Answer: 3, 1, 4, 2

Rationale: Asking the client if he'll discuss the hallucinations promotes trust, an essential first step in communicating with hallucinating clients. When the client relates his hallucinations, the nurse should observe for nonverbal cues, such as the client's eyes looking around the room. Asking the client about these observations will help promote understanding of the symptoms, increase trust, and decrease the client's perception that the nurse can read his mind. Asking the client if he has recently taken drugs or alcohol helps determine the source of the current experience. Once trust is established, the client will be more comfortable discussing the history of his hallucinations, such as when the voices started. This step will be beneficial in helping him manage in the present.

Critical thinking strategy: Focus on actions that build a therapeutic relationship.

Client needs category: Psychosocial integrity

Client needs subcategory: None

Cognitive level: Application

Integrated process: Nursing process/implementation

Reference: Boyd, pages 290–296.

---

8. A client who is taking medication to control his schizophrenia asks the nurse to explain the causes of the disorder. The nurse knows that an overactive dopamine system in the brain is one of the leading causes of schizophrenia and tells the client that excessive dopamine activity is responsible for his symptoms. Which symptoms is she referring to? Select all that apply.

☐ **1.** Hallucinations

☐ **2.** Withdrawn behavior

☐ **3.** Grandiosity

☐ **4.** Delusional thinking

☐ **5.** Excessive tearfulness

☐ **6.** Hypotension

Answer: 1, 3, 4

Rationale: Hallucinations, grandiosity, and delusional thinking are attributable to the effects of excessive dopamine activity. Withdrawn behavior isn't associated with dopamine. Excessive tearfulness and hypotension aren't commonly associated with schizophrenia or dopamine activity.

Critical thinking strategy: Focus on the effects of dopamine on the brain, and review the signs and symptoms of schizophrenia.

Client needs category: Psychosocial integrity

Client needs subcategory: None

Cognitive level: Analysis

Integrated process: Teaching and learning

Reference: Boyd, pages 281–289

9. A client with a diagnosis of undifferentiated schizophrenia is admitted to the inpatient unit after developing water intoxication. Which of the following nursing interventions are appropriate? Select all that apply.

☐ **1.** Medicate the client at night.

☐ **2.** Provide gum for the client.

☐ **3.** Lock the unit's kitchen and bathroom.

☐ **4.** Weigh the client every day.

☐ **5.** Monitor the client's intake and output.

☐ **6.** Maintain a structured environment.

Answer: 2, 4, 5, 6

Rationale: It's appropriate for the nurse to monitor intake and output, weigh the client daily, and encourage the client to chew gum rather than drink water. The nurse also provides a structured environment as a way to distract and divert the client away form obtaining fluids. Medicating the client at night and locking the unit's kitchen and bathroom shouldn't be necessary.

Critical thinking strategy: Remember that nursing actions must be appropriate and realistic.

Client needs category: Physiological integrity

Client needs subcategory: Reduction of risk potenital

Cognitive level: Application

Integrated process: Nursing process/implementation

Reference: Boyd, pages 283–284

Substance abuse, eating disorders, and impulse control disorders

1. During her assessment of a client who has been diagnosed with bulimia nervosa, the nurse knows to check for certain characteristics that accompany binge eating. Indentify the characteristics that are most applicable. Select all that apply.

☐ **1.** Guilt

☐ **2.** Dental caries

☐ **3.** Self-induced vomiting

☐ **4.** Weight loss

☐ **5.** Normal weight

☐ **6.** Introverted behavior

Answer: 1, 2, 3, 5

Rationale: Guilt, dental caries, self-induced vomiting, and normal weight are associated with bulimia nervosa. Weight loss and introverted behavior are associated with anorexia nervosa.

Critical thinking strategy: Review bulimia nervosa, and remember that binge eating is often followed by purging or other compensatory behaviors.

Client needs category: Psychosocial integrity

Client needs subcategory: None

Cognitive level: Analysis

Integrated process: Nursing process/assessment

Reference: Boyd, pages 526–528

2. Clients with opioid addiction who are in withdrawal typically present with which of the following signs and symptoms? Select all that apply.

☐ **1.** Abdominal cramps

☐ **2.** Dry, warm skin

☐ **3.** Rhinorrhea

☐ **4.** Dilated pupils

☐ **5.** Hypersomnia

☐ **6.** Feelings of hunger

Answer: 1, 3, 4

Rationale: Opioid withdrawal commonly manifests as abdominal cramps, rhinorrhea, dilated pupils, and anorexia (not hunger). Insomnia (not hypersomnia), and diaphoresis (not dry, warm skin), are also common.

Critical thinking strategy: Focus on the withdrawal effects of opioids on the various body systems.

Client needs category: Physiological integrity

Client needs subcategory: Pharmacological and parenteral therapies

Cognitive level: Analysis

Integrated process: Nursing process/assessment

Reference: Boyd, page 553

---

3. During her shift in the emergency department, a nurse assesses a client who may be under the influence of amphetamines. Which of the following symptoms are indicative of amphetamine use? Select all that apply.

☐ **1.** Depressed affect

☐ **2.** Diaphoresis

☐ **3.** Shallow respirations

☐ **4.** Hypotension

☐ **5.** Tremors

☐ **6.** Dilated pupils

Answer: 2, 3, 5, 6

Rationale: A client under the influence of amphetamines may present with euphoria, diaphoresis, shallow respirations, dilated pupils, dry mouth, anorexia, tachycardia, hypertension, hyperthermia, tremors, seizures, and altered mental status. Depressed affect and hypotension aren't associated with amphetamine use.

Critical thinking strategy: Recall the overall effect of amphetamines on the body.

Client needs category: Physiological integrity

Client needs subcategory: Pharmacological and parenteral therapies

Cognitive level: Application

Integrated process: Nursing process/assessment

Reference: Boyd, page 542

4. A nurse is caring for an anorexic client with a nursing diagnosis of *Imbalanced nutrition: Less than body requirements related to dysfunctional eating patterns.* Which of the following interventions would be supportive for this client? Select all that apply.

☐ **1.** Provide small, frequent meals.

☐ **2.** Monitor weight gain.

☐ **3.** Allow the client to skip meals until the antidepressant levels are therapeutic.

☐ **4.** Encourage the client to keep a journal.

☐ **5.** Monitor the client during meals and for 1 hour afterward.

☐ **6.** Encourage the client to eat three substantial meals per day.

Answer: 1, 2, 4, 5

Rationale: Because they're engaged in self-starvation, clients with anorexia rarely can tolerate large meals three times per day. Small, frequent meals may be tolerated better and they provide a way to gradually increase daily caloric intake. The nurse should monitor the client's weight carefully because a client with anorexia may try to hide her weight loss. The nurse should also monitor the client during meals and for 1 hour afterward to ensure that she consumes all of her food and doesn't attempt to purge. The client may be afraid to express her feelings; keeping a journal can serve as an outlet for these feelings, which can assist recovery. A client with anorexia is already underweight and shouldn't be permitted to skip meals.

Critical thinking strategy: Focus on the goal of gaining weight and how it's best achieved.

Client needs category: Psychosocial integrity

Client needs subcategory: None

Cognitive level: Analysis

Integrated process: Caring

Reference: Boyd, pages 517–525

---

5. When assessing a client diagnosed with impulse control disorder, the nurse observes violent, aggressive, and assaultive behavior. Which assessment data is the nurse also likely to find? Select all that apply.

☐ **1.** The client functions well in other areas of his life.

☐ **2.** The degree of aggressiveness is out of proportion to the stressor.

☐ **3.** The violent behavior is usually justified by a stressor.

☐ **4.** The client has a history of parental alcoholism and a chaotic, abusive family life.

☐ **5.** The client has no remorse about the inability to control his behavior.

Answer: 1, 2, 4

Rationale: A client with an impulse control disorder who displays violent, aggressive, and assaultive behavior generally functions well in other areas of his life. The degree of aggressiveness is out of proportion to the stressor, and he frequently has a history of parental alcoholism and a chaotic family life. The client often verbalizes sincere remorse and guilt for the aggressive behavior.

Critical thinking strategy: Remember this disorder is characterized by irresistible impulsivity.

Client needs category: Psychosocial integrity

Client needs subcategory: None

Cognitive level: Application

Integrated process: Nursing process/assessment

Reference: Boyd, page 474

6. A nurse is caring for a client with borderline personality disorder. Which of the following interventions are appropriate for clients with this disorder? Select all that apply.

- ☐ **1.** Providing antianxiety medications
- ☐ **2.** Providing emotional consistency
- ☐ **3.** Exploring anger in appropriate ways
- ☐ **4.** Encouraging independence as soon as possible
- ☐ **5.** Promoting gradual separation and individuation
- ☐ **6.** Ensuring the client's safety

Answer: 2, 3, 5, 6

Rationale: In clients with borderline personalities, the primary goal is to ensure a safe environment. As the client begins to learn how to manage his behavior, suicide still remains a risk. A key intervention includes providing emotional support that's consistent. The client needs to learn how to manage anger effectively and typically begins needing less support as he separates and develops his individual coping behaviors. Antianxiety drugs are reserved for clinical emergencies.

Critical thinking strategy: Focus on interventions that feature client safety and behavior management.

Client needs category: Psychosocial integrity

Client needs subcategory: None

Cognitive level: Application

Integrated process: Nursing process/implementation

Reference: Boyd, pages 448–457

---

7. A client is prescribed chlordiazepoxide (Librium) as needed to control the symptoms of alcohol withdrawal. Which of the following symptoms may indicate the need for an additional dose of this medication? Select all that apply.

- ☐ **1.** Tachycardia
- ☐ **2.** Mood swings
- ☐ **3.** Elevated blood pressure and temperature
- ☐ **4.** Piloerection
- ☐ **5.** Tremors
- ☐ **6.** Increasing anxiety

Answer: 1, 3, 5, 6

Rationale: Benzodiazepines such as chlordiazepoxide are usually administered based on elevations in heart rate, blood pressure, and temperature as well as on the presence of tremors and increasing anxiety. Mood swings are expected during the withdrawal period and aren't an indication for further medication administration. Piloerection (goosebumps, or a feeling of hair of the skin standing on end) isn't a symptom of alcohol withdrawal.

Critical thinking strategy: Review the clinical manifestations of alcohol withdrawal.

Client needs category: Physiological integrity

Client needs subcategory: Pharmacological and parenteral therapies

Cognitive level: Analysis

Integrated process: Nursing process/evaluation

Reference: Boyd, pages 123, 545

8. The nurse is assessing a 25-year-old man who is a polysubstance abuser, with cocaine being his drug of choice. Which of the following physiological symptoms is suggestive of cocaine intoxication? Select all that apply.

☐ **1.** Respiratory depression

☐ **2.** Psychomotor agitation

☐ **3.** Cardiac arrhythmias

☐ **4.** Dilated pupils

☐ **5.** Projectile vomiting

☐ **6.** Slurred speech

Rationale: The most common physiological symptoms observed in a client experiencing cocaine intoxication are respiratory depression, cardiac arrhythmias, psychomotor agitation, and dilated pupils. Projectile vomiting and slurred speech aren't associated with cocaine intoxication.

Critical thinking strategy: Remember that cocaine intoxication tends to affect the central nervous system.

Client needs category: Physiological integrity

Client needs subcategory: Physiological adaptation

Cognitive level: Analysis

Integrated process: Nursing process/evaluation

Reference: Boyd, pages 547–548

PART SEVEN

Comprehensive tests

Comprehensive test 1

1. Which action should a nurse take when administering a new blood pressure medication to a client?

☐ **1.** Administer the medication to the client without explanation.

☐ **2.** Inform the client about the new medication only if he asks about it.

☐ **3.** Inform the client about the new medication, including its name, use, and the reason for the change in medication.

☐ **4.** Administer the medication, and inform the client that the physician will later explain the medication.

Answer: 3

Rationale: It's important for the nurse to inform the client about the medication, including its name, use, and the reason for the medication change, because teaching the client about his treatment regimen promotes compliance. The other responses are inappropriate.

Critical thinking strategy: Recall that explaining new medications helps with compliance and preventing errors.

Client needs category: Safe, effective care environment

Client needs subcategory: Management of care

Cognitive level: Application

Integrated process: Teaching and learning

---

2. A client arrives at the emergency department with chest and stomach pain and a report of black, tarry stools for several months. Which order should the nurse anticipate?

☐ **1.** Cardiac monitor, oxygen, creatine kinase, and lactate dehydrogenase (LD) levels

☐ **2.** Prothrombin time (PT), partial thromboplastin time (PTT), fibrinogen, and fibrin split product values

☐ **3.** ECG, complete blood count, testing for occult blood, and comprehensive serum metabolic panel

☐ **4.** EEG, alkaline phosphatase and aspartate aminotransferase levels, and basic serum metabolic panel

---

Answer: 3

Rationale: An ECG evaluates the complaint of chest pain, laboratory tests determine anemia, and the test for occult blood determines blood in the stool. Cardiac monitoring, oxygen, and creatine kinase and LD levels are appropriate for a primary cardiac problem. A basic metabolic panel and alkaline phosphatase and aspartate aminotransferase levels assess liver function. PT, PTT, fibrinogen, and fibrin split products are measured to verify bleeding dyscrasias. An EEG evaluates brain electrical activity.

Critical thinking strategy: Recall the possible causes of the described symptoms

Client needs category: Physiological integrity

Client needs subcategory: Reduction of risk potential

Cognitive level: Analysis

Integrated process: Nursing process/planning

3. Following the initial care of a client with asthma and impending anaphylaxis from hypersensitivity to a drug, the nurse should take which emergency treatment step next?

☐ **1.** Administer beta-adrenergic blockers.

☐ **2.** Administer bronchodilators.

☐ **3.** Obtain serum electrolyte levels.

☐ **4.** Have the client lie flat in the bed.

Rationale: Bronchodilators would help open the client's airway and improve his oxygenation status. Beta-adrenergic blockers aren't indicated in the management of asthma because they may cause bronchospasm. Obtaining laboratory values wouldn't be done on an emergency basis, and having the client lie flat in bed could worsen his ability to breathe.

Critical thinking strategy: Remember the ABCs of emergency care, and determine which step would best accomplish this.

Client needs category: Physiological integrity

Client needs subcategory: Physiological adaptation

Cognitive level: Analysis

Integrated process: Nursing process/implementation

---

4. A 19-year-old client with a mild concussion is discharged from the emergency department. Before discharge, he complains of a headache. When offered acetaminophen, his mother tells the nurse the headache is severe and she would like her son to have something stronger. Which response by the nurse is appropriate?

☐ **1.** "Your son had a mild concussion; acetaminophen is strong enough."

☐ **2.** "Maybe the physician will prescribe aspirin instead."

☐ **3.** "Opioids are avoided after a head injury because they may hide a worsening condition."

☐ **4.** "Stronger medications may lead to vomiting, which increases the intracranial pressure (ICP)."

Rationale: Opioids may mask changes in the level of consciousness (LOC) that indicate increased ICP; therefore, it shouldn't be given. Saying acetaminophen is strong enough ignores the mother's question and, therefore, isn't appropriate. Aspirin is contraindicated in conditions that may involve bleeding, such as traumatic injuries, and for children or young adults with viral illnesses due to the danger of Reye's syndrome. Stronger medications may not necessarily lead to vomiting but will sedate the client, thereby masking changes in his LOC.

Critical thinking strategy: Determine the relationship between analgesics and the changes in level of consciousness following a concussion.

Client needs category: Physiological integrity

Client needs subcategory: Reduction of risk potential

Cognitive level: Application

Integrated process: Teaching and learning

5. Clients with osteoarthritis may be on bed rest for prolonged periods. Which nursing interventions would be appropriate for these clients?

☐ **1.** Encourage coughing and deep breathing, and limit fluid intake.

☐ **2.** Provide only passive range of motion (ROM), and decrease stimulation.

☐ **3.** Have the client lie as still as possible, and give adequate pain medication.

☐ **4.** Turn the client every 2 hours, and encourage coughing and deep breathing.

Answer: 4

Rationale: Appropriate interventions for a bedridden client include turning every 2 hours, providing adequate nutrition, and encouraging coughing and deep breathing. Hydration, active and passive ROM, and adequate pain medication are also appropriate nursing measures. To prevent contractures, the client shouldn't limit his fluid intake or lie as still as possible.

Critical thinking strategy: Focus on the effects of bed rest on different body systems.

Client needs category: Safe, effective care environment

Client needs subcategory: Management of care

Cognitive level: Application

Integrated process: Nursing process/implementation

---

6. A nurse is providing nutritional teaching for a client with a family history of colon cancer. Which food choice by the client demonstrates that he understands the correct diet to follow?

☐ **1.** Vegetarian chili

☐ **2.** Hot dogs and sauerkraut

☐ **3.** Egg salad on rye bread

☐ **4.** Spaghetti and meat sauce

Answer: 1

Rationale: A high-fiber, low-fat food, such as vegetarian chili, increases gastric motility and decreases the chance of constipation, helping to reduce the risk of colon cancer. The other choices aren't representative of a high-fiber, low-fat diet.

Critical thinking strategy: Recall dietary guidelines for preventing colon cancer.

Client needs category: Health promotion and maintenance

Client needs subcategory: None

Cognitive level: Application

Integrated process: Teaching and learning

7. Adequate fluid replacement, vasopressin replacement, and correction of underlying intracranial pathology are objectives of therapy for which disease process?

☐ **1.** Diabetes mellitus

☐ **2.** Diabetes insipidus

☐ **3.** Diabetic ketoacidosis

☐ **4.** Syndrome of inappropriate antidiuretic hormone secretion (SIADH)

Rationale: Maintaining adequate fluid, replacing vasopressin, and correcting underlying intracranial problems (typically lesions, tumors, or trauma affecting the hypothalamus or pituitary gland) are the main objectives in treating diabetes insipidus. Diabetes mellitus doesn't involve vasopressin deficiencies or an intracranial disorder, but rather a disturbance in the production or use of insulin. Diabetic ketoacidosis results from severe insulin insufficiency. An excess of vasopressin leads to SIADH, causing the client to retain fluid.

Critical thinking strategy: Focus on pathologies that can lead to disturbances with body fluids and vasopressin release, and review endocrine disorders.

Client needs category: Physiological integrity

Client needs subcategory: Pharmacological and parenteral therapies

Cognitive level: Analysis

Integrated process: Nursing process/analysis

---

8. In which group is it most important for a client to understand the importance of an annual Papanicolaou test?

☐ **1.** Clients with a history of recurrent candidiasis

☐ **2.** Clients who were pregnant before age 20

☐ **3.** Clients infected with the human papillomavirus (HPV)

☐ **4.** Clients with a long history of oral contraceptive use

Rationale: HPV causes genital warts, which are associated with an increased incidence of cervical cancer. Recurrent candidiasis, pregnancy before age 20, and use of oral contraceptives don't increase the risk of cervical cancer.

Critical thinking strategy: Recall the diagnostic findings associated with a Papanicolaou test.

Client needs category: Health promotion and maintenance

Client needs subcategory: None

Cognitive level: Analysis

Integrated process: Nursing process/analysis

9. Which instruction should the nurse give to a client taking nystatin (Mycostatin) oral solution?

☐ **1.** Take the drug right after meals.

☐ **2.** Take the drug right before meals.

☐ **3.** Mix the drug with small amounts of food.

☐ **4.** Take half the dose before and half after a meal.

Rationale: Nystatin oral solution should be swished around the mouth after eating for the best contact with mucous membranes. Taking the drug before or with meals doesn't allow for optimal contact with mucous membranes.

Critical thinking strategy: Focus on the reason for using this medication.

Client needs category: Physiological integrity

Client needs subcategory: Pharmacological and parenteral therapies

Cognitive level: Application

Integrated process: Teaching and learning

---

10. A newly admitted client is extremely hostile toward a staff member he has just met, without apparent reason. According to Freudian theory, the nurse should suspect that the client is exhibiting which phenomena?

☐ **1.** Intellectualization

☐ **2.** Transference

☐ **3.** Triangulation

☐ **4.** Splitting

Rationale: Transference is the unconscious assignment of negative or positive feelings evoked by a significant person in the client's past to another person. Intellectualization is a defense mechanism in which the client avoids dealing with emotions by focusing on facts. Triangulation refers to conflicts involving three family members. Splitting is a defense mechanism commonly seen in clients with personality disorders in which the world is perceived as all good or all bad.

Critical thinking strategy: Recall the characteristics of defense mechanisms and relate them to the behaviors described.

Client needs category: Psychosocial integrity

Client needs subcategory: None

Cognitive level: Analysis

Integrated process: Nursing process/analysis

11. After repeated office visits, physical examinations, and diagnostic tests for assorted complaints, a client is referred to a psychiatrist. The client later tells a friend, "I can't imagine why my doctor wants me to see a psychiatrist." Which statement is the most likely explanation for the client's statement?

☐ **1.** The client probably believes psychiatrists are only for "crazy" people.

☐ **2.** The client probably doesn't understand the correlation of symptoms and stress.

☐ **3.** The client probably believes his physician has made an error in diagnosis.

☐ **4.** The client probably believes his physician wants to get rid of him as a client.

Answer: 3

Rationale: The client with hypochondriasis is preoccupied with bodily functions or physical sensations. Despite repeated physical examinations, diagnostic tests, and reassurance from physicians, he continues to have concerns about bodily disease. Consequently, the hypochondriac client typically believes that physicians and other health care professionals have poor insight whenever they view his concern about having a serious illness as excessive or unreasonable. The other responses aren't valid.

Critical thinking strategy: Remember to choose an answer that best explains the thought process of a client with hypochondriasis.

Client needs category: Psychosocial integrity

Client needs subcategory: None

Cognitive level: Analysis

Integrated process: Caring

---

12. A client at 42 weeks' gestation is 3 cm dilated and 30% effaced, with membranes intact and the fetus at +2 station. Fetal heart rate (FHR) is 140 beats/minute. After 2 hours, the nurse notes that, for the past 10 minutes, the external fetal monitor has been displaying a FHR of 190 beats/minute. The client states that her baby has been extremely active. Uterine contractions are strong, occurring every 3 to 4 minutes and lasting 40 to 60 seconds. Which finding would indicate fetal hypoxia?

☐ **1.** Abnormally long uterine contractions

☐ **2.** Abnormally strong uterine intensity

☐ **3.** Excessively frequent contractions, with rapid fetal movement

☐ **4.** Excessive fetal activity and fetal tachycardia

Answer: 4

Rationale: Fetal tachycardia and excessive fetal activity are the first signs of fetal hypoxia. The duration of uterine contractions is within normal limits. Uterine intensity can be mild to strong yet still within normal limits. The frequency of contractions is within normal limits for the active phase of labor.

Critical thinking strategy: Recall the signs of fetal hypoxia, and relate them to FHR.

Client needs category: Physiological integrity

Client needs subcategory: Reduction of risk potential

Cognitive level: Analysis

Integrated process: Nursing process/assessment

13. When attempting to interact with a neonate experiencing drug withdrawal, the nurse recognizes which behavior as a sign of the neonate's willingness to interact?

☐ **1.** Gaze aversion

☐ **2.** Hiccups

☐ **3.** Quiet, alert state

☐ **4.** Yawning

Answer: 3

Rationale: When caring for a neonate experiencing drug withdrawal, the nurse needs to be alert for signs of distress from the neonate. Stimuli should be introduced one at a time when the neonate is in a quiet, alert state. Gaze aversion, yawning, sneezing, hiccups, and body arching are distress signals that the neonate can't handle stimuli at that time.

Critical thinking strategy: Focus on behaviors that aren't related to drug withdrawal.

Client needs category: Psychosocial integrity

Client needs subcategory: None

Cognitive level: Analysis

Integrated process: Nursing process/assessment

---

14. A paradoxical pulse occurs in a client who had coronary artery bypass graft (CABG) surgery 2 days ago. Which surgical complication should the nurse suspect?

☐ **1.** Left-sided heart failure

☐ **2.** Aortic regurgitation

☐ **3.** Complete heart block

☐ **4.** Pericardial tamponade

Answer: 4

Rationale: A paradoxical pulse (a palpable decrease in pulse amplitude on quiet inspiration) signals pericardial tamponade, a complication of CABG surgery. Left-sided heart failure can cause pulsus alternans (a pulse amplitude alteration from beat to beat, with a regular rhythm). Aortic regurgitation may cause a bisferious pulse (an increased arterial pulse with a double systolic peak). Complete heart block may cause a bounding pulse (a strong pulse with increased pulse pressure).

Critical thinking strategy: Focus on what the term *paradoxical* means and which area of the cardiovascular system it's related to.

Client needs category: Physiological integrity

Client needs subcategory: Physiological adaptation

Cognitive level: Application

Integrated process: Nursing process/planning

15. A client had coronary artery bypass graft (CABG) surgery 3 days ago. Which condition should the nurse suspect when the client's platelet count decreases from 230,000 µl to 5,000 µl?

☐ **1.** Pancytopenia

☐ **2.** Idiopathic thrombocytopenic purpura (ITP)

☐ **3.** Disseminated intravascular coagulation (DIC)

☐ **4.** Heparin-associated thrombosis and thrombocytopenia (HATT)

Answer: 4

Rationale: HATT may occur after CABG surgery due to heparin use during surgery. Pancytopenia is a reduction in all blood cells. Although ITP and DIC cause platelet aggregation and bleeding, neither is common in a client after revascularization surgery.

Critical thinking strategy: Focus on the type of surgery in relation to the change in platelet count.

Client needs category: Physiological integrity

Client needs subcategory: Physiological adaptation

Cognitive level: Application

Integrated process: Nursing process/evaluation

---

16. A comatose client needs a nasopharyngeal airway for suctioning. After the airway is inserted, he gags and coughs. Which action should the nurse take?

☐ **1.** Remove the airway and insert a shorter one.

☐ **2.** Reposition the airway.

☐ **3.** Leave the airway in place until the client gets used to it.

☐ **4.** Remove the airway and attempt suctioning without it.

Answer: 1

Rationale: If the client gags or coughs after nasopharyngeal airway placement, the tube may be too long. The nurse should remove it and insert a shorter one. Simply repositioning the airway won't solve the problem. The client won't get used to the tube because it's the wrong size. Suctioning without a nasopharyngeal airway causes trauma to the natural airway.

Critical thinking strategy: Focus on the symptoms in relation to the anatomy of the respiratory system.

Client needs category: Physiological integrity

Client needs subcategory: Reduction of risk potential

Cognitive level: Application

Integrated process: Nursing process/implementation

17. Why should the nurse administer vasopressin I.M. to a client after a hypophysectomy?

☐ **1.** To treat growth failure

☐ **2.** To prevent syndrome of inappropriate antidiuretic hormone secretion (SIADH)

☐ **3.** To reduce cerebral edema and lower intracranial pressure

☐ **4.** To replace antidiuretic hormone (ADH) normally secreted from the pituitary

Answer: 4

Rationale: After hypophysectomy, or removal of the pituitary gland, the body can't synthesize ADH. Somatropin or growth hormone, not vasopressin, is used to treat growth failure. SIADH results from excessive ADH secretion. Mannitol or corticosteroids are used to reduce cerebral edema.

Critical thinking strategy: Recall the area of the body affected by the surgery

Client needs category: Physiological integrity

Client needs subcategory: Pharmacological and parenteral therapies

Cognitive level: Application

Integrated process: Nursing process/implementation

---

18. A client is demonstrating his understanding of touchdown weight bearing prior to discharge. The nurse would be satisfied with which demonstration?

☐ **1.** Bearing full weight on the affected extremity

☐ **2.** Bearing 30% to 50% of weight on the affected extremity

☐ **3.** Bearing no weight on the extremity but allowing the extremity to touch the floor

☐ **4.** Bearing no weight on the extremity and keeping the extremity elevated at all times

Answer: 3

Rationale: Touchdown weight bearing involves bearing no weight on the extremity but allowing the affected extremity to touch the floor. Full weight bearing allows for full weight to be put on the affected extremity. Partial weight bearing allows for 30% to 50% weight bearing on the affected extremity. Non-weight bearing refers to bearing no weight on the affected extremity.

Critical thinking strategy: Focus on the term *touchdown,* and review guidelines for the amount of weight bearing and extremity activity allowed.

Client needs category: Safe, effective care environment

Client needs subcategory: Management of care

Cognitive level: Application

Integrated process: Teaching and learning

19. Which consideration is the nurse's highest priority when preparing to administer a medication to a client with liver cancer?

☐ **1.** Frequency of the medication

☐ **2.** Purpose of the medication

☐ **3.** Necessity of the medication

☐ **4.** Metabolism of the medication

Rationale: The rate and ability of the liver to metabolize medications will be altered in a client with liver cancer. Therefore, it's essential to know how each medication is metabolized. The other considerations are important but not as vital.

Critical thinking strategy: Focus on normal drug metabolism and the pathophysiology of liver cancer, and remember to prioritize choices.

Client needs category: Physiological integrity

Client needs subcategory: Reduction of risk potential

Cognitive level: Comprehension

Integrated process: Nursing process/planning

---

20. Sodium and water retention in a client with Cushing's syndrome contribute to which common disorder?

☐ **1.** Hypoglycemia and dehydration

☐ **2.** Hypotension and hyperglycemia

☐ **3.** Pulmonary edema and dehydration

☐ **4.** Hypertension and heart failure

Rationale: In Cushing's syndrome, increased mineralocorticoid activity results in sodium and water retention, which commonly contributes to hypertension and heart failure. Hypoglycemia and dehydration are uncommon in a client with Cushing's syndrome. Diabetes mellitus and hyperglycemia may develop, but hypotension isn't part of the disease process. Pulmonary edema and dehydration also aren't complications of Cushing's syndrome.

Critical thinking strategy: Focus on the effects water and sodium retention on various body systems.

Client needs category: Physiological integrity

Client needs subcategory: Physiological adaptation

Cognitive level: Analysis

Integrated process: Nursing process/evaluation

21. Which of the following instructions is most applicable when teaching a client about vaginal irrigation?

☐ **1.** Insert the nozzle about 3″ (8 cm) into the vagina.

☐ **2.** Direct the tip of the nozzle toward the sacrum.

☐ **3.** Instill the solution in a constant flow over 5 to 10 minutes.

☐ **4.** Raise the solution at least 25″ (63.5 cm) above the hip level.

Answer: 2

Rationale: The normal position of the vagina slants up and back toward the sacrum. Directing the tip of the nozzle toward the sacrum allows it to follow the normal slant of the vagina and minimizes tissue trauma. The nozzle should be inserted about 2″ (5 cm). The fluid can be instilled intermittently and, for best therapeutic results, over 20 to 30 minutes. The container should be no higher than 25″ above hip level to avoid forcing fluid and bacteria through the cervical os into the uterus.

Critical thinking strategy: Recall the anatomy of the female reproductive system.

Client needs category: Safe, effective care environment

Client needs subcategory: Safety and infection control

Cognitive level: Application

Integrated process: Teaching and learning

---

22. Which technique is correct for obtaining a wound culture from a surgical site?

☐ **1.** Thoroughly irrigate the wound before collecting the culture.

☐ **2.** Use a sterile swab to wipe the crusty area around the outside of the wound.

☐ **3.** Gently roll a sterile swab from the center of the wound outward to collect drainage.

☐ **4.** Use one sterile swab to collect drainage from several possible infected sites along the incision.

Answer: 3

Rationale: Rolling a swab from the center outward is the correct way to culture a wound. Irrigating the wound washes away drainage, debris, and many of the microorganisms colonizing or infecting the wound. The outside of the wound may be colonized with microorganisms from this wound or another wound, or from normal microorganisms found on the client's skin. These may grow in culture and confuse the interpretation of results. All of the sources of drainage from an incision or a surgical wound may not be infected, or they may be infected with different microorganisms; consequently, each swab should be used on only one site.

Critical thinking strategy: Focus on the wound area where the most microorganisms would be obtained.

Client needs category: Safe, effective care environment

Client needs subcategory: Safety and infection control

Cognitive level: Knowledge

Integrated process: Nursing process/implementation

23. Which individual counseling approach should be used to assist a client with a phobic disorder?

☐ **1.** Have the client keep a daily journal.

☐ **2.** Help the client identify the source of the anxiety.

☐ **3.** Teach the client effective ways to problem-solve.

☐ **4.** Develop strategies to prevent the client from using substances.

Rationale: By understanding the source of the anxiety, the client will understand how this anxiety has been displaced as a phobic response. Keeping a journal is an effective method in many situations; however, its use is limited in the treatment of phobias. Problem solving is a more useful technique for clients with obsessive-compulsive disorder than for clients with phobias. People with phobias don't tend to self-medicate like clients with other psychiatric disorders.

Critical thinking strategy: Review the defining characteristics of phobic disorders, and focus on the optimal therapeutic approach.

Client needs category: Psychosocial integrity

Client needs subcategory: None

Cognitive level: Application

Integrated process: Caring

---

24. A client with antisocial personality disorder is trying to manipulate the health care team. Which strategy is important for the staff to use?

☐ **1.** Focus on how to teach the client more effective behaviors for meeting basic needs.

☐ **2.** Help the client verbalize underlying feelings of hopelessness and learn coping skills.

☐ **3.** Remain calm and don't emotionally respond to the client's manipulative actions.

☐ **4.** Help the client eliminate the intense desire to have everything in life turn out perfectly.

Rationale: The best strategy to use with a client trying to manipulate staff is to stay calm and refrain from responding emotionally. Negative reinforcement of inappropriate behavior increases the chance it will be repeated. Later, it may be possible to address how to meet the client's basic needs. Clients with antisocial personality disorder don't tend to experience feelings of hopelessness or to desire life events to turn out perfectly. In most cases, these clients negate responsibility for their behavior.

Critical thinking strategy: Focus on the strategy that doesn't reinforce the client's behavior.

Client needs category: Psychosocial integrity

Client needs subcategory: None

Cognitive level: Analysis

Integrated process: Caring

25. A child is admitted to the hospital for an asthma exacerbation. The nursing history reveals this client was exposed to chickenpox 1 week ago. When would this client require isolation, if he were to remain hospitalized?

☐ **1.** Isolation isn't required.

☐ **2.** Immediate isolation is required.

☐ **3.** Isolation would be required 10 days after exposure.

☐ **4.** Isolation would be required 12 days after exposure.

Answer: 2

Rationale: The incubation period for chickenpox is 2 to 3 weeks, usually 13 to 17 days. A client is commonly isolated 1 week after exposure to avoid the risk of an earlier breakout. A person is infectious from 1 day before eruption of lesions to 6 days after the vesicles have formed crusts.

Critical thinking strategy: Recall the incubation period for chicken pox, and relate this to the timing of isolation.

Client needs category: Safe, effective care environment

Client needs subcategory: Safety and infection control

Cognitive level: Application

Integrated process: Nursing process/planning

---

26. Which diet is recommended for a child with cystic fibrosis?

☐ **1.** Fat-restricted

☐ **2.** High-calorie

☐ **3.** Low-protein

☐ **4.** Sodium-restricted

Answer: 2

Rationale: A well-balanced high-calorie, high-protein diet is recommended for a child with cystic fibrosis due to the impaired intestinal absorption. Fat restriction isn't required because digestion and absorption of fat in the intestine are impaired. The child usually increases his enzyme intake along with the consumption of high-fat foods. Low-sodium foods can lead to hyponatremia; therefore, high-sodium foods are recommended, especially during hot weather or when the child has a fever.

Critical thinking strategy: Focus on the disease process of cystic fibrosis in relation to children's nutritional needs.

Client needs category: Safe, effective care environment

Client needs subcategory: Management of care

Cognitive level: Application

Integrated process: Nursing process/planning

27. A child has just returned to the pediatric unit following ventriculoperitoneal shunt placement for hydrocephalus. Which intervention should a nurse perform first?

☐ **1.** Assess intake and output.

☐ **2.** Place the child on the side opposite the shunt.

☐ **3.** Offer fluids because the child has a dry mouth.

☐ **4.** Administer pain medication by mouth as ordered.

Answer: 2

Rationale: Following shunt placement surgery, the child should be placed on the side opposite of the surgical site to prevent pressure on the shunt valve. Intake and output will also need to be assessed, but that isn't the nurse's priority. The child is usually on nothing-by-mouth status until the nasogastric tube is removed and bowel sounds return. Pain medication should be administered by an I.V. route initially postoperatively.

Critical thinking strategy: Focus on the immediate postoperative period, and review ventriculoperitoneal shunt care.

Client needs category: Physiological integrity

Client needs subcategory: Basic care and comfort

Cognitive level: Application

Integrated process: Nursing process/planning

---

28. Which information should a nurse provide to the parents of a child undergoing diagnostic testing for muscular dystrophy?

☐ **1.** Genitals will be covered by a lead apron.

☐ **2.** Local anesthetic will be used for the test.

☐ **3.** Electrode wires will be attached to the scalp.

☐ **4.** A fiber-optic endoscope will be inserted into a joint.

Answer: 2

Rationale: A muscle biopsy, used to confirm the diagnosis of muscular dystrophy, shows the degeneration of muscle fibers and infiltration of fatty tissue. It's typically performed using a local anesthetic. Genitals are covered by a lead apron during an X-ray examination, which is used to detect osseous, not muscular, problems. Electrode wires are attached to the scalp during an electroencephalography to observe brain wave activity; this test isn't used to diagnose muscular dystrophy. Arthroscopy, also not used to test for muscular dystrophy, involves the insertion of a fiber-optic scope into a joint.

Critical thinking strategy: Focus on the term *muscular*, eliminating options involving other body areas; recall diagnostic test procedures.

Client needs category: Physiological integrity

Client needs subcategory: Basic care and comfort

Cognitive level: Application

Integrated process: Teaching and learning

29. A young child has just had surgical repair of a cleft palate. Which instruction should be included in the discharge teaching to his parents?

☐ **1.** Continue a normal diet.

☐ **2.** Continue using arm restraints at home.

☐ **3.** Don't allow the child to drink from a cup.

☐ **4.** Establish good mouth care and proper brushing.

Answer: 2

Rationale: Arm restraints are also used at home to keep the child's hands away from the mouth until the palate is healed. A soft diet is recommended; no food harder than mashed potatoes can be eaten. Fluids are best taken from a cup. Proper mouth care is encouraged after the palate is healed.

Critical thinking strategy: Focus on the child's age and immediate home care needs, and recall postoperative interventions following cleft palate repair.

Client needs category: Physiological integrity

Client needs subcategory: Physiological adaptation

Cognitive level: Application

Integrated process: Teaching and learning

---

30. Which comment made by the mother of a neonate at her 2-week office visit should alert the nurse to suspect congenital hypothyroidism?

☐ **1.** "My baby is unusually quiet and good."

☐ **2.** "My baby seems to be a yellowish color."

☐ **3.** "After feedings, my baby pulls her legs up and cries."

☐ **4.** "My baby seems to really look at my face during feeding time."

Answer: 1

Rationale: Parental remarks about an unusually "quiet and good" neonate together with any of the early physical manifestations should lead to a suspicion of hypothyroidism, which requires a referral for specific tests. If a neonate begins to look yellow in color, hyperbilirubinemia may be the cause. If the neonate is pulling her legs up and crying after feedings, she might be showing signs of colic. Neonates like looking at the human face and should show interest in this when 2-weeks-old.

Critical thinking strategy: Focus on the pathophysiology of congenital hypothyroidism

Client needs category: Health promotion and maintenance

Client needs subcategory: None

Cognitive level: Application

Integrated process: Nursing process/evaluation

31. In teaching a group of parents about monitoring for urinary tract infection (UTI) in preschoolers, the nurse should mention which finding as most indicative of the need to have a child evaluated?

☐ **1.** The child voids only twice in any 6-hour period.

☐ **2.** The child exhibits incontinence after being toilet trained.

☐ **3.** The child has difficulty sitting still for more than a 30-minute period.

☐ **4.** The child's urine smells strongly of ammonia after standing for more than 2 hours.

Answer: 2

Rationale: A child who exhibits incontinence after being toilet trained should be evaluated for UTI. Most urine smells strongly of ammonia after standing for more than 2 hours, so this doesn't necessarily indicate UTI. The other options aren't reasons for parents to suspect problems with their child's urinary system.

Critical thinking strategy: Focus on the signs and symptoms of urinary tract infection and relate to a preschool-age child.

Client needs category: Safe, effective care environment

Client needs subcategory: Management of care

Cognitive level: Application

Integrated process: Teaching and learning

---

32. Providing adequate nutrition is essential for a burn client. Which statement best describes the nutritional needs of a child who has burns?

☐ **1.** A child needs 100 cal/kg during hospitalization.

☐ **2.** The hypermetabolic state after a burn injury leads to poor healing.

☐ **3.** Caloric needs can be lowered by controlling environmental temperature.

☐ **4.** Maintaining a hypermetabolic rate will lower the child's risk for infection.

Answer: 2

Rationale: A burn injury causes a hypermetabolic state that leads to protein and lipid catabolism, which affects wound healing. Caloric intake should be 1½ to 2 times the basal metabolic rate, with a minimum of 1.5 to 2 g/kg of body weight of protein daily. Keeping the temperature within a normal range lets the body function efficiently and use calories for healing and normal physiological processes. If the temperature is too warm or cold, energy must be used for warming or cooling, taking energy away from tissue repair. High metabolic rates increase the risk for infection.

Critical thinking strategy: Consider the nutritional needs related to metabolism and wound healing.

Client needs category: Physiological integrity

Client needs subcategory: Basic care and comfort

Cognitive level: Analysis

Integrated process: Nursing process/evaluation

33. A charge nurse is preparing client care assignments for the next shift. A client who underwent femoral-popliteal bypass surgery is scheduled to return from the postanesthesia care unit. Which staff member should receive this client?

☐ **1.** Registered nurse with 1 year of experience

☐ **2.** Licensed practical nurse (LPN) with 5 years of experience

☐ **3.** Nursing assistant with 15 years of experience

☐ **4.** Charge nurse with 10 years of experience

Answer: 1

Rationale: Because this client requires frequent neurovascular assessments, a registered nurse should receive him. An LPN, although she's experienced and can collect data, doesn't have the education to perform the physical assessment required by this client. The nursing assistant lacks the necessary assessment skills. The charge nurse needs to be available to direct the care of other clients.

Critical thinking strategy: Focus on the postoperative needs of the client to determine staff assignments.

Client needs category: Safe, effective care environment

Client needs subcategory: Management of care

Cognitive level: Analysis

Integrated process: Nursing process/planning

---

34. According to a standard staging classification of Hodgkin's disease, which criterion reflects stage II?

☐ **1.** Involvement of extralymphatic organs or tissues

☐ **2.** Involvement of a single lymph node region or structure

☐ **3.** Involvement of two or more lymph node regions or structures

☐ **4.** Involvement of lymph node regions or structures on both sides of the diaphragm

Answer: 3

Rationale: Stage II involves two or more lymph node regions. Stage I involves only one lymph node region; stage III involves nodes on both sides of the diaphragm; and stage IV involves extralymphatic organs or tissues.

Critical thinking strategy: Recall the criteria for stage II classification.

Client needs category: Physiological integrity

Client needs subcategory: Physiological adaptation

Cognitive level: Analysis

Integrated process: Nursing process/assessment

35. A healthy client comes to the clinic for a routine examination. When auscultating his lower lung lobes, the nurse should expect to hear which type of breath sound?

☐ **1.** Bronchial

☐ **2.** Tracheal

☐ **3.** Vesicular

☐ **4.** Bronchovesicular

Rationale: Vesicular breath sounds are soft, low-pitched sounds normally heard over the lower lobes of the lung. They're prolonged on inhalation and shortened on exhalation. Bronchial breath sounds are loud, high-pitched sounds normally heard next to the trachea; discontinuous, they're loudest during exhalation. Tracheal breath sounds are harsh, discontinuous sounds heard over the trachea during inhalation or exhalation. Bronchovesicular breath sounds are medium-pitched, continuous sounds that occur during inhalation or exhalation and are best heard over the upper third of the sternum and between the scapulae.

Critical thinking strategy: Focus on the anatomy of the lungs, and review breath sound characteristics.

Client needs category: Health promotion and maintenance

Client needs subcategory: None

Cognitive level: Application

Integrated process: Nursing process/assessment

---

36. The nurse is preparing to do a 12-lead ECG on a client. Indicate the correct area where the V₂ electrode should be placed on the figure below.

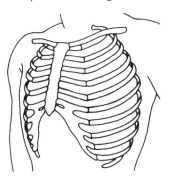

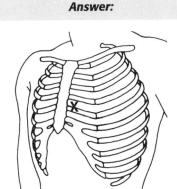

Rationale: The V₂ electrode should be placed over the fourth intercostal space, at the left sternal border.

Critical thinking strategy: Focus on the anatomy of chest, and review the correct placement of electrodes for a 12-lead ECG.

Client needs category: Safe, effective care environment

Client needs subcategory: Management of care

Cognitive level: Application

Integrated process: Nursing process/application

37. A client is scheduled for chemonucleolysis with chymopapain to relieve the pain of a herniated disk. Which factor should be assessed before the procedure?

☐ **1.** Allergy to meat tenderizers

☐ **2.** Allergy to shellfish

☐ **3.** Ability to lie flat during the procedure

☐ **4.** Range of motion (ROM) on the affected side

Rationale: Chymopapain, derived from papaya, is an ingredient in meat tenderizers. Sensitivity to this substance may preclude its use in a client. Allergy to shellfish may be a contraindication to tests using iodine-based dyes. The client may be positioned on his side in a "C" position to allow access to the intervertebral area. Full ROM isn't needed for this procedure.

Critical thinking strategy: Recall the pharmacologic use of chymopapain, and review the chemonucleolysis procedure.

Client needs category: Physiological integrity

Client needs subcategory: Pharmacological and parenteral therapies

Cognitive level: Application

Integrated process: Nursing process/assessment

---

38. A client is ready to be discharged after arthroscopic knee surgery. Which information would the nurse expect the physician to write on the discharge instructions?

☐ **1.** "Ice and elevate the extremity for 12 hours after discharge."

☐ **2.** "Infection shouldn't be a problem because of the small incision size."

☐ **3.** "Swelling and coolness of the joint and limb are normal right after surgery."

☐ **4.** "Take acetaminophen with codeine every 4 hours as necessary for pain relief."

Rationale: Mild to moderate pain is normal after this type of surgery and can be relieved by oral opioid analgesics. To minimize swelling, the client should ice and elevate the extremity for at least 24 hours after surgery. Infection is a potential problem after an invasive procedure, regardless of the incision size. Swelling and coolness of the joint and limb may indicate complications from tourniquet use during surgery.

Critical thinking strategy: Focus on postoperative management, and review the potential complications of arthroscopy.

Client needs category: Physiological integrity

Client needs subcategory: Basic care and comfort

Cognitive level: Application

Integrated process: Teaching and learning

39. Which parameter is measured with the dexamethasone suppression test?

☐ **1.** The amount of dexamethasone in the system

☐ **2.** Cortisol levels after the system is challenged

☐ **3.** Changes in certain body chemicals, which are altered in depression

☐ **4.** Cortisol levels before and after the system is challenged with a synthetic steroid

---

Answer: 4

Rationale: The dexamethasone suppression test measures cortisol levels before and after the system is challenged with a synthetic steroid. The dexamethasone suppression test doesn't measure dexamethasone or body chemicals altered in depression. Dexamethasone is used to challenge the cortisol level.

Critical thinking strategy: Focus on the action of dexamethasone and the definition of *suppression*.

Client needs category: Health promotion and maintenance

Client needs subcategory: None

Cognitive level: Knowledge

Integrated process: Nursing process/analysis

---

40. During a routine physical examination, a firm mass is palpated in the right breast of a 35-year-old female client. Which assessment or client history finding would suggest breast cancer rather than fibrocystic disease?

☐ **1.** History of early menarche

☐ **2.** Cyclic change in mass size

☐ **3.** History of anovulatory cycles

☐ **4.** Increased vascularity of the breast

Answer: 4

Rationale: Increase in breast size or vascularity is consistent with breast cancer. Early menarche as well as late menopause or a history of anovulatory cycles is associated with fibrocystic disease. Masses associated with fibrocystic disease of the breast are firm, most commonly located in the upper outer quadrant of the breast, and increase in size prior to menstruation. They may be bilateral in a mirror image and are typically well demarcated and freely moveable.

Critical thinking strategy: Focus on the pathophysiology and clinical manifestations of breast cancer and fibrocystic disease.

Client needs category: Health promotion and maintenance

Client needs subcategory: None

Cognitive level: Application

Integrated process: Nursing process/analysis

41. A client with disseminated herpes zoster is given I.V. hydrocortisone (Solu-Cortef). Which laboratory value would the nurse expect to be elevated as a result of this therapy?

☐ **1.** Calcium

☐ **2.** Glucose

☐ **3.** Magnesium

☐ **4.** Potassium

Answer: 2

Rationale: Corticosteroids increase blood sugar and tend to lower serum potassium and calcium levels. Their effect on magnesium isn't substantial.

Critical thinking strategy: Recall the action of corticosteroids in the body, and review laboratory values.

Client needs category: Physiological integrity

Client needs subcategory: Pharmacological and parenteral therapies

Cognitive level: Analysis

Integrated process: Nursing process/evaluation

---

42. Which precaution must be taken when giving phenytoin (Dilantin) to a client with a nasogastric (NG) tube for feeding?

☐ **1.** Check the phenytoin level after giving the drug to monitor for toxicity.

☐ **2.** Elevate the head of the bed before giving phenytoin through the NG tube.

☐ **3.** Give phenytoin 1 hour before or 2 hours after NG tube feedings to ensure absorption.

☐ **4.** Verify proper placement of the NG tube by placing the end of the tube in a glass of water and observing for bubbles.

Answer: 3

Rationale: Nutritional supplements and milk interfere with the absorption of phenytoin, decreasing its effectiveness. Phenytoin levels are typically checked before giving the drug, and the drug is withheld for elevated levels to avoid compounding toxicity. The head of the bed should be elevated when giving any drug or solution, so this isn't specific to phenytoin administration. The nurse verifies NG tube placement by checking for stomach contents before giving drugs and feedings.

Critical thinking strategy: Focus on safety precautions specific to nasogastric tubes and phenytoin administration.

Client needs category: Physiological integrity

Client needs subcategory: Pharmacological and parenteral therapies

Cognitive level: Application

Integrated process: Nursing process/planning

43. A client is undergoing peritoneal dialysis. The dialysate dwell time is completed, and the clamp is opened to allow the dialysate to drain. The nurse notes that drainage has stopped and that only 500 ml has drained; the amount of dialysate instilled was 1,500 ml. Which intervention should be done first?

☐ **1.** Change the client's position.

☐ **2.** Call the physician.

☐ **3.** Check the catheter for kinks or obstruction.

☐ **4.** Clamp the catheter and instill more dialysate at the next exchange time.

44. A client has been hospitalized with a diagnosis of conversion-disorder blindness. Which statement best explains this manifestation?

☐ **1.** The client is suppressing her true feelings.

☐ **2.** The client's anxiety has been relieved through her physical symptoms.

☐ **3.** The client is acting indifferent because she doesn't want to show her actual fear.

☐ **4.** The client's needs are being met, so she doesn't need to be anxious.

45. Discharge teaching for the family of a school-age child with idiopathic thrombocytopenia should include restriction of which activity?

☐ **1.** Swimming

☐ **2.** Bicycle riding

☐ **3.** Computer games

☐ **4.** Exposure to large crowds

Answer: 2

Rationale: When routine blood counts reveal the platelet level is 100,000/mm^3 or less, the child shouldn't engage in contact sports, bicycle or scooter riding, climbing, or other activities that could lead to injury (especially to the head). Swimming releases energy, builds muscle, and allows the child to compete without risking injury, as long as she follows normal safety precautions. Computer games don't cause physical injury. It isn't necessary for this child to avoid large crowds because idiopathic thrombocytopenia doesn't suppress the immune system.

Critical thinking strategy: Focus on the definition of *thrombocytopenia,* and review the function and action of platelets.

Client needs category: Safe, effective care environment

Client needs subcategory: Safety and infection control

Cognitive level: Application

Integrated process: Teaching and learning

---

46. A toddler in respiratory distress is admitted to the pediatric intensive care unit. When he refuses to keep his oxygen face mask on, his mother tries to help. Which action by the nurse is most appropriate?

☐ **1.** Giving the child his favorite toy to play with

☐ **2.** Asking the mother read the child's favorite book to him

☐ **3.** Administering a strong sedative so the child will sleep

☐ **4.** Telling the child that the face mask will help him breathe better

---

Answer: 2

Rationale: Having the mother read the child's favorite book will ease his anxiety and provide comfort to the child. Although giving the child a favorite toy is also appropriate, the child needs his mother's comfort because the face mask is frightening. Sedation is contraindicated because it can mask signs of respiratory distress. A toddler is too young to understand that something will make him feel better.

Critical thinking strategy: Focus on the child's age and the circumstances surrounding hospitalization, and prioritize comfort measures.

Client needs category: Safe, effective care environment

Client needs subcategory: Management of care

Cognitive level: Application

Integrated process: Nursing process/implementation

47. Which assignment made by a charge nurse would be appropriate?

☐ **1.** A registered nurse (RN) assigned to an infant newly diagnosed with bacterial meningitis

☐ **2.** A student nurse assigned to an adolescent with cystic fibrosis who is receiving several medications

☐ **3.** A licensed practical nurse (LPN) or a licensed vocational nurse (LVN) assigned to a newly admitted child with acute leukemia who is receiving a blood transfusion

☐ **4.** A nursing assistant assigned to a transferred client with a head injury and frequent seizures

Rationale: An RN would be appropriately assigned to care for an infant with meningitis. The RN would make frequent assessments and provide a high level of care. Student nurses may not be allowed to give medications without supervision, and it may be easier for the RN or LPN to provide care to this client. In many institutions, LPNs (or LVNs) aren't allowed to monitor clients receiving blood or blood products. A client transferred to the unit with a head injury would need frequent assessments that only an RN or an LPN would be able to provide.

Critical thinking strategy: Consider the client's needs, and relate them to the skill level of the staff members.

Client needs category: Safe, effective care environment

Client needs subcategory: Management of care

Cognitive level: Application

Integrated process: Nursing process/planning

---

48. A 6-year-old boy is admitted to a pediatric unit for treatment of osteomyelitis. The nurse knows that the peak incidence in children is between ages 1 and 12 and that boys are affected two to three times more commonly than girls. Which organism most commonly causes osteomyelitis?

☐ **1.** *Staphylococcus epidermidis*

☐ **2.** *Escherichia coli* O157.H7

☐ **3.** *Pneumocystis carinii*

☐ **4.** *S. aureus*

Rationale: *S. aureus* is the most common causative pathogen of osteomyelitis; the usual source of the infection is an upper respiratory infection. *S. epidermidis* is a microorganism found on the skin of healthy individuals. *E. coli* O157.H7, which is in uncooked meat, can cause a severe case of diarrhea. *P. carinii* causes pneumonia in clients with human immunodeficiency virus or acquired immunodeficiency syndrome but doesn't normally cause healthy individuals to become ill.

Critical thinking strategy: Recall the location and the effects of the listed microorganisms, and relate this to osteomyelitis.

Client needs category: Physiological integrity

Client needs subcategory: Physiological adaptation

Cognitive level: Application

Integrated process: Nursing process/analysis

49. The nurse is preparing to teach a client about his prescribed spironolactone (Aldactone) to monitor for adverse effects of the drug. The nurse should instruct the client about which of the following adverse effects? Select all that apply.

☐ **1.** Confusion

☐ **2.** Fatigue

☐ **3.** Hypertension

☐ **4.** Leg cramps

☐ **5.** Weakness

Answer: 1, 2, 5

Rationale: Confusion, fatigue, and weakness are signs of hyperkalemia, an adverse effect of spironolactone. Spironolactone is used to treat hypertension, so it wouldn't produce this effect. Leg cramps are an adverse effect of hypokalemia.

Critical thinking strategy: Focus on the mechanism of action of spironolactone, and review the adverse effects of the drug.

Client needs category: Physiological integrity

Client needs subcategory: Pharmacological therapies

Cognitive level: Analysis

Integrated process: Teaching and learning

---

50. Which structural defect involves a portion of an organ protruding through an abnormal opening?

☐ **1.** Cleft lip

☐ **2.** Cleft palate

☐ **3.** Gastroschisis

☐ **4.** Tracheoesophageal fistula

Answer: 3

Rationale: Gastroschisis is a herniation of the bowel through an abnormal opening in the abdominal wall. Cleft lip and palate are facial malformations, not herniations. Tracheoesophageal fistula is a malformation of the trachea and esophagus.

Critical thinking strategy: Focus on the definitions of the terms listed in relation to the anatomy of the gastrointestinal tract.

Client needs category: Physiological integrity

Client needs subcategory: Physiological adaptation

Cognitive level: Knowledge

Integrated process: Nursing process/analysis

51. A client has received dietary instructions as part of his treatment plan for diabetes type 1. Which statement by the client should alert the nurse that he needs additional instructions?

☐ **1.** "I'll need a bedtime snack because I take an evening dose of NPH insulin."

☐ **2.** "I can eat whatever I want as long as I cover the calories with sufficient insulin."

☐ **3.** "I can have an occasional low-calorie drink as long as I include it in my meal plan."

☐ **4.** "I should eat meals as scheduled, even if I'm not hungry, to prevent hypoglycemia."

Answer: 2

Rationale: The goal of dietary therapy in diabetes mellitus is to attain and maintain ideal body weight. Each client is prescribed a specific caloric intake and insulin regimen to help accomplish this goal.

Critical thinking strategy: Review the goals of dietary therapy for type 1 diabetes mellitus.

Client needs category: Physiological integrity

Client needs subcategory: Basic care and comfort

Cognitive level: Analysis

Integrated process: Teaching and learning

---

52. If both kidneys are affected in a child with Wilms' tumor, the nurse should understand that treatment prior to surgery might include which of the following?

☐ **1.** Peritoneal dialysis

☐ **2.** Abdominal gavage

☐ **3.** Radiation and chemotherapy

☐ **4.** Antibiotics and I.V. fluid therapy

Answer: 3

Rationale: If both kidneys are involved, the child may be treated with radiation therapy or chemotherapy preoperatively to shrink the tumor, allowing more conservative therapy. Peritoneal dialysis would be needed only if the kidneys aren't functioning. Abdominal gavage wouldn't be indicated. Antibiotics aren't needed because Wilms' tumor isn't an infection.

Critical strategy thinking: Recall that the diagnosis involves tumors, and review the choices based on this information.

Client needs category: Safe, effective care environment

Client needs subcategory: Management of care

Cognitive level: Application

Integrated process: Nursing process/analysis

53. Topical treatment with 2.5% hydrocortisone (Cortane) is prescribed for a 6-month-old infant with eczema. The mother is instructed to use the cream for no longer than 1 week. Why is this time limit appropriate?

☐ **1.** The drug loses its efficacy after prolonged use.

☐ **2.** This reduces adverse effects, such as skin atrophy and fragility.

☐ **3.** If no improvement is seen after 1 week, a stronger concentration will be prescribed.

☐ **4.** If no improvement is seen after 1 week, an antibiotic will be prescribed.

Answer: 2

Rationale: Hydrocortisone cream should be used for brief periods to decrease such adverse effects as atrophy of the skin. The drug doesn't lose efficacy after prolonged use. A stronger concentration may not be prescribed if no improvement is seen, and an antibiotic would be inappropriate in this instance.

Critical thinking strategy: Recall how hydrocortisone affects various body systems

Client needs category: Physiological integrity

Client needs subcategory: Pharmacological and parenteral therapies

Cognitive level: Application

Integrated process: Teaching and learning

---

54. A 23-year-old client develops cardiac tamponade when the car he was driving hits a telephone pole; he wasn't wearing a seatbelt. The nurse helps the physician perform pericardiocentesis. Which outcome would indicate that pericardiocentesis has been effective?

☐ **1.** Neck vein distention

☐ **2.** Pulsus paradoxus

☐ **3.** Increased blood pressure

☐ **4.** Muffled heart sounds

Answer: 3

Rationale: Cardiac tamponade is associated with decreased cardiac output, which in turn reduces blood pressure. By removing a small amount of blood, pericardiocentesis increases blood pressure. Neck vein distention, pulsus paradoxus, and muffled heart sounds indicate persistent cardiac tamponade, meaning pericardiocentesis hasn't been effective.

Critical thinking strategy: Recall the disease process of cardiac tamponade.

Client needs category: Physiological integrity

Client needs subcategory: Physiological adaptation

Cognitive level: Application

Integrated process: Nursing process/evaluation

55. Which assessment finding is expected in a child with acute rheumatic fever?

☐ **1.** Leukocytosis

☐ **2.** Normal electrocardiogram

☐ **3.** High fever lasting 5 or more days

☐ **4.** Normal erythrocyte sedimentation rate

Rationale: Leukocytosis can be seen as an immune response triggered by colonization of the pharynx with group A streptococci. The electrocardiogram will show a prolonged PR interval as a result of carditis. The inflammatory response will cause an elevated erythrocyte sedimentation rate. A low-grade fever is a minor manifestation. A high fever lasting 5 or more days may present with Kawasaki disease.

Critical thinking strategy: Recall the disease process and pathophysiology of rheumatic fever.

Client needs category: Physiological integrity

Client needs subcategory: Physiological adaptation

Cognitive level: Application

Integrated process: Nursing process/assessment

---

56. Which substance is associated with abnormal values early in the course of multiple myeloma?

☐ **1.** Immunoglobulins

☐ **2.** Platelets

☐ **3.** Red blood cells (RBCs)

☐ **4.** White blood cells (WBCs)

Rationale: Multiple myeloma is characterized by malignant plasma cells that produce an increased amount of immunoglobulin that isn't functional. As more malignant plasma cells are produced, there's less space in the bone marrow for RBC production. In late stages, platelets and WBCs are reduced as the bone marrow is infiltrated by malignant plasma cells.

Critical thinking strategy: Review the pathophysiology of multiple myeloma and its effect on various cells of the body.

Client needs category: Health promotion and maintenance

Client needs subcategory: None

Cognitive level: Analysis

Integrated process: Nursing process/analysis

57. A 20-year-old client with cystic fibrosis is being discharged with a high-frequency chest wall oscillating vest. Which statement by the client indicates that she understands how to use the vest?

☐ **1.** "I'll wear the vest for 5 minutes each time a treatment is due."

☐ **2.** "I'll lie down to use the vest."

☐ **3.** "I'll require help in applying the vest."

☐ **4.** "I can be in any position to use the vest."

Rationale: The vest system doesn't require special positioning or breathing to be effective. In most cases, treatments last 15 to 20 minutes and clients can manage therapy without any assistance.

Critical thinking strategy: Recall the purpose of the vest and relate this to the selections.

Client needs category: Physiological integrity

Client needs subcategory: Basic care and comfort

Cognitive level: Analysis

Integrated process: Teaching and learning

---

58. Which intervention is most appropriate to include in a bladder program for a client in rehabilitation for a spinal cord injury?

☐ **1.** Insert an indwelling urinary catheter.

☐ **2.** Schedule intermittent catheterization every 2 to 4 hours.

☐ **3.** Perform a straight catheterization every 8 hours while the client is awake.

☐ **4.** Perform Credé's maneuver to the lower abdomen before the client voids.

Rationale: Intermittent catheterization should begin every 2 to 4 hours early in treatment. When residual volume is less than 400 ml, the schedule may advance to every 4 to 6 hours. Indwelling catheters may predispose the client to infection and are removed as soon as possible. Credé's maneuver is applied after voiding to enhance bladder emptying.

Critical thinking strategy: Focus on the type of injury in relation to bladder function.

Client needs category: Physiological integrity

Client needs subcategory: Basic care and comfort

Cognitive level: Application

Integrated process: Teaching and learning

59. Which condition is characterized by osteopenia and renal calculi?

☐ **1.** Hyperparathyroidism

☐ **2.** Hypoparathyroidism

☐ **3.** Hypopituitarism

☐ **4.** Hypothyroidism

Rationale: Hyperparathyroidism is characterized by osteopenia and renal calculi secondary to overproduction of parathyroid hormone. The hallmark symptom of hypoparathyroidism is tetany from hypocalcemia. Hypopituitarism presents with extreme weight loss and atrophy of all endocrine glands. Symptoms of hypothyroidism include hair loss, weight gain, and cold intolerance.

Critical thinking strategy: Focus on the pathophysiology of the disorders mentioned, and review the clinical manifestations of each.

Client needs category: Physiological integrity

Client needs subcategory: Physiological adaptation

Cognitive level: Comprehension

Integrated process: Nursing process/analysis

---

60. A client arrives to the emergency department with suspected appendicitis. The admitting nurse performs an assessment. Order the following steps according to the sequence in which they are performed. Use all of the options.

1.	Percuss all four abdominal quadrants.
2.	Obtain a health history.
3.	Inspect the abdomen, noting the shape, contours, and any visible peristalsis or pulsations.
4.	Auscultate bowel sounds in all four quadrants
5.	Gently palpate all four quadrants, saving the painful area for last.

Answer: 2, 3, 4, 1, 5

Rationale: The first step in the data collection process is to obtain a health history. Then, the nurse should visually inspect the abdomen. Of the three remaining steps, it's important to auscultate before percussing or palpating the client's abdomen. Touching or palpating the abdomen before listening may actually change the bowel sounds, leading to faulty data.

Critical thinking strategy: Focus on basic assessment techniques, and consider the client's diagnosis.

Client needs category: Physiological integrity

Client needs subcategory: Physiological adaption

Cognitive level: Analysis

Integrated process: Nursing process/assessment

61. A mother infected with human immunodeficiency virus (HIV) asks the nurse about the possibility of breast-feeding her neonate. Which response by the nurse would be most appropriate?

- ☐ **1.** "Breast-feeding isn't an option."
- ☐ **2.** "Breast-feeding would be best for your baby."
- ☐ **3.** "Breast-feeding is only an option if the mother is taking zidovudine (Retrovir)."
- ☐ **4.** "Breast-feeding is an option if milk is expressed and fed by a bottle."

Answer: 1

Rationale: Mothers infected with HIV are unable to breast-feed because the virus has been isolated in breast milk and could be transmitted to the infant. Taking zidovudine doesn't prevent transmission. The risk of breast-feeding isn't associated with direct contact with the breast but with the possibility of the HIV contained in the breast milk.

Critical thinking strategy: Recall how HIV is transmitted

Client needs category: Health promotion and maintenance

Client needs subcategory: None

Cognitive level: Application

Integrated process: Teaching and learning

---

62. A child with a diagnosis of meningococcal meningitis develops signs of sepsis and a purpuric rash over both lower extremities. The primary health care provider should be notified immediately because these signs could be indicative of which complication?

- ☐ **1.** A severe allergic reaction to the antibiotic regimen with impending anaphylaxis
- ☐ **2.** Onset of the syndrome of inappropriate antidiuretic hormone secretion (SIADH)
- ☐ **3.** Meningococcemia
- ☐ **4.** Adhesive arachnoiditis

Answer: 3

Rationale: Meningococcemia is a serious complication usually associated with meningococcal infection. A client with a severe allergic reaction and impending anaphylaxis would most likely have signs and symptoms of respiratory distress, gastrointestinal problems (abdominal pain, cramps, diarrhea), hypotension, hives, itching, and anxiety. SIADH can be an acute complication, but it wouldn't be accompanied by the purpuric rash. Adhesive arachnoiditis occurs in the chronic phase of the disease and leads to obstructed flow of cerebrospinal fluid.

Critical thinking strategy: Focus on the symptoms in relation to the pathophysiology of meningococcal meningitis

Client needs category: Physiological integrity

Client needs subcategory: Reduction of risk potential

Cognitive level: Application

Integrated process: Nursing process/evaluation

63. When a 6-month-old infant is admitted for intestinal obstruction, which assessment finding should alert the nurse to a potential problem?

☐ **1.** Presence of the Moro reflex

☐ **2.** The child's playing with his feet

☐ **3.** Eruption of the first tooth

☐ **4.** Rolling from stomach to back

Rationale: By 6 months of age, the Moro (startle) reflex should no longer be observed. Playing with the feet, eruption of the first tooth, and rolling from the stomach to back are all normal for a 6-month-old infant.

Critical thinking strategy: Consider the infant's age, and review the choices in relation to developmental milestones.

Client needs category: Health promotion and maintenance

Client needs subcategory: None

Cognitive level: Analysis

Integrated process: Nursing process/assessment

---

64. Which assessment finding should alert the nurse to change the intranasal route for vasopressin administration?

☐ **1.** Mucous membrane irritation

☐ **2.** Severe coughing

☐ **3.** Nosebleeds

☐ **4.** Pneumonia

Rationale: Mucous membrane irritation caused by a cold or allergy renders the intranasal route unreliable. Severe coughing, pneumonia, or nosebleeds shouldn't interfere with the intranasal route.

Critical thinking strategy: Focus on the route of administration and consider which assessment finding would interfere with the drug's absorption.

Client needs category: Physiological integrity

Client needs subcategory: Pharmacological and parenteral therapies

Cognitive level: Application

Integrated process: Nursing process/analysis

65. A nurse is developing a teaching plan for a client who will undergo a stapedectomy for treatment of otosclerosis. Which information should the plan include?

☐ **1.** Ringing in the ears is common after surgery.

☐ **2.** Vertigo and dizziness are common after surgery.

☐ **3.** Hearing should return immediately after surgery.

☐ **4.** Excessive drainage is common after surgery.

Answer: 2

Rationale: Vertigo is the most common complication of stapedectomy. The client should move slowly to avoid triggering or worsening vertigo and should ask for assistance with ambulation. Ringing in the ears (tinnitus) rarely follows this surgery and should be reported to the physician. Hearing typically decreases after surgery because of ear packing and tissue swelling, but commonly returns over the next 2 to 6 weeks. Usually, postoperative drainage and pain are minimal; excessive drainage should be reported.

Critical thinking strategy: Recall the physiology and function of the stapes.

Client needs category: Physiological integrity

Client needs subcategory: Reduction of risk potential

Cognitive level: Application

Integrated process: Teaching and learning

---

66. A 17-year-old client with diabetes has a decreased level of consciousness and a fingerstick glucose level of 39 mg/dl. Her family reports that she has been skipping meals in an effort to lose weight. Which nursing intervention is most appropriate?

☐ **1.** Placing a Salem sump tube and providing tube feedings

☐ **2.** Administering a 500-ml bolus of normal saline solution

☐ **3.** Administering 1 ampule of 50% dextrose solution

☐ **4.** Calling the physician for orders

Answer: 3

Rationale: Administering 50% dextrose solution helps preserve and restore the client's physiologic integrity. Providing a feeding tube is appropriate only in a less urgent situation; during the time it takes to insert a nasogastric tube, administer a feeding, and wait for digestion to occur, the client may suffer permanent brain damage and seizures from severe hypoglycemia. A blood pressure drop wasn't mentioned; a bolus of normal saline solution would correct only the client's fluid status, not her glucose level. Calling the physician would delay treatment at a time when rapid intervention is crucial.

Critical thinking strategy: Think about treatment choices in terms of low blood glucose and lack of nutrition.

Client needs category: Physiological integrity

Client needs subcategory: Pharmacological and parenteral therapies

Cognitive level: Application

Integrated process: Nursing process/implementation

67. A client is diagnosed with genitourinary tuberculosis, which can infect the kidney, ureter, bladder, testes, and epididymis. Which statement about genitourinary tuberculosis is true?

☐ **1.** It isn't infectious and can't be passed from one person to another.

☐ **2.** It can't be passed sexually from partner to partner.

☐ **3.** It's a late manifestation of respiratory tuberculosis.

☐ **4.** It's an early manifestation of an autoimmune disorder.

Answer: 3

Rationale: Genitourinary tuberculosis is usually a late manifestation of respiratory tuberculosis and can occur if the disease spreads through the bloodstream from the lungs. *Bacillus* in the urine is infectious, and urine should be handled cautiously. A condom should be used during sex to prevent spread of the infection.

Critical thinking strategy: Review the pathophysiology of tuberculosis

Client needs category: Physiological integrity

Client needs subcategory: Physiological adaptation

Cognitive level: Knowledge

Integrated process: Nursing process/analysis

---

68. A client having an acute asthmatic attack is admitted to the emergency room. The health care provider writes an order for *epinephrine 1:1,000 injection 0.3 ml subcutaneous stat.* The nurse reads in the unit's drug reference that epinephrine 1:1,000 contains 1 mg/ml. Instructions direct the nurse to dilute each mg of the 1:1,000 concentration with 10 ml of normal saline, resulting in a solution that contains 0.1 mg/1 ml. How many milligrams of epinephrine will be administered to the client after the nurse has added the diluent? Record your answer using three decimal places.

_____ milligrams

Answer: 0.003

Rationale: Using the ratio-and-proportion method, calculate the correct dosage by using the following formula:

Dose on hand/quantity on hand $= X$/Dose prescribed

$$0.1 \text{ mg}/1 \text{ ml} = X \text{ mg}/ 0.3 \text{ ml}$$

$$\frac{0.1 \text{ mg}}{1 \text{ ml}} = \frac{X \text{ mg}}{0.3 \text{ ml}}$$

$$X = 0.003 \text{ mg}$$

Critical thinking strategy: Focus on client safety when administering medications, and review dosage calculations formulas.

Client needs category: Physiological integrity

Client needs subcategory: Reduction of risk potential

Cognitive level: Application

Integrated process: Nursing process/planning

69. Which method is considered the definitive treatment for hypopituitarism due to growth hormone deficiency?

☐ **1.** Treatment with desmopressin acetate (DDAVP)

☐ **2.** Replacement of antidiuretic hormone (ADH)

☐ **3.** Treatment with testosterone or estrogen

☐ **4.** Replacement with biosynthetic growth hormone

Rationale: The definitive treatment for growth hormone deficiency, replacement with biosynthetic growth hormone, is successful in 80% of affected children. DDAVP is used to treat diabetes insipidus. ADH deficiency causes diabetes insipidus and isn't related to hypopituitarism. Testosterone or estrogen may be given during adolescence for normal sexual maturation, but neither is the definitive treatment for hypopituitarism.

Critical thinking strategy: Focus on the hormone mentioned in the stem of the question, then use the process of elimination to select an answer.

Client needs category: Physiological integrity

Client needs subcategory: Pharmacological and parenteral therapies

Cognitive level: Application

Integrated process: Nursing process/analysis

---

70. When providing discharge teaching for a client with uric acid calculi, the nurse should include an instruction to avoid which type of diet?

☐ **1.** Low-calcium

☐ **2.** Low-oxalate

☐ **3.** High-oxalate

☐ **4.** High-purine

Rationale: To control uric acid calculi, the client should follow a low-purine diet, which excludes high-purine foods such as organ meats. The other diets don't control uric acid calculi.

Critical thinking strategy: Focus on the cause of uric acid calculi, and review dietary guidelines.

Client needs category: Physiological integrity

Client needs subcategory: Reduction of risk potential

Cognitive level: Application

Integrated process: Teaching and learning

71. Which description about the development of sequelae in infants with bacterial meningitis is most accurate?

☐ **1.** They usually occur during the first 2 months of life.

☐ **2.** They only occur in children with meningococcal meningitis.

☐ **3.** They primarily involve the fourth ventricle of the brain.

☐ **4.** They tend to affect the ocular nerves, leading to retinal damage.

Answer: 1

Rationale: In infants with bacterial meningitis who are younger than 2 months old, communicating hydrocephalus and the effects of cerebritis on the immature brain lead to the frequent occurrence of sequelae. Sequelae are least common in children with meningococcal meningitis. Meningitis affects the meninges (the connective tissue layers of the brain), not the ventricles, and it primarily affects the nerves for hearing, not vision.

Critical thinking strategy: Recall the pathophysiology of bacterial meningitis.

Client needs category: Physiological integrity

Client needs subcategory: Physiological adaptation

Cognitive level: Application

Integrated process: Nursing process/analysis

---

72. When assessing a neonate diagnosed with diabetes insipidus, which finding would indicate the need for intervention?

☐ **1.** Edema

☐ **2.** Increased head circumference

☐ **3.** Weight gain

☐ **4.** Weight loss

Answer: 4

Rationale: Diabetes insipidus usually presents gradually. Weight loss from a large loss of fluid occurs. Edema isn't evident in the neonate with diabetes insipidus. There should be an increase in his head circumference with treatment. A normal neonate should gain weight as he grows.

Critical thinking strategy: Recall the pathophysiology of diabetes insipidus and relate this to the findings

Client needs category: Physiological integrity

Client needs subcategory: Reduction of risk potential

Cognitive level: Application

Integrated process: Nursing process/assessment

73. Which instruction should be included in client teaching specifically related to anticonvulsant drug efficacy?

☐ **1.** Wear a medical identification bracelet.

☐ **2.** Maintain a seizure frequency chart.

☐ **3.** Avoid potentially hazardous activities.

☐ **4.** Discontinue the drug immediately if adverse effects are suspected.

Answer: 2

Rationale: Ongoing evaluation of therapeutic effects can be accomplished by maintaining a seizure frequency chart that indicates the date, time, and nature of all seizure activity. These data may be helpful in making dosage alterations and specific drug selection. Avoidance of hazardous activities and wearing a medical identification bracelet are ways to minimize dangers related to seizure activity, but these factors don't affect drug efficacy. Anticonvulsant drugs should never be discontinued abruptly because of the risk of developing status epilepticus.

Critical thinking strategy: Recall the pathophysiology of epilepsy, and review the uses and adverse effects of anticonvulsants.

Client needs category: Physiological integrity

Client needs subcategory: Pharmacological and parenteral therapies

Cognitive level: Application

Integrated process: Teaching and learning

---

74. Which statement by the parent of a child being treated for pinworms indicates that further teaching is needed?

☐ **1.** "I'll make my child wash his hands well before meals."

☐ **2.** "I'll warn my child to avoid sharing hairbrushes and hats to prevent spreading pinworms to others."

☐ **3.** "I'll give my child only one dose of medication."

☐ **4.** "I'll keep my child's nails short."

Answer: 2

Rationale: Sharing hairbrushes and hats reduces the spread of lice, not pinworms. Hands should be washed well before food preparation and eating to avoid ingesting eggs that may be under the fingernails from scratching the itchy infested perianal area. Only a single dose of medication, such as mebendazole, is needed to treat pinworms. Keeping the fingernails short reduces the risk of carrying eggs under the nails.

Critical thinking strategy: Recall the cause and transmission of pinworms, and review the life cycle of the causative organism.

Client needs category: Safe, effective care environment

Client needs subcategory: Safety and infection control

Cognitive level: Application

Integrated process: Teaching and learning

75. The nurse is caring for a homeless client with pneumonia. Laboratory testing reveals the following results: blood urea nitrogen (BUN) 180 mg/dl, creatinine 30 mg/dl, potassium 6.2 mEq/L, and hemoglobin 6.2%. Based on the physician's order below, which drug order should the nurse question?

Physician orders	
12/21/09 0900	Gentamicin 180 mg I.V. piggyback every 8 hours
	Erythropoietin 50 units/kg subcutaneously Monday, Wednesday, and Friday
	Aluminum hydroxide gel 500 mg P.O. four times daily
	Ferrous sulfate 325 mg P.O. three times daily ———————— Garry Reynolds, MD

☐ **1.** Gentamicin

☐ **2.** Erythropoietin

☐ **3.** Aluminum hydroxide gel

☐ **4.** Ferrous sulfate

Answer: 1

Rationale: Based on the high BUN, creatinine, and potassium levels, the client is in renal failure. Gentamicin is nephrotoxic and can exacerbate the renal failure. Ferrous sulfate and erythropoietin would be given to treat the client's anemia. Aluminum hydroxide gel would also be appropriate because it binds with phosphate, which is elevated in renal failure.

Critical thinking strategy: Focus on what the laboratory results indicate and why each medication would be prescribed for this client.

Nursing process step: Implementation

Client needs category: Physiological integrity

Client needs subcategory: Reduction of risk potential

Cognitive level: Analysis

Integrated process: Nursing process/analysis

Comprehensive test 2

1. Which medication may be prescribed to prevent a thromboembolic stroke?

☐ **1.** Acetaminophen

☐ **2.** Streptokinase (Streptase)

☐ **3.** Ticlopidine (Ticlid)

☐ **4.** Methylprednisolone (Medrol)

Answer: 3

Rationale: Ticlopidine inhibits platelet aggregation by interfering with adenosine diphosphate release in the coagulation cascade and, therefore, is used to prevent thromboembolic stroke. Aspirin, not acetaminophen, interferes with platelet aggregation. Streptokinase is used with evolving myocardial infarctions and strokes to dissolve existing clots. Methylprednisolone, a steroid with anticoagulant properties, isn't used to treat thromboembolic stroke.

Critical thinking strategy: Recall the pathophysiology of thromboembolic stroke, and review the indications for the medications listed.

Client needs category: Physiological integrity

Client needs subcategory: Pharmacological and parenteral therapies

Cognitive level: Application

Integrated process: Nursing process/analysis

2. A client's electrocardiogram (ECG) is showing ST elevation in leads V_2, V_3, and V_4. Which artery is most likely occluded?

☐ **1.** Circumflex artery

☐ **2.** Internal mammary artery

☐ **3.** Left anterior descending artery

☐ **4.** Right coronary artery

Answer: 3

Rationale: The client's ECG changes suggest an anterior-wall myocardial infarction. The left anterior descending artery is the primary source of blood for the anterior wall of the heart. The circumflex artery supplies the lateral wall of the heart, the internal mammary artery supplies the anterior chest wall and breasts, and the right coronary artery supplies the inferior wall of the heart.

Critical thinking strategy: Focus on the relationship between the heart's electrical conduction system and the specific coronary arteries mentioned.

Client needs category: Physiological integrity

Client needs subcategory: Physiological adaptation

Cognitive level: Analysis

Integrated process: Nursing process/evaluation

---

3. Which of the following may cause an acquired immune deficiency?

☐ **1.** Age

☐ **2.** Genetics

☐ **3.** Environment

☐ **4.** Medical treatments

Answer: 4

Rationale: Immune deficiencies may result from medical treatments, such as medications, radiation, or transplants. Immune function may decline with age, but it isn't considered the cause of acquired immune deficiency. Genetics and environment haven't been shown to be factors in acquired immune deficiency.

Critical thinking strategy: Focus on the word *acquired* when considering the answer.

Client needs category: Physiological integrity

Client needs subcategory: Physiological adaptation

Cognitive level: Analysis

Integrated process: Nursing process/analysis

4. A nurse teaches a group of police officers about the spread of tuberculosis (TB). Which statement by an officer indicates that teaching has been effective?

☐ **1.** "I could get TB by being in close proximity for a brief time with someone who has the disease."

☐ **2.** "I could get TB if I inhale infected droplets when an infected individual coughs."

☐ **3.** "I could get TB if I search the home of someone infected with TB."

☐ **4.** "I could get TB if I come in contact with blood from an infected person."

Answer: 2

Rationale: TB infection typically occurs from inhaling infected droplets after a person with TB coughs. Transmission usually requires close, frequent, and prolonged contact. Human immunodeficiency virus, not TB, is spread through contact with an infected person's blood.

Critical thinking strategy: Recall the transmission of TB

Client needs category: Safe, effective care environment

Client needs subcategory: Safety and infection control

Cognitive level: Analysis

Integrated process: Teaching and learning

---

5. The nurse determines that a client understands his risk for compartment syndrome if he knows to report which early symptom following treatment for a tibial fracture?

☐ **1.** Heat

☐ **2.** Paraesthesia

☐ **3.** Skin pallor

☐ **4.** Swelling

Answer: 2

Rationale: Paresthesia is the earliest sign of compartment syndrome. Pain, heat, and swelling are also signs but occur after paresthesia. Skin pallor isn't a sign of compartment syndrome.

Critical thinking strategy: Focus on the word *early*, and review the signs of compartment syndrome.

Client needs category: Physiological integrity

Client needs subcategory: Physiological adaptation

Cognitive level: Analysis

Integrated process: Teaching and learning

6. Which action should be included in the immediate management of acute gastritis?

☐ **1.** Advising the client to reduce work-related stress

☐ **2.** Preparing the client for gastric resection

☐ **3.** Treating the underlying cause of disease

☐ **4.** Administering enteral tube feedings

Answer: 3

Rationale: Discovering and treating the cause of gastritis is the most beneficial approach in the immediate management phase. Reducing the amount of stress and reducing or eliminating oral intake until the symptoms are gone are important in the recovery phase. A gastric resection is considered only when serious erosion has occurred.

Critical thinking strategy: Focus on the word *immediate*, and prioritize the management of this condition.

Client needs category: Safe, effective care environment

Client needs subcategory: Safety and infection control

Cognitive level: Analysis

Integrated process: Nursing process/planning

---

7. A client comes to the emergency department complaining of dull, deep bone pain that's unrelated to movement. The nurse knows whether or not to assess this client for a possible fracture based on which of the following statements?

☐ **1.** The client has the classic symptoms of a fracture.

☐ **2.** Fracture pain is sharp and related to movement.

☐ **3.** Fracture pain is sharp and unrelated to movement.

☐ **4.** Fracture pain is dull, deep, and related to movement.

Answer: 2

Rationale: Fracture pain is sharp and related to movement. Pain that's dull, deep, and unrelated to movement isn't typical of a fracture.

Critical thinking strategy: Focus on the client's specific symptoms, and review the pathophysiology of a fracture, particularly with respect to pain.

Client needs category: Health promotion and maintenance

Client needs subcategory: None

Cognitive level: Analysis

Integrated process: Nursing process/assessment

8. Surgical management of ulcerative colitis may be performed to treat which complication?

☐ **1.** Gastritis

☐ **2.** Bowel herniation

☐ **3.** Bowel outpouching

☐ **4.** Bowel perforation

> ### *Answer: 4*
>
> **Rationale:** Bowel perforation, obstruction, or hemorrhage and toxic megacolon are common complications of ulcerative colitis that may require surgery. Gastritis and herniation aren't associated with irritable bowel diseases, and outpouching of the bowel wall is diverticulosis.
>
> **Critical thinking strategy:** Recall the pathophysiology of ulcerative colitis and the anatomy of the gastrointestinal system
>
> **Client needs category:** Safe, effective care environment
>
> **Client needs subcategory:** Safety and infection control
>
> **Cognitive level:** Application
>
> **Integrated process:** Nursing process/planning

---

9. A client who is started on metformin (Glucophage) and glyburide (DiaBeta) would have initially presented with which symptoms?

☐ **1.** Polydipsia, polyuria, and weight loss

☐ **2.** Weight gain, tiredness, and bradycardia

☐ **3.** Irritability, diaphoresis, and tachycardia

☐ **4.** Diarrhea, abdominal pain, and weight loss

> ### *Answer: 1*
>
> **Rationale:** Symptoms of hyperglycemia include polydipsia, polyuria, and weight loss. Metformin and sulfonylureas are commonly ordered medications. Weight gain, tiredness, and bradycardia are symptoms of hypothyroidism. Irritability, diaphoresis, and tachycardia are symptoms of hypoglycemia. Symptoms of Crohn's disease include diarrhea, abdominal pain, and weight loss.
>
> **Critical thinking strategy:** Focus on the action of these medications, and correlate the action with the specific symptoms presented.
>
> **Client needs category:** Physiological integrity
>
> **Client needs subcategory:** Reduction of risk potential
>
> **Cognitive level:** Analysis
>
> **Integrated process:** Nursing process/assessment

10. Which statement best explains why it's important to empty the bowel before treatment with intracavitary radiation for cancer of the cervix?

☐ **1.** Feces in the bowel increase the risk of ileus.

☐ **2.** An empty bowel allows the applicator to be positioned with little or no discomfort.

☐ **3.** Bowel movements increase the risk of inadvertent contamination of the vagina and urethra.

☐ **4.** Pressure changes in the pelvis associated with bowel movements can alter the position of the applicator and the radiation source.

Answer: 4

Rationale: A position change of the radioactive implant could deliver more radiation to healthy tissue and less to the malignant lesion. This increases the risk of injury to healthy tissue and decreases the effectiveness of treatment on the cancer. Feces in the bowel increase the likelihood of a bowel movement, which can change the position of the applicator and radiation source. Feces in the bowel don't increase the risk of ileus or inadvertent contamination of the vagina and urethra from a bowel movement. Applicators are usually inserted under anesthesia in the operating room.

Critical thinking strategy: Recall the effect of radiation therapy on all body tissues.

Client needs category: Physiological integrity

Client needs subcategory: Reduction of risk potential

Cognitive level: Analysis

Integrated process: Nursing process/analysis

---

11. The assessment of a client on the first day after thoracotomy shows a temperature of 100° F (37.8° C); heart rate, 96 beats/minute; blood pressure, 136/86 mm Hg; and shallow respirations at 24 breaths/minute, with rhonchi at the bases. The client complains of incisional pain. Which nursing action has priority?

☐ **1.** Medicate the client for pain.

☐ **2.** Help the client get out of bed.

☐ **3.** Give ibuprofen (Motrin) as ordered to reduce the fever.

☐ **4.** Encourage the client to cough and deep-breathe.

Answer: 1

Rationale: Although the interventions are incorporated in the client's care plan, the priority is to relieve the client's pain and make him comfortable. This would give the client energy and stamina to achieve the other objectives.

Critical thinking strategy: Prioritize the interventions according to the most beneficial action for the client.

Client needs category: Physiological integrity

Client needs subcategory: Basic care and comfort

Cognitive level: Application

Integrated process: Nursing process/assessment

12. After telling a nurse to "pray for me," a client gives away personal possessions and shows a sudden calmness. The nurse recognizes that this behavior may signal which condition?

☐ **1.** Major depression

☐ **2.** Panic attack

☐ **3.** Suicidal ideation

☐ **4.** Severe anxiety

Answer: 3

Rationale: Verbal clues to suicidal ideation include such statements as "Pray for me" and "I won't be here when you get back." Nonverbal clues include giving away personal possessions, a sudden calmness, and risk-taking behaviors. The nurse should recognize the combination of these signs as indicating suicidal ideation—not depression, panic, or anxiety. Clients with major depression generally don't exhibit suicidal behavior until their outlook on their problems begins to improve (an improvement in behavior should raise suspicion, especially if accompanied by sudden calmness).

Critical thinking strategy: Focus on the client's actions and words, and use the process of elimination to select the answer.

Client needs category: Psychosocial integrity

Client needs subcategory: None

Cognitive level: Comprehension

Integrated process: Caring

---

13. Which nursing intervention is appropriate to include when planning care for a client with panic disorder?

☐ **1.** Identify childhood trauma.

☐ **2.** Monitor nutritional intake.

☐ **3.** Institute suicide precautions.

☐ **4.** Monitor episodes of disorientation.

Answer: 3

Rationale: Clients with panic disorder are at risk for suicide because they can be impulsive. Childhood trauma is associated with posttraumatic stress disorder, not panic disorder. Nutritional problems don't typically accompany panic disorder. Clients aren't typically disoriented; they may have a temporary altered sense of reality, but that lasts only for the duration of the attack.

Critical thinking strategy: Recall the thought process behind panic disorder, and review its characteristic signs and symptoms.

Client needs category: Psychosocial integrity

Client needs subcategory: None

Cognitive level: Application

Integrated process: Nursing process/planning

14. A single 24-year-old client is admitted with acute schizophrenic reaction. Which method is the most appropriate therapy for this type of schizophrenia?

☐ **1.** Counseling to produce insight into behavior

☐ **2.** Biofeedback to reduce agitation associated with schizophrenia

☐ **3.** Drug therapy to reduce symptoms associated with acute schizophrenia

☐ **4.** Electroconvulsive therapy to treat the mood component of schizophrenia

---

Answer: 3

Rationale: Drug therapy is usually successful in normalizing behavior and reducing or eliminating hallucinations, delusions, disordered thinking, affect flattening, apathy, and asociality. Counseling wouldn't be appropriate at this time. Electroconvulsive therapy might be considered for schizoaffective disorder, which has a mood component; it's also one of the treatments of choice for clinical depression. Biofeedback reduces anxiety and modifies behavioral responses, but it isn't a major component in treating schizophrenia.

Critical thinking strategy: Focus on the defining characteristics of schizophrenia, and review how each treatment might benefit the client.

Client needs category: Psychosocial integrity

Client needs subcategory: None

Cognitive level: Application

Integrated process: Nursing process/planning

---

15. A client recovering from alcohol addiction asks the nurse how he should to talk to his children about the impact of his addiction on them. Which response is most appropriate?

☐ **1.** "Try to limit references to the addiction, and focus on the present."

☐ **2.** "Talk about all the hardships you've had in working to remain sober."

☐ **3.** "Tell them you're sorry, and emphasize that you're doing so much better now."

☐ **4.** "Talk to them by acknowledging the difficulties and pain your drinking caused."

Answer: 4

Rationale: Part of the healing process for the family is to acknowledge the pain, embarrassment, and overall difficulties the client's drinking problem caused family members. The first option facilitates the client's ability to deny the problem. The second option prevents the client from acknowledging the difficulties the children endured. The third option might lead the client to believe only a simple apology is needed. The addiction must be addressed, and the children's pain acknowledged.

Critical thinking strategy: Think about which statement will be most helpful in the healing process of the family.

Client needs category: Psychosocial integrity

Client needs subcategory: None

Cognitive level: Application

Integrated process: Caring

16. A 26-year-old man is reported missing after being the victim of a violent crime. Two months later, a family member finds him working in a city 100 miles from his home. The man doesn't recognize the family member or recall being the victim of a crime. He most likely has which condition?

☐ **1.** Depersonalization disorder

☐ **2.** Dissociative amnesia

☐ **3.** Dissociative fugue

☐ **4.** Dissociative identity disorder

Answer: 3

Rationale: Dissociative fugue is characterized by sudden, unexpected travel from home or usual surroundings after a traumatic event. During the episode, the person may assume a new identity and not recognize people from his past. Depersonalization disorder is the sudden loss of the sense of one's own reality. Dissociative amnesia doesn't involve flight from work or home. Dissociative identity disorder is the coexistence of two or more personalities in one person.

Critical thinking strategy: Focus on the client's state of mind and the specifics of his situation, and relate them to the disorders mentioned.

Client needs category: Psychosocial integrity

Client needs subcategory: None

Cognitive level: Knowledge

Integrated process: Nursing process/analysis

---

17. Clients with gestational diabetes are usually managed by which therapy?

☐ **1.** Dietary control of carbohydrates, fats, and proteins

☐ **2.** Metformin (Glucophage)

☐ **3.** Ultra-lente (long-acting) insulin

☐ **4.** Metformin (Glucophage) and ultra-lente (long-acting) insulin

Answer: 1

Rationale: Clients with gestational diabetes are usually managed by dietary control of carbohydrates, fats, and proteins alone to control their glucose intolerance. Oral hypoglycemic drugs such as Metformin are contraindicated in pregnancy and are considered teratogenic. Long-acting insulin such as ultra-lente usually isn't needed for blood glucose control in the client with gestational diabetes.

Critical thinking strategy: Focus on the term *gestational,* and consider the effects the therapies may have on the fetus as well as the mother.

Client needs category: Health promotion and maintenance

Client needs subcategory: None

Cognitive level: Application

Integrated process: Nursing process/analysis

18. During a vaginal examination of a client in labor, the nurse palpates the fetus's larger, diamond-shaped fontanel positioned toward the anterior portion of the client's pelvis. Which statement best describes this situation?

☐ **1.** The client can expect a brief, intense labor with possible lacerations.

☐ **2.** The client is at risk for uterine rupture and needs constant monitoring.

☐ **3.** The client may need interventions to ease back pain and change the fetal position.

☐ **4.** The fetus will be delivered using forceps or a vacuum extractor.

Rationale: The fetal position is occiput posterior, a position that commonly produces intense back pain during labor. Most of the time, the fetus rotates during labor to occiput anterior position. Positioning the client on her side can facilitate this rotation. An occiput posterior position would most likely result in prolonged labor. Occiput posterior alone doesn't create a risk of uterine rupture. The fetus would be delivered with forceps or vacuum extractor only if its presenting part doesn't rotate and descend spontaneously.

Critical thinking strategy: Review the position of the fetus's fontanels, and relate this to the anatomy of the female reproductive system.

Client needs category: Safe, effective care environment

Client needs subcategory: Management of care

Cognitive level: Analysis

Integrated process: Nursing process/analysis

---

19. A nurse should expect to observe which behavior in a client on the 4th postpartum day?

☐ **1.** The client asks many questions about the baby's care.

☐ **2.** The client wants to relate her birth experience.

☐ **3.** The client asks the nurse to select her meals for her.

☐ **4.** The client asks the nurse to help her bathe herself.

Rationale: The taking-hold phase usually lasts from days 3 to 10 postpartum. During this stage, the mother strives for independence and autonomy; she also becomes curious and interested in the care of the baby and is most ready to learn. During the taking-in phase, which usually lasts 2 to 3 days, the mother is passive and dependent and expresses her own needs. During this taking-in phase, the client may ask the nurse to help her with self-care, wants to talk about the birth experience, and lets others make decisions for her.

Critical thinking strategy: Focus on the transition phases of the postpartum period and when each phase occurs.

Client needs category: Psychosocial integrity

Client needs subcategory: None

Cognitive level: Application

Integrated process: Nursing process/evaluation

20. Which action best explains the main role of surfactant in the neonate?

☐ **1.** Assists with ciliary body maturation in the upper airways

☐ **2.** Helps maintain a rhythmic breathing pattern

☐ **3.** Promotes clearing mucus from the respiratory tract

☐ **4.** Helps the lungs remain expanded after the initiation of breathing

Rationale: Surfactant works by reducing surface tension in the lung. It allows the lung to remain slightly expanded, decreasing the amount of work required for inspiration. Surfactant hasn't been shown to influence ciliary body maturation, regulate the neonate's breathing pattern, or clear the respiratory tract.

Critical thinking strategy: Recall the anatomy and physiology of the neonatal respiratory system.

Client needs category: Health promotion and maintenance

Client needs subcategory: None

Cognitive level: Knowledge

Integrated process: Nursing process/evaluation

---

21. A 6-month-old infant is admitted to the pediatric unit for a 2-week course of antibiotics. His parents can visit only on weekends. Which action indicates that the nurse understands the infant's emotional needs?

☐ **1.** The nurse places the infant in a four-bed unit.

☐ **2.** The nurse places the infant in a room away from other children.

☐ **3.** The nurse assigns the infant to a different nurse each day.

☐ **4.** The nurse assigns the infant to the same nurse as often as possible.

Rationale: Building a sense of trust is crucial with an infant at this stage of growth and development. Consistent caregivers will promote a sense of trust. Placing him in a four-bed unit isn't the best choice because a 6-month-old child doesn't play with other children. Placing him in a room away from other children would isolate him from others, which is neither necessary nor helpful.

Critical thinking strategy: Focus on the child's age, developmental level, and emotional needs.

Client needs category: Safe, effective care environment

Client needs subcategory: Management of care

Cognitive level: Application

Integrated process: Caring

22. Gastric glands in the fundus and body of the stomach secrete intrinsic factor and hydrochloric acid. Why are these substances needed? Select all that apply.

☐ **1.** Vitamin B_{12} absorption

☐ **2.** Emulsifying fats

☐ **3.** Dissolving food fibers

☐ **4.** Killing microorganisms

☐ **5.** Activating the enzyme pepsin

☐ **6.** Vitamin B_6 absorption

Answer: 1, 3, 4, 5

Rationale: Intrinsic factor is needed for vitamin B_{12} absorption, and hydrochloric acid is needed for dissolving food fibers, killing microorganisms, and activating the enzyme pepsin. Vitamin B_6, an essential nutrient, must be replaced daily because it's water soluble and eliminated in urine. Bile is the substance secreted from the gallbladder to emulsify fats as they are consumed.

Critical thinking strategy: Review the anatomy and physiology of the gastrointestinal system.

Client needs category: Physiological integrity

Client needs subcategory: Physiological adaptation

Cognitive level: Analysis

Integrated process: Nursing process/analysis

---

23. A client with a ventricular septal repair is receiving dopamine (Intropin) postoperatively. Which response is expected?

☐ **1.** Decreased heart rate

☐ **2.** Decreased urine output

☐ **3.** Increased cardiac output

☐ **4.** Decreased cardiac contractility

Answer: 3

Rationale: Dopamine stimulates beta 1- and beta 2-adrenergic receptors. It's a selective cardiac stimulant that increases cardiac output, heart rate, and cardiac contractility. Urine output increases in response to dilation of the blood vessels leading to the mesentery and kidneys.

Critical thinking strategy: Recall the action of the medication in relation to the cardiovascular system.

Client needs category: Physiological integrity

Client needs subcategory: Pharmacological and parenteral therapies

Cognitive level: Knowledge

Integrated process: Nursing process/evaluation

24. Which communicable disease requires isolating an infected child from pregnant women?

☐ **1.** Pertussis

☐ **2.** Roseola

☐ **3.** Rubella

☐ **4.** Scarlet fever

Answer: 3

Rationale: Rubella (German measles) has a teratogenic effect on the fetus. An infected child must be isolated from pregnant women. Pertussis, roseola, and scarlet fever don't have any teratogenic effects on the fetus.

Critical thinking strategy: Consider the effect communicable diseases have on a developing fetus.

Client needs category: Safe, effective care environment

Client needs subcategory: Safety and infection control

Cognitive level: Application

Integrated process: Nursing process/implementation

---

25. A 2-year-old child with status asthmaticus is admitted to the pediatric unit and begins to receive continuous treatment with albuterol, given by nebulizer. Which adverse effect is common with this drug?

☐ **1.** Bradycardia

☐ **2.** Lethargy

☐ **3.** Tachycardia

☐ **4.** Tachypnea

Answer: 3

Rationale: Albuterol is a rapid-acting bronchodilator. Common adverse effects include tachycardia, nervousness, tremors, insomnia, irritability, and headache.

Critical thinking strategy: Recall the action and adverse effects of albuterol.

Client needs category: Physiological integrity

Client needs subcategory: Pharmacological and parenteral therapies

Cognitive level: Knowledge

Integrated process: Nursing process/evaluation

26. At the scene of a trauma, which nursing intervention is appropriate for a child with a suspected fracture?

☐ **1.** Avoid moving the child.

☐ **2.** Sit the child up to facilitate breathing.

☐ **3.** Move the child to a safe place immediately.

☐ **4.** Immobilize the extremity and then move child to a safe place.

Answer: 4

Rationale: At the scene of a trauma, the nurse should immobilize the extremity of a child with a suspected fracture and then move him to a safe place. If the child is already in a safe place, don't attempt to move him. Never try to sit the child up; this could worsen the fracture.

Critical thinking strategy: Consider the best way to prevent further damage to the affected area, and focus on safety.

Client needs category: Safe, effective care environment

Client needs subcategory: Safety and infection control

Cognitive level: Application

Integrated process: Nursing process/planning

---

27. Which physiologic change should the nurse anticipate as a diabetic child becomes more physically active during the day?

☐ **1.** Increased need for food

☐ **2.** Decreased need for food

☐ **3.** Decreased risk of insulin shock

☐ **4.** Increased risk of hyperglycemia

Answer: 1

Rationale: If a child is more active at one time of the day than another, his food intake or insulin can be adjusted to meet this increased activity pattern. Ideally, food intake should be increased when a diabetic child is more physically active. The child would have an increased risk of insulin shock and a decreased risk of hyperglycemia when he's more physically active.

Critical thinking strategy: Recall the relationship between blood glucose and calories and exercise.

Client needs category: Safe, effective care environment

Client needs subcategory: Management of care

Cognitive level: Application

Integrated process: Nursing process/evaluation

28. When providing discharge information to the parents of a child with a hypospadias repair, which area is essential to cover?

☐ **1.** Care of the circumcision

☐ **2.** Techniques for providing tub baths

☐ **3.** Care for the indwelling catheter or stent

☐ **4.** Encouragement of voiding every 2 hours

Answer: 3

Rationale: The parents should be taught to care for the indwelling catheter or stent and irrigation techniques, if indicated. The child with hypospadias shouldn't be circumcised because the foreskin may be needed during surgical repair. To prevent infection, tub baths should be avoided until the stent has been removed. Following surgical repair, the child will have an indwelling urinary catheter, so encouraging the child to void isn't appropriate.

Critical thinking strategy: Focus on the type of surgery and the child's postoperative needs.

Client needs category: Safe, effective care environment

Client needs subcategory: Management of care

Cognitive level: Analysis

Integrated process: Teaching and learning

---

29. A teenager asks advice about getting a tattoo. Which statement about tattoos is a common misconception?

☐ **1.** Human immunodeficiency syndrome (HIV) is a possible risk factor.

☐ **2.** Hepatitis B is a possible risk factor.

☐ **3.** Tattoos are easily removed with laser surgery.

☐ **4.** Allergic response to pigments is a possible risk factor.

Answer: 3

Rationale: Removing a tattoo isn't an easy process, and most people are left with a significant scar. Also, the cost is expensive and not covered by insurance. Because of the moderate amount of bleeding with a tattoo, both hepatitis B and HIV are potential risks if proper techniques aren't followed. Allergic reactions are possible when establishments don't use Food and Drug Administration-approved pigments for tattoo coloring. Reactions can also occur in clients who are hypersensitive to the pigments or tools used.

Critical thinking strategy: Remember to focus on the selection that is a misperception and eliminate the selections that are facts

Client needs category: Health promotion and maintenance

Client needs subcategory: Safety and infection control

Cognitive level: Knowledge

Integrated process: Teaching and learning

30. The nurse is teaching a client about the patho-physiology of asthma. Place in chronological order the sequence of an asthma attack. Use all of the options.

| **1.** Inflammation |
| **2.** Mucus production |
| **3.** Airflow limitation |
| **4.** Trigger by stimulus |
| **5.** Acute asthma attack |
| **6.** Breathlessness |

Rationale: Asthma is triggered by a stimulus. The stimulus may be environmental, stress-related, or medication-related. Inflammation in the airways occurs as a response to the stimulus, followed by an increase in mucus production. The presence of inflammation and mucus narrow the bronchi, causing limited airflow. At this point, the client experiences breathlessness, chest tightness, and wheezing—all symptoms of an acute asthma attack.

Critical thinking strategy: Recall the causes and pathophysiology of asthma.

Client needs category: Physiological integrity

Client needs subcategory: Physiological adaptation

Cognitive level: Application

Integrated process: Teaching and learning

---

31. The nurse-manager of a 20-bed coronary care unit isn't on duty when a staff nurse makes a serious medication error that results in a client's overdose. The client nearly dies. Which statement accurately reflects the accountability of the nurse-manager?

☐ **1.** The nurse-manager should receive a call at home from the on-duty nursing supervisor, apprising her of the problem as soon as possible.

☐ **2.** Because the nurse-manager is off duty and not accountable for incidents that occur in her absence, she needn't be notified.

☐ **3.** The nurse-manager only needs to be informed of the incident when she reports to work on her next scheduled day.

☐ **4.** Although the nurse-manager is off-duty and not responsible for what happened, the nursing supervisor should call the nurse-manger only if time permits.

Answer: 1

Rationale: The nurse-manager is accountable for what happens on the unit 24 hours per day, 7 days per week. If a serious problem occurs, the nurse-manager should be notified as soon as possible. None of the other choices accurately reflect the nurse-manager's accountability in this situation.

Critical thinking strategy: Focus on the time factor and the nurse-manager's responsibilities.

Client needs category: Safe, effective care environment

Client needs subcategory: Safety and infection control

Cognitive level: Analysis

Integrated process: Communication and documentation

32. Which is the most common symptom of myocardial infarction (MI)?

☐ **1.** Chest pain

☐ **2.** Dyspnea

☐ **3.** Edema

☐ **4.** Palpitations

Rationale: The most common symptom of an MI is chest pain, resulting from deprivation of oxygen to the heart. Dyspnea is the second most common symptom, related to an increase in metabolic needs of the body during an MI. Edema is a later sign of heart failure, commonly seen after an MI. Palpitations may result from reduced cardiac output, producing arrhythmias.

Critical thinking strategy: Recall the pathophysiology of MI.

Client needs category: Safe, effective care environment

Client needs subcategory: Management of care

Cognitive level: Analysis

Integrated process: Nursing process/analysis

---

33. A chest X-ray shows a client's lungs to be clear. His Mantoux test is positive, with 10 mm of induration. His previous test was negative. Why are these test results possible?

☐ **1.** He had tuberculosis (TB) in the past and no longer has it.

☐ **2.** He was successfully treated for TB, but skin tests always stay positive.

☐ **3.** He's a seroconverter, meaning the TB has gotten to his bloodstream.

☐ **4.** He's a tuberculin converter, which means he has been infected with TB since his last skin test.

Rationale: A tuberculin converter's skin test will be positive, meaning he has been exposed to and infected with TB and now has a cell-mediated immune response to the skin test. The client's blood and X-ray results may stay negative. It doesn't mean the infection has advanced to the active stage. Because his X-ray is negative, he should be monitored every 6 months to see if he develops changes in his chest X-ray or pulmonary examination. Being a seroconverter doesn't mean the TB has gotten into his bloodstream; it means it can be detected by a blood test.

Critical thinking strategy: Recall the purpose of the Mantoux test, and review the disease course following exposure to TB.

Client needs category: Physiological integrity

Client needs subcategory: Physiological adaptation

Cognitive level: Application

Integrated process: Nursing process/analysis

34. A client at the eye clinic is newly diagnosed with glaucoma. The nurse should stress the need to take medication as prescribed because noncompliance may lead to which condition?

☐ **1.** Diplopia

☐ **2.** Permanent vision loss

☐ **3.** Progressive loss of peripheral vision

☐ **4.** Pupillary constriction

Answer: 2

Rationale: Without treatment, glaucoma may progress to irreversible blindness. Treatment won't restore visual damage but will halt disease progression. Blurred or foggy vision, not diplopia, is typical in glaucoma. Central vision loss, not peripheral loss, is typical in glaucoma. Miotics, which constrict the pupil, are used in the treatment of glaucoma to permit the outflow of aqueous humor.

Critical thinking strategy: Focus on the pathophysiology of glaucoma.

Client needs category: Physiological integrity

Client needs subcategory: Pharmacological and parenteral therapies

Cognitive level: Application

Integrated process: Teaching and learning

---

35. A client with newly diagnosed chronic obstructive pulmonary disease (COPD) comes to the clinic for a routine examination. The nurse teaches him strategies for preventing airway irritation and infection. Which statement by the client indicates that teaching was successful?

☐ **1.** "I should avoid enclosed, crowded areas during the summer."

☐ **2.** "I'm glad I only need to get the flu vaccine."

☐ **3.** "I should use products with aerosol sprays."

☐ **4.** "I should avoid using powders."

Answer: 4

Rationale: A client with COPD should avoid exposure to powders, dust, and smoke from cigarettes, pipes, and cigars. He should stay indoors when the humidity, temperature, and pollen counts are high; and he should avoid aerosol sprays. He should also obtain immunizations against pneumococcal pneumonia as well as influenza.

Critical thinking strategy: Consider the complications that can occur with COPD.

Client needs category: Health promotion and maintenance

Client needs subcategory: None

Cognitive level: Analysis

Integrated process: Teaching and learning

36. Which measure would be included in teaching the client with multiple sclerosis (MS) to avoid exacerbation of the disease?

☐ **1.** Patching the affected eye

☐ **2.** Sleeping 8 hours each night

☐ **3.** Taking hot baths for relaxation

☐ **4.** Drinking 1½ to 2 qt (1.5 to 2 L) of fluid daily

Answer: 2

Rationale: MS is exacerbated by exposure to stress, fatigue, and heat. Clients should balance activity with rest. Patching the affected eye may result in improvement in vision and balance but won't prevent exacerbation of the disease. Adequate hydration will help prevent urinary tract infections secondary to a neurogenic bladder.

Critical thinking strategy: Review the pathophysiology of MS.

Client needs category: Physiological integrity

Client needs subcategory: Reduction of risk potential

Cognitive level: Application

Integrated process: Teaching and learning

---

37. A high-protein diet is ordered for a client recovering from a fracture. High protein is ordered for which reason?

☐ **1.** Protein promotes gluconeogenesis.

☐ **2.** Protein has anti-inflammatory properties.

☐ **3.** Protein promotes cell growth and bone union.

☐ **4.** Protein decreases pain medication requirements.

Answer: 3

Rationale: High-protein intake promotes cell growth and bone union. Protein doesn't promote gluconeogenesis, exert anti-inflammatory properties, or decrease pain medication requirements.

Critical thinking strategy: Recall the main effect of proteins on the body.

Client needs category: Physiological integrity

Client needs subcategory: Basic care and comfort

Cognitive level: Application

Integrated process: Nursing process/planning

38. The victim of a motor vehicle accident is brought into the trauma center with substernal injuries. He is in a great deal of pain. The nurse assesses the client's pain level as a 9 on 0-to-10 pain scale and notifies the physician, who orders *morphine sulfate gr ½ I.M. stat.* The only available morphine is morphine sulfate in a 20-ml vial, labeled 15 mg per ml. How many milliliters of pain medication should the nurse administer? Record your answer using a whole number.

_____ milliliters

Answer: 2

Rationale: Calculate the dosage by converting grains to milligrams:

$$1 \text{ gr}: 60 \text{ mg} :: \tfrac{1}{2} \text{ gr} : X \text{ mg} = 30 \text{ mg.}$$

Then use the ratio-and-proportion method to determine the amount of milliliters to administer:

$$15 \text{ mg}: 1 \text{ ml} :: 30 \text{ mg}: X \text{ ml}$$

$$\frac{15 \times X}{15} = \frac{30}{15}$$

$$X = 2 \text{ ml}$$

Critical thinking strategy: Recall dosage calculations using ratios and proportions, and review equivalents for the apothecaries' system.

Client needs category: Physiological integrity

Client needs subcategory: Pharmacological and parenteral therapies

Cognitive level: Application

Integrated process: Nursing process/planning

---

39. A client with which condition may be likely to develop rectal cancer?

☐ **1.** Adenomatous polyps

☐ **2.** Diverticulitis

☐ **3.** Hemorrhoids

☐ **4.** Peptic ulcer disease

Answer: 1

Rationale: A client with adenomatous polyps has a higher risk for developing rectal cancer than others do. Clients with diverticulitis are more likely to develop colon cancer. Hemorrhoids don't increase the chance of any type of cancer. Clients with peptic ulcer disease have a higher incidence of gastric cancer.

Critical thinking strategy: Focus on the causes of rectal cancer.

Client needs category: Health promotion and maintenance

Client needs subcategory: None

Cognitive level: Analysis

Integrated process: Nursing process/analysis

40. Which disorder is suggested by polydipsia and large amounts of waterlike urine with a specific gravity of 1.003?

☐ **1.** Diabetes mellitus

☐ **2.** Diabetes insipidus

☐ **3.** Diabetic ketoacidosis

☐ **4.** Syndrome of inappropriate antidiuretic hormone secretion (SIADH)

Answer: 2

Rationale: Diabetes insipidus is characterized by a great thirst (polydipsia) and large amounts of dilute, waterlike urine with a specific gravity of 1.001 to 1.005. Diabetes mellitus presents with polydipsia, polyuria, and polyphagia, but the client also has hyperglycemia. Diabetic ketoacidosis presents with weight loss, polyuria, and polydipsia, and the client has severe acidosis. A client with SIADH can't excrete dilute urine; he retains fluid and develops a sodium deficiency.

Critical thinking strategy: Focus on the listed value of the urine specific gravity.

Client needs category: Physiological integrity

Client needs subcategory: Physiological adaptation

Cognitive level: Analysis

Integrated process: Nursing process/analysis

---

41. Which instruction about skin care at the stoma site should be given to a client with an ileal conduit?

☐ **1.** Change the appliance at bedtime.

☐ **2.** Leave the stoma open to air while changing the appliance.

☐ **3.** Clean the skin around the stoma with mild soap and water, and dry it thoroughly.

☐ **4.** Cut the faceplate or wafer of the appliance no more than 4 mm larger than the stoma.

Answer: 3

Rationale: Cleaning the skin around the stoma with mild soap and water and drying it thoroughly helps keep the area clean from urine, which can irritate the skin. The appliance should be changed early in the morning, when urine output is less, to decrease the amount of urine in contact with the skin. The stoma should be covered with a gauze pad when changing the appliance to prevent seepage of urine onto the skin. The faceplate or wafer of the appliance shouldn't be more than 3 mm larger than the stoma to reduce the skin area in contact with urine.

Critical thinking strategy: Focus on the most effective intervention that maintains skin integrity.

Client needs category: Physiological integrity

Client needs subcategory: Basic care and comfort

Cognitive level: Application

Integrated process: Teaching and learning

42. A client with facial lacerations requires hospitalization for 1 week. During assessment, the nurse notes scabs on the wounds. This finding corresponds to which phase of wound healing?

☐ **1.** Contraction phase

☐ **2.** Inflammatory phase

☐ **3.** Proliferative phase

☐ **4.** Remodeling phase

Answer: 3

Rationale: During the proliferative phase of wound healing, which lasts from the 4th to 21st day after injury, granulation tissue appears (scabs form) and the wound edges start to pull together. Contraction, the third phase of wound healing, may begin around the 7th day and involves a significant decrease in the wound surface. The inflammatory phase, the first healing phase, immediately follows the injury and lasts 4 to 6 days; it involves control of bleeding and release of chemicals needed for healing. The remodeling phase, the final phase, may lead to scar flattening and correction of any deformities that occurred during the third phase.

Critical thinking strategy: Recall what occurs during the different phases of wound healing.

Client needs category: Physiological integrity

Client needs subcategory: Basic care and comfort

Cognitive level: Analysis

Integrated process: Nursing process/evaluation

---

43. The phrase *gravida 4, para 2* indicates which prenatal history?

☐ **1.** A client has been pregnant four times and had two miscarriages.

☐ **2.** A client has been pregnant four times had two children born after 20 weeks' gestation.

☐ **3.** A client had been pregnant four times and had two cesarean deliveries.

☐ **4.** A client has been pregnant four times and had two spontaneous abortions.

Answer: 2

Rationale: *Gravida* refers to the number of times a client had been pregnant; *para* refers to the number of viable children born after 20 weeks' gestation. Therefore, the client who is gravida 4, para 2 has been pregnant four times and had two live-born children.

Critical thinking strategy: Focus on the meaning of the terms *gravida* and *para*.

Client needs category: Health promotion and maintenance

Client needs subcategory: None

Cognitive level: Knowledge

Integrated process: Nursing process/assessment

44. Which nursing action is required before a client in labor receives an epidural?

☐ **1.** Give a fluid bolus of 500 ml.

☐ **2.** Check for maternal pupil dilation.

☐ **3.** Assess maternal reflexes.

☐ **4.** Assess maternal gait.

Rationale: One of the major adverse effects of epidural administration is hypotension. Therefore, a 500-ml fluid bolus is usually administered to help prevent hypotension in the client who wishes to receive an epidural for pain relief. Assessments of maternal reflexes, pupil response, and gait aren't necessary.

Critical thinking strategy: Focus on the adverse effects of epidural administration.

Client needs category: Physiological integrity

Client needs subcategory: Reduction of risk potential

Cognitive level: Analysis

Integrated process: Nursing process/implementation

---

45. When caring for a breast-feeding client who delivers by cesarean section, the nurse should teach the client to do what?

☐ **1.** Delay breast-feeding until 24 hours after delivery.

☐ **2.** Breast-feed frequently during the day and every 4 to 6 hours at night.

☐ **3.** Use the cradle-hold position to avoid incisional discomfort.

☐ **4.** Use the football-hold position to avoid incisional discomfort.

Rationale: When breast-feeding after a cesarean delivery, the client should be encouraged to hold her neonate in a football-holding position to avoid incisional discomfort. Breast-feeding should be initiated as soon after birth as possible. The mother should be encouraged to breast-feed her infant every 2 to 3 hours throughout the night as well as during the day to increase her milk supply.

Critical thinking strategy: Focus on comfort measures following surgery.

Client needs category: Physiological integrity

Client needs subcategory: Basic care and comfort

Cognitive level: Analysis

Integrated process: Teaching and learning

46. Pneumonias can be classified by four etiologic processes. Which causative agent is responsible for bacterial pneumonia?

- ☐ **1.** *Mycoplasma*
- ☐ **2.** Parainfluenza virus
- ☐ **3.** Pneumococcus
- ☐ **4.** Respiratory syncytial virus (RSV)

Answer: 3

Rationale: *Streptococcus pneumoniae,* commonly known as pneumococcus, is the most common causative agent of bacterial pneumonia, accounting for about 90% of all cases. *Mycoplasma* is a causative agent of primary atypical pneumonia. Parainfluenza virus and RSV are leading causes of viral pneumonias.

Critical thinking strategy: Focus on the term *bacterial,* and review the different types of pneumonia and their causative organisms.

Client needs category: Physiological integrity

Client needs subcategory: Physiological adaptation

Cognitive level: Knowledge

Integrated process: Nursing process/assessment

---

47. Which condition indicates to a nurse that a sterile field has been contaminated?

- ☐ **1.** Sterile objects are held above the waist of the nurse.
- ☐ **2.** Sterile packages are opened with the first edge away from the nurse.
- ☐ **3.** The outer inch of the sterile towel hangs over the side of the table.
- ☐ **4.** Wetness in the sterile cloth on top of the non-sterile table has been noted.

Answer: 4

Rationale: Moisture outside the sterile package contaminates the sterile field because fluid can be wicked into the sterile field. Bacteria tend to settle, so there's less contamination above waist level and away from the nurse. The outer inch of the drape is considered contaminated but doesn't indicate that the sterile field itself has been contaminated.

Critical thinking strategy: Review the basics of infection control and sterile field procedures.

Client needs category: Safe, effective care environment

Client needs subcategory: Management of care

Cognitive level: Application

Integrated process: Nursing process/assessment

48. Which intervention should be the nurse's priority when treating a client experiencing chest pain while walking?

☐ **1.** Have the client sit down.

☐ **2.** Get the client back to bed.

☐ **3.** Obtain an electrocardiogram (ECG).

☐ **4.** Administer sublingual nitroglycerin.

Answer: 1

Rationale: The priority intervention is to decrease the client's oxygen consumption; this would be accomplished by having the client sit down. When the client's condition is stabilized, he can be returned to bed. An ECG can be obtained after the client is sitting down. After the ECG, sublingual nitroglycerin would be administered.

Critical thinking strategy: Consider the importance of preserving cardiac tissue when prioritizing interventions.

Client needs category: Physiological integrity

Client needs subcategory: Basic care and comfort

Cognitive level: Analysis

Integrated process: Nursing process/implementation

---

49. Which sign or symptom of increased intracranial pressure (ICP) after head trauma would the nurse expect to appear first?

☐ **1.** Bradycardia

☐ **2.** Large amounts of very dilute urine

☐ **3.** Restlessness and confusion

☐ **4.** Widened pulse pressure

Answer: 3

Rationale: The earliest symptom of increased ICP is a change in mental status. Bradycardia, widened pulse pressure, and bradypnea occur later. The client may void large amounts of very dilute urine if there's damage to the posterior pituitary.

Critical thinking strategy: Review the signs and symptoms of increased ICP in relation to their timing.

Client needs category: Physiological integrity

Client needs subcategory: Physiological adaptation

Cognitive level: Analysis

Integrated process: Nursing process/assessment

50. Which discharge instructions should be given to a client after surgical repair of a hip fracture?

☐ **1.** "Don't flex the hip more than 30 degrees, don't cross your legs, and get help putting on your shoes."

☐ **2.** "Don't flex the hip more than 60 degrees, don't cross your legs, and get help putting on your shoes."

☐ **3.** "Don't flex the hip more than 90 degrees, don't cross your legs, and get help putting on your shoes."

☐ **4.** "Don't flex the hip more than 120 degrees, don't cross your legs, and get help putting on your shoes."

Rationale: Discharge instructions should include not flexing the hip more than 90 degrees, not crossing the legs, and getting help to put on shoes. These restrictions prevent dislocation of the new prosthesis.

Critical thinking strategy: Think about the amount of flexion each amount of degree requires and relate this to postsurgical activity

Client needs category: Safe, effective care environment

Client needs subcategory: Management of care

Cognitive level: Application

Integrated process: Teaching and learning

---

51. Which process best describes the mechanism of action of medications used to treat peptic ulcer disease, such as ranitidine (Zantac)?

☐ **1.** Neutralize acid

☐ **2.** Reduce acid secretions

☐ **3.** Stimulate gastrin release

☐ **4.** Protect the mucosal barrier

Ranitidine (Zantac) is a histamine-2 receptor antagonist that reduces acid secretion by inhibiting gastrin secretion. Antacids neutralize acid, and mucosal barrier fortifiers protect the mucosal barrier.

Critical thinking strategy: Recall the pathophysiology of peptic ulcer disease, and review the actions of medications used to treat it.

Client needs category: Physiological integrity

Client needs subcategory: Pharmacological and parenteral therapies

Cognitive level: Application

Integrated process: Nursing process/implementation

52. While performing a cervical examination on a pregnant client, a nurse's fingertips feel pulsating tissue. What would be the most appropriate nursing intervention?

☐ **1.** Leave the client, and call the physician.

☐ **2.** Put the client in a semi-Fowler's position.

☐ **3.** Ask the client to push with the next contraction.

☐ **4.** Leave the fingers in place, and press the nurse's call light.

Answer: 4

Rationale: When the umbilical cord precedes the fetal presenting part, it's known as a prolapsed cord. Leaving the fingers in place and calling for assistance is the safest intervention for the fetus because it keeps the fetus off the cord, thereby reducing cord compression. The nursing staff can contact the physician to alert him of the situation. The client will probably need a cesarean delivery because of the risk of fetal demise from the fetus's pressing against the cord during delivery. Placing the client in semi-Fowler's position would increase fetal pressure on the umbilical cord. Asking the client to push with the next contraction is contraindicated because it would also force the presenting part against the cord, causing severe bradycardia and possible fetal demise.

Critical thinking strategy: Focus on the safety of the fetus.

Client needs category: Physiological integrity

Client needs subcategory: Reduction of risk potential

Cognitive level: Application

Integrated process: Nursing process/implementation

---

53. Which activity is recommended to prevent foreign body aspiration in children during meals?

☐ **1.** Insist that children are seated.

☐ **2.** Give children toys to play with.

☐ **3.** Allow children to watch television.

☐ **4.** Allow children to eat in a separate room.

Answer: 1

Rationale: Children should remain seated while eating. The risk of aspiration increases if a child is running, jumping, or talking with food in his mouth. Television and toys are a dangerous distraction to toddlers and young children and should be avoided. Children need constant supervision and should be monitored while eating snacks and meals.

Critical thinking strategy: Focus on activities that can lead to aspiration of food.

Client needs category: Safe, effective care environment

Client needs subcategory: Safety and infection control

Cognitive level: Application

Integrated process: Nursing process/implementation

54. Which drug is most commonly used to treat cardiogenic shock?

☐ **1.** Dopamine

☐ **2.** Enalapril (Vasotec)

☐ **3.** Furosemide (Lasix)

☐ **4.** Metoprolol (Lopressor)

Answer: 1

Rationale: Dopamine, a sympathomimetic drug, improves myocardial contractility and blood flow through vital organs by increasing perfusion pressure. Enalapril is an angiotensin-converting enzyme inhibitor that directly lowers blood pressure. Furosemide is a diuretic and doesn't have a direct effect on contractility or tissue perfusion. Metoprolol is a beta-adrenergic blocker that slows heart rate and lowers blood pressure; neither is a desired effect in the treatment of cardiogenic shock.

Critical thinking strategy: Recall the classifications of the listed medications, and review the pathophysiology of cardiogenic shock.

Client needs category: Physiological integrity

Client needs subcategory: Pharmacological and parenteral therapies

Cognitive level: Application

Integrated process: Nursing process/analysis

---

55. When caring for a client with quadriplegia, which nursing intervention takes priority?

☐ **1.** Forcing fluids to prevent renal calculi

☐ **2.** Maintaining skin integrity

☐ **3.** Obtaining adaptive devices for more independence

☐ **4.** Preventing atelectasis

Answer: 4

Rationale: Clients with quadriplegia have paralysis or weakness of the diaphragm and the abdominal or intercostal muscles. Maintenance of airway and breathing take top priority. Although forcing fluids, maintaining skin integrity, and obtaining adaptive devices for more independence are all important interventions, preventing atelectasis has more priority.

Critical thinking strategy: Focus on the ABCs (airway, breathing, and circulation) when prioritizing nursing interventions.

Client needs category: Physiological integrity

Client needs subcategory: Reduction of risk potential

Cognitive level: Application

Integrated process: Nursing process/planning

56. A client is being discharged from the emergency department after cast application for a tibial fracture. A serious complication of this injury is identified with the nursing diagnosis *Impaired gas exchange: Fat embolus related to long bone fracture.* Based on this diagnosis, which instruction should the nurse provide?

☐ **1.** "Cough and deep-breathe at least every 2 hours."

☐ **2.** "Keep your leg elevated, and apply ice for the first 24 to 48 hours."

☐ **3.** "Call the physician at once if you experience apprehensiveness, shortness of breath, fever, or palpitations."

☐ **4.** "Restrict your fluid intake to 1 liter per day."

Answer: 3

Rationale: Fat embolism is a complication of a long-bone fracture. Signs and symptoms include apprehension, altered mental status, respiratory distress, tachycardia, tachypnea, fever, and petechiae over the neck, upper arms, and chest. Coughing and deep-breathing exercises can help prevent other complications of a long-bone fracture but have no effect on fat emboli. The client should also be instructed to drink plenty of fluids to stay well hydrated; this will help prevent embolic complications.

Critical thinking strategy: Recall the signs and symptoms of fat embolism.

Client needs category: Physiological integrity

Client needs subcategory: Reduction of risk potential

Cognitive level: Application

Integrated process: Teaching and learning

---

57. A client comes to the clinic for a follow-up appointment after diagnostic tests show he has gastroesophageal reflux disease. Which instruction should the nurse provide?

☐ **1.** "Lie down and rest after each meal."

☐ **2.** "Avoid alcohol and caffeine."

☐ **3.** "Drink 16 ounces of water with each meal."

☐ **4.** "Eat three well-balanced meals every day."

Answer: 2

Rationale: A client with gastroesophageal reflux disease should avoid alcohol, caffeine and foods that increase acidity, all of which can cause epigastric pain. To further prevent reflux, the client should remain upright for 2 to 3 hours after eating; avoid eating for 2 to 3 hours before bedtime; avoid bending and wearing tight clothing; avoid drinking large fluid volumes with meals; and eat small, frequent meals to help reduce gastric acid secretion.

Critical thinking strategy: Focus on ways to reduce gastric acidity.

Client needs category: Physiological integrity

Client needs subcategory: Reduction of risk potential

Cognitive level: Application

Integrated process: Teaching and learning

58. Hydrocortisone given I.V. is the proper treatment for which disease?

☐ **1.** Addison's disease

☐ **2.** Cushing's syndrome

☐ **3.** Hyperthyroidism

☐ **4.** Hypoparathyroidism

Answer: 1

Rationale: I.V. hydrocortisone is the proper treatment for Addison's disease because it replaces glucocorticoid deficiency. Cushing's syndrome is associated with excessive amounts of glucocorticoids. Hyperthyroidism and hypoparathyroidism aren't treated with hydrocortisone.

Critical thinking strategy: Focus on the pathophysiology of the diseases listed in relation to hydrocortisone use.

Client needs category: Physiological integrity

Client needs subcategory: Pharmacological and parenteral therapies

Cognitive level: Knowledge

Integrated process: Nursing process/evaluation

---

59. A nurse should include which in-home management instruction for a child who's receiving desmopressin acetate (DDAVP) for symptomatic control of diabetes insipidus?

☐ **1.** Give DDAVP only when urine output begins to decrease.

☐ **2.** Clean the skin with alcohol before applying a DDAVP dermal patch.

☐ **3.** Increase the DDAVP dose if polyuria occurs just before the next scheduled dose.

☐ **4.** Call the physician for an alternate route for administering DDAVP when the child has an upper respiratory infection (URI) or allergic rhinitis.

Answer: 4

Rationale: Excessive nasal mucus associated with URI or allergic rhinitis may interfere with DDAVP absorption when the drug is given intranasally. Use only clear water to clean the skin. Soaps, oils, lotions, alcohol, or other products may irritate the skin under the patch. Parents should be instructed to contact the physician for advice in changing the administration route during times when nasal mucus may be increased. The DDAVP dose should remain unchanged, even if the child has polyuria just before the next dose. This is to avoid overmedicating the child.

Critical thinking strategy: Focus on administration routes for DDAVP.

Client needs category: Safe, effective care environment

Client needs subcategory: Management of care

Cognitive level: Application

Integrated process: Teaching and learning

60. A 22-year-old client complains of substernal chest pain and states that his heart feels like "it's racing out of my chest." He reports no history of cardiac disorders. The nurse attaches him to a cardiac monitor and notes sinus tachycardia with a rate of 136 beats/minute. Breath sounds are clear, and the respiratory rate is 26 breaths/minute. Which drug should the nurse question the client about using?

☐ **1.** Barbiturates

☐ **2.** Opioids

☐ **3.** Cocaine

☐ **4.** Benzodiazepines

Answer: 3

Rationale: Because of the client's age and negative medical history, the nurse should question him about cocaine use. Barbiturate overdose may trigger respiratory depression and a slow pulse. Opioids can cause marked respiratory depression, while benzodiazepines can cause drowsiness and confusion. Cocaine increases myocardial oxygen consumption and can cause coronary artery spasm, leading to tachycardia, ventricular fibrillation, myocardial ischemia, and myocardial infarction.

Critical thinking strategy: Focus on the client's signs and symptoms, and review the adverse effects of the medications listed.

Client needs category: Physiological integrity

Client needs subcategory: Physiological adaptation

Cognitive level: Analysis

Integrated process: Nursing process/assessment

---

61. The nurse is reading the progress notes for a client who has a pressure ulcer. Based on the nurse's note in the chart below, what stage pressure ulcer does this client have?

Progress notes	
7/9/09 0800	Client admitted to unit from long-term care facility with a pressure ulcer on coccyx approximately 2 cm x 1 cm x 0.5 cm. No drainage noted. Base has deep pink granulation tissue without visible subcutaneous tissue. Skin surrounding ulcer pink, with intact, well-defined edges. ——————— Rebecca Stellato, RN

☐ **1.** Stage I

☐ **2.** Stage II

☐ **3.** Suspected deep-tissue injury

☐ **4.** Unstageable

Answer: 2

Rationale: A Stage II pressure ulcer has visible skin breaks and possible discoloration. Penetrating to the subcutaneous fat layer, the sore is painful and visibly swollen. The ulcer may be characterized as an abrasion, blister, or shallow crater. In a stage I pressure ulcer, the skin is red and intact and doesn't blanche with external pressure; it feels warm and firm. In suspected deep-tissue injury, the skin is purple or maroon but intact; a blood-filled blister may be present. In an unstageable pressure ulcer, the ulcer destroys tissue from the skin to possibly the bone; the base of the ulcer is covered by slough, eschar, or both.

Critical thinking strategy: Focus on the signs and symptoms, and review the pathophysiology of pressure ulcers, anatomy of skin, and stages of pressure ulcers.

Client needs category: Physiological integrity

Client needs subcategory: Physiological adaptation

Cognitive level: Analysis

Integrated process: Nursing process/assessment

62. For a client with damage to the caudate nucleus, putamen, and globus pallidus, which condition should be monitored?

☐ **1.** Eye movement

☐ **2.** Modulation of sounds

☐ **3.** Motor movement

☐ **4.** Muscle synergy

Answer: 3

Rationale: Motor movement is regulated by the basal ganglia, which consists of the caudate nucleus, putamen, and globus pallidus. Eye movement is controlled by several different cranial nerves. Modulation of sounds occurs from the occipital lobe. The cerebellum regulates muscle synergy.

Critical thinking strategy: Review the anatomy and physiology of the neurologic system.

Client needs category: Safe, effective care environment

Client needs subcategory: Management of care

Cognitive level: Application

Integrated process: Nursing process/assessment

---

63. A client in skeletal traction complains of pain even though he received an analgesic 1 hour ago. The nurse wants to offer an alternative pain-management measure. Which measure can she implement within her scope of practice?

☐ **1.** Acupressure and shiatsu

☐ **2.** Hypnosis and therapeutic touch

☐ **3.** Relaxation and imagery

☐ **4.** Swedish massage and the Feldenkrais method

Answer: 3

Rationale: Relaxation and imagery are effective adjuncts to pharmacologic pain management that the nurse can implement without a physician's order. Although the other therapies may promote pain management, they require special training or certification.

Critical thinking strategy: Consider which of the answers may require special training, and eliminate them as possibilities.

Client needs category: Physiological integrity

Client needs subcategory: Basic care and comfort

Cognitive level: Application

Integrated process: Caring

64. A 30-year-old client experiences weight loss, abdominal distention, crampy abdominal pain, and intermittent diarrhea after the birth of her second child. Diagnostic tests reveal gluten-induced enteropathy. Which foods must she eliminate from her diet permanently?

☐ **1.** Milk and dairy products

☐ **2.** Protein-containing foods

☐ **3.** Cereal grains (except rice and corn)

☐ **4.** Carbohydrates

Answer: 3

Rationale: To manage gluten-induced enteropathy, the client must eliminate gluten, which means avoiding all cereal grains except rice and corn. In initial disease management, clients eat a high-calorie, high-protein diet with mineral and vitamin supplements to help normalize the nutritional status. Lactose intolerance is sometimes an associated problem, so milk and dairy products are limited until improvement occurs. Cereal grains are the only carbohydrates this client must eliminate.

Critical thinking strategy: Focus on which food group contains gluten.

Client needs category: Physiological integrity

Client needs subcategory: Basic care and comfort

Cognitive level: Application

Integrated process: Teaching and learning

---

65. The serum calcium level of a client with hyperthyroidism is 14.6 mg/dl. Which treatment should the nurse anticipate?

☐ **1.** Withholding fluids

☐ **2.** Starting oral calcium supplements

☐ **3.** Giving vitamin D supplements

☐ **4.** Administering I.V. fluids at 200 ml/hour

Answer: 4

Rationale: Normal calcium levels are 8.5 to 10.5 mg/dl, so a level of 14.6 mg/dl is dangerously high. To decrease the calcium level, intake of calcium should be reduced and calcium excretion should be promoted by administering I.V. and oral fluids and diuretics. Giving vitamin D would increase the calcium level.

Critical thinking strategy: Recall normal values for serum calcium.

Client needs category: Physiological integrity

Client needs subcategory: Physiological adaptation

Cognitive level: Analysis

Integrated process: Nursing process/planning

66. A 10-year-old child monitors and adjusts his own insulin. Which response reflects an understanding of appropriate adjustment of insulin dosage when the child has the flu?

☐ **1.** "I won't take my insulin because I'm too sick to eat right now."

☐ **2.** "I'll take my usual dose of regular and NPH insulin."

☐ **3.** "I'll do a fingerstick test first, then figure out how much insulin to take."

☐ **4.** "I'll do a fingerstick test and record the results."

Answer: 3

Rationale: Because of the stress of illness, serum glucose will likely be elevated during an episode of the flu. Appropriate adjustment of insulin dosage based on a fingerstick reading will help prevent the child from becoming hypoglycemic or ketoacidotic.

Critical thinking strategy: Consider what effect illness will have on serum glucose levels.

Client needs category: Physiological integrity

Client needs subcategory: Physiological adaptation

Cognitive level: Analysis

Integrated process: Teaching and learning

---

67. The selection of a nursing care delivery system (NCDS) is critical to the success of a nursing area. Which factor is essential to the evaluation of an NCDS?

☐ **1.** Determining how planned absences, such as vacation time, will be scheduled so that all staff are treated fairly

☐ **2.** Identifying who will be responsible for making client care decisions

☐ **3.** Deciding what type of dress code will be implemented

☐ **4.** Identifying salary ranges for various types of staff

Answer: 2

Rationale: Determining who has responsibility for making decisions regarding client care is an essential element of all client care delivery systems. Dress code, salary, and scheduling planned staff absences are important to any organizations, but they aren't actually determined by the NCDS.

Critical thinking strategy: Focus on the definition of type of delivery system discussed.

Client needs category: Safe, effective care environment

Client needs subcategory: Management of care

Cognitive level: Application

Integrated process: Communication and documentation

68. During the postpartum period, what does a firm fundus indicate?

☐ **1.** A firm tumor at the top of the uterus

☐ **2.** Contraction of the uterus

☐ **3.** Continuing labor contractions

☐ **4.** Bladder distention

Answer: 2

Rationale: A firm postpartum fundus means that the uterus has contracted and is constricting blood vessels, thereby decreasing lochial flow. A uterine tumor doesn't necessarily cause a firm fundus. The client wouldn't experience labor contractions during the postpartum period. Bladder distention restricts the uterus from contracting downward, resulting in a soft, boggy uterus and increased vaginal bleeding.

Critical thinking strategy: Focus on the term *postpartum* in relation to the condition of the fundus.

Client needs category: Physiological integrity

Client needs subcategory: Physiological adaptation

Cognitive level: Knowledge

Integrated process: Nursing process/assessment

---

69. A client with a subarachnoid hemorrhage is prescribed a 1,000-mg loading dose of phenytoin (Dilantin) I.V. Which consideration is most important when administering this dose?

☐ **1.** Therapeutic drug levels should be maintained between 20 and 30 mg/ml.

☐ **2.** Rapid phenytoin administration can cause cardiac arrhythmias.

☐ **3.** Phenytoin should be mixed with dextrose in water before administration.

☐ **4.** Phenytoin should be administered through an I.V. catheter in the client's hand.

Answer: 2

Rationale: Phenytoin I.V. shouldn't be given at a rate exceeding 50 mg/minute because rapid administration can depress the myocardium, causing arrhythmias. Therapeutic drug levels range from 10 to 20 mg/ml. Phenytoin shouldn't be mixed in solution for administration. However, because it's compatible with normal saline solution, it can be injected through an I.V. line containing normal saline solution. When given through an I.V. catheter in the hand, phenytoin may cause purple glove syndrome.

Critical thinking strategy: Recall the adverse effects of this medication on various body systems.

Client needs category: Physiological integrity

Client needs subcategory: Pharmacological and parenteral therapies

Cognitive level: Application

Integrated process: Nursing process/planning

70. A client has a percutaneous endoscopic gastrostomy tube in place for tube feedings. Before starting a continuous feeding, the nurse should place the client in which position?

☐ **1.** Semi-Fowler

☐ **2.** Supine

☐ **3.** Reverse Trendelenburg

☐ **4.** High-Fowler

Answer: 1

Rationale: To prevent aspiration of stomach contents, the nurse should place the client in a semi-Fowler position. The supine and reverse Trendelenburg positions may cause aspiration. High-Fowler position isn't necessary and may not be as well tolerated as semi-Fowler's in this situation.

Critical thinking strategy: Focus on the importance of maintaining the airway during a tube feeding.

Client needs category: Physiological integrity

Client needs subcategory: Reduction of risk potential

Cognitive level: Application

Integrated process: Nursing process/implementation

---

71. After undergoing a thyroidectomy, a client develops hypocalcemia and tetany. Which medication should the nurse anticipate administering?

☐ **1.** Calcium gluconate

☐ **2.** Potassium chloride

☐ **3.** Sodium bicarbonate

☐ **4.** Sodium phosphorus

Answer: 1

Rationale: Immediate treatment for a client who develops hypocalcemia and tetany after thyroidectomy is calcium gluconate. Potassium chloride and sodium bicarbonate aren't indicated. Sodium phosphorus wouldn't be given because the client's phosphorus levels are already elevated.

Critical thinking strategy: Focus on the physiology of the thyroid gland and definition of *hypocalcemia.*

Client needs category: Physiological integrity

Client needs subcategory: Pharmacological and parenteral therapies

Cognitive level: Application

Integrated process: Nursing process/planning

72. Which instruction is most applicable to a client who was just diagnosed with chronic pyelonephritis?

☐ **1.** Remain on bed rest for up to 2 weeks.

☐ **2.** Expect to take an analgesic on a regular basis for the next 6 months.

☐ **3.** Expect to provide a urine specimen for culturing every 2 weeks for up to 6 months.

☐ **4.** Expect to be on an antibiotic for several weeks or even months.

Answer: 4

Rationale: Chronic pyelonephritis is a long-term condition, often requiring antibiotic treatment for several weeks or months and close monitoring to prevent permanent kidney damage. Bed rest and analgesics may be prescribed during the acute stage, but they're not usually required long-term. A urine culture is typically ordered 2 weeks after stopping antibiotics to ensure that the infection has been eradicated.

Critical thinking strategy: Focus on treatment modalities related to long-term inflammatory conditions.

Client needs category: Physiological integrity

Client needs subcategory: Reduction of risk potential

Cognitive level: Application

Integrated process: Teaching and learning

---

73. A nurse completes her discharge teaching for a client being treated for a sexually transmitted infection (STI) and provides him with a copy of written instructions. Which comment would indicate that the client has understood the instructions?

☐ **1.** "I don't need condoms because I'm not allergic to penicillin. Besides, I can always come in for a shot at the first sign of infection."

☐ **2.** "I'll notify my sex partners and avoid having unprotected sex from now on."

☐ **3.** "I'll just be careful not to have intercourse with someone who has an STI."

☐ **4.** "I guess there's not much anyone can do to prevent it. If you're going to get it, you're going to get it."

Answer: 2

Rationale: The nurse would know that the client understands the teaching when he can describe preventive behaviors and good, safe health practices. The other options indicate that the client doesn't understand the need to take preventive measures.

Critical thinking strategy: Review the pathophysiology of STIs and how they are transmitted.

Client needs category: Safe, effective care environment

Client needs subcategory: Safety and infection control

Cognitive level: Analysis

Integrated process: Teaching and learning

74. When assessing a client with necrotizing entero-colitis, the nurse should expect which finding?

☐ **1.** Abdominal distention and gastric retention

☐ **2.** Gastric retention and guaiac-negative stools

☐ **3.** Metabolic alkalosis and abdominal distention

☐ **4.** Guaiac-negative stools and metabolic alkalosis

Answer: 1

Rationale: Necrotizing enterocolitis is an ischemia disorder of the gut. The cause is unknown, but it's more common in preterm neonates who have had a hypoxic episode. The neonate's intestines become di-lated and necrotic, and the abdomen becomes ex-tremely distended. Paralytic ileus develops, causing gastric retention. These retained gastric contents, along with any passed stool, will be guaiac-positive. The neonate also develops metabolic acidosis, not meta-bolic alkalosis.

Critical thinking strategy: Review the pathophysiol-ogy of necrotizing enterocolitis.

Client needs category: Physiological integrity

Client needs subcategory: Physiological adaptation

Cognitive level: Comprehension

Integrated process: Nursing process/analysis

---

75. A child has been diagnosed with mumps, a viral infection that involves the parotid glands. Indicate on the illustration below where would you expect to see swelling.

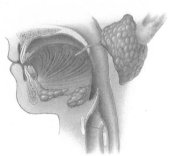

Answer:

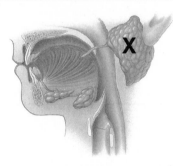

Rationale: The parotid glands are one of three pair of salivary glands located below and in front of the ears.

Critical thinking strategy: Recall the anatomy of the head and neck and the location of the salivary glands.

Client needs category: Physiological integrity

Client needs subcategory: Physiological adaptation

Cognitive level: Analysis

Integrated process: Nursing process/assessment

Selected references

Boyd, M.A. *Psychiatric Nursing: Contemporary Practice*, 4th ed. Philadelphia: Lippincott Williams & Wilkins, 2008.

Craven, R.F., et al. *Fundamentals of Nursing: Human Health and Function,* 6th ed. Philadelphia: Lippincott Williams & Wilkins, 2009.

Dosage Calculations Made Incredibly Easy, 3rd ed. Philadelphia: Lippincott Williams & Wilkins, 2005.

Nursing2009 Drug Handbook. Philadelphia: Lippincott Williams & Wilkins, 2008.

Pillitteri, A. *Maternal & Child Health Nursing: Care of the Childbearing and Childrearing Family,* 5th ed. Philadelphia: Lippincott Williams & Wilkins, 2007.

Smeltzer, S.C., et al. *Brunner & Suddarth's Textbook of Medical-Surgical Nursing,* 11th ed. Philadelphia: Lippincott Williams & Wilkins, 2008.

Taylor, C.R., et al. *Fundamentals of Nursing: The Art and Science of Nursing Care,* 6th ed. Philadelphia: Lippincott Williams & Wilkins, 2008.